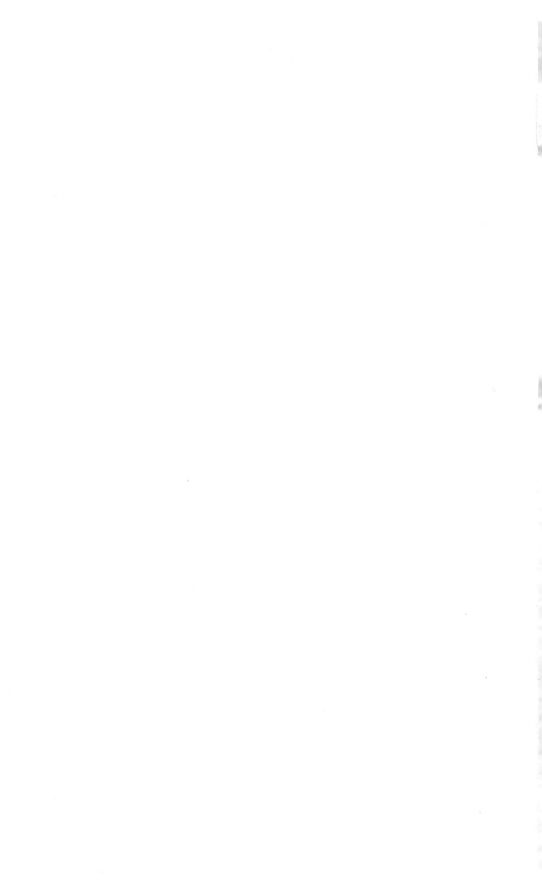

Rationalizing Epidemics

Rationalizing Epidemics

Meanings and Uses of American Indian Mortality since 1600

DAVID S. JONES

HARVARD UNIVERSITY PRESS

Cambridge, Massachusetts
London, England

Copyright © 2004 by the President and Fellows of Harvard College
All rights reserved
Printed in the United States of America

Library of Congress Cataloging-in-Publication Data

Jones, David Shumway.
    Rationalizing epidemics : meanings and uses of American Indian mortality
since 1600 / David Shumway Jones.
        p.   cm.
    Includes bibliographical references and index.
    ISBN 0-674-01305-0 (cloth : alk. paper)
        1. Indians of North America—Mortality—History.
        2. Indians of North America—Diseases—Epidemiology—History.
        I. Title.
RA408.I49J66   2004
614.4′2′08997—dc22   2003067538

To the memory of Alexa Caronna Jones,
who inspired me to finish it.

Contents

Figures

Acknowledgments

This book could not have happened without the kindness and generosity of many people. Allan Brandt taught me most of what I know about the history of medicine. He first suggested approaching American Indian epidemics from the perspective of health disparities and has provided crucial direction at every juncture. Arthur Kleinman introduced me to the field of medical anthropology and the important interplay between local contexts and international structures. David Barnes helped me clarify many of my ideas. Their combined influence appears on every page of this work.

Many others have provided expertise and advice on specific issues, including Joyce Chaplin, John Coatsworth, Anne Harrington, Nancy Krieger, John Krige, Everett Mendelsohn, Charles Rosenberg, and Barbara Gutmann Rosenkrantz. My colleagues at Harvard's Department of the History of Science provided insight, support, and guidance throughout, including Karen Flood, Lara Friedenfelds, Michael Gordin, Jeremy Greene, Eric Kupferberg, Rachel Schneller, Rena Selya, Nadav Talal, Elly Truitt, Conevery Bolton Valencius, Nick Weiss, and especially Nick King and Deborah Weinstein. Friends and colleagues outside of the department have also endured my ideas and frustrations over the years, including Lara Goitein, Debbie Gordon, Eric Morrow, Roy Perlis, Alan Schooley, and Kimberly Schooley.

Robert Martensen inspired my first interest in the history of medicine and has been endlessly supportive ever since. David Spanagel introduced me to the field of history of science and gave me many opportunities to experiment with my ideas. Leon Eisenberg, Byron Good, Martha Gardner, Jeff Peppercorn, Scott Podolsky, Joel Roselin, and the other members of the Department of Social Medicine at Harvard Medical School have helped me to balance the perspectives of two very different worlds. David Josephs, Michelle Healy, and the other members of the medical staff at Crownpoint Hospital introduced me to contemporary health care on the Navajo Reservation.

The research could not have taken place without the assistance of librarians and archivists at the New York Weill Cornell Medical Center Archives, especially Adele Lerner and James Gehrlich, the National Archives and Records Administration, and the many libraries of Harvard University. The editors, staff, and anonymous reviewers at Harvard University Press provided crucial assistance in the final preparation of this book, especially Ann Downer-Hazell, Sara Davis, Sheila Barrett, Kate Brick, and Jay Boggis.

Generous funding was provided by the Department of the History of Science and the Graduate School of Arts and Sciences, Harvard University; the Department of Social Medicine, Harvard Medical School; and the Medical Scientist Training Program of the National Institutes of Health.

My family, especially my parents, provided inexhaustible enthusiasm and support for my decision to pursue both history and medicine.

None of this could have been possible without the love and support of my wife, Elizabeth Caronna.

Rationalizing Epidemics

Introduction

IN A SIMPLER WORLD suffering would elicit compassion from those who observe it. But the world is complicated, and suffering instead elicits diverse reactions from its observers. Consider responses to epidemics that devastated American Indian populations after European arrival in North America.

During the fall of 1837, traders of Pratte, Chouteau, and Company despaired in their remote posts along the Missouri River: the "whole country north and south is one solid mass of Buffaloes, and sorry to say, no Indians to kill them." It was a crisis the traders had created. Smallpox had followed them up the river the previous June, spread quickly among the Mandan, Assiniboine, and Blackfeet, and left devastation in its wake. Some traders had tried to contain the epidemic through quarantine and inoculation. All worried about the loss of trade, fearing that the company's losses would be "immense in fact incalculable as our most profitable Indians have died." Events did not turn out as expected. As surviving Indians sold furs that had belonged to those who had died, the traders reaped a record yield. Even though they feared that these furs might carry smallpox, the traders shipped them to markets in New York City. Andrew Culbertson later confessed that the furs "were purchased and shipped down the river with an utter neglect of any precaution to prevent the re-transmission of the disease." Surprised when

1

smallpox did not break out back east, he could only conclude that "the ways of Providence are mysterious and past finding out."[1]

Epidemics among American Indians have always generated similarly complex responses. In 1634 John Winthrop saw smallpox among the Massachusett as an opportunity for claiming new land: "God hathe hereby cleered our title to this place." He did, however, praise colonists who cared for the dying Indians. In 1885 Valentine T. McGillycuddy seemed resigned that the Sioux, "in obedience to the law of the survival of the fittest," would be driven to extinction by tuberculosis. Despite his fatalism, he worked to improve health services on the Pine Ridge Reservation. When Walsh McDermott sought patients for antibiotic research in 1952, he found the tuberculosis-stricken Navajo: his team had been "looking for an ethnic situation in which we could test the drug and this provided exactly that situation." But instead of simply exploiting the Navajo as a research population, McDermott worked to achieve their "total health."[2]

This book is an attempt to describe and understand these responses to the suffering caused by disease. Although the four examples are widely separated in time, each raises similar questions. How did colonists, traders, and physicians explain outbreaks of disease among American Indians? How did they account for the increased burden of smallpox and tuberculosis experienced by Indians compared to other populations? How did Indians, Europeans, and Americans respond to the epidemics and to the disparities in health status? How did epidemics simultaneously elicit empathy and opportunism? How have health disparities between American Indians and Americans persisted for hundreds of years? These common concerns link the different cases into a coherent and important analysis.[3]

The questions could be answered in a variety of ways. Some historians have studied specific epidemics, charting their causes and consequences to show how economic and political interests shape responses to disease. Others have studied various tribes, exploring how they responded to the many challenges, including disease, that followed European settlement of the Americas. Still others have traced the evolution of medical theory and practice. A different approach, focusing specifically on health disparities, brings these different perspectives together to address the full scope of the problem.

Health disparities have puzzled observers for centuries. Throughout history people have recognized that some populations are healthier or sicker than others. This recognition has triggered a crucial and enduring phenomenon: the rationalization of epidemics. Observers have to explain patterns in the disease environment: why epidemics strike when they do and why they strike some populations more severely than others. Epidemics must be made understandable, meaningful, and rational. Even as societies struggle to assign meaning to health disparities, epidemics demand responses from the populations they strike. Some people work to mitigate the effects of epidemics, while others seek to profit from victims' losses. Individual choices reflect intersections of medical theory, economic necessity, racial ideology, political opportunism, and the lived experiences of everyday life. As health disparities are made rational, interventions are rationalized.

The ways in which societies rationalize epidemics have been constrained only by the limits of human imagination. Nonetheless, striking patterns have endured sweeping changes in the meanings of disease. Observers always generate an overabundance of potential explanations. Confronted with such diversity, observers must choose which mechanisms are most meaningful to them. Their choices, which assign responsibility for the disease, have social and political utility. Disparities can be seen as proof of natural hierarchy, as products of misbehavior, or as evidence of social injustice. These assessments motivate or undermine interventions, influencing whether observers prevent an epidemic's spread, treat its victims, or exploit its opportunities. Even as epidemics emerge as the product of specific social structures, they enable actions that reproduce those structures. This book seeks to understand those choices.

Plagues

The suffering caused by disease after European arrival in the Americas took many forms. Colonists described plagues, poxes, fevers, fluxes, and a "very strange disease" among the American Indians they encountered. Terrible epidemics persisted as a striking continuity across centuries of social, economic, and political change. Smallpox struck the coast of New England in the winter of 1634 with mortality that approached 90 percent. When smallpox appeared among the tribes of the Missouri Valley in 1837, it seemed "to mock and glory in its very de-

structiveness." By the 1890s tuberculosis had become "the great de-
stroyer" of Indian tribes. It plagued Indian reservations deep into the
twentieth century, long after it had receded from the general population of the United States.[4]

These diseases have left deep scars in historical records. They appear
in journals, letters, adventure stories, government reports, and medical
investigations. Historians have written extensively about American Indian epidemics, which receive at least passing mention in all histories
of American Indians and early America. Historians have even developed a theory of "virgin soil epidemics" to explain the devastation
wrought by European epidemics on Indians. These historians have
elucidated changing patterns of Indian disease since the colonial period. Specific social forces—malnutrition, migration, and social disrup-
tion—conspired to leave American Indians vulnerable to disease. As
social conditions changed, so too did epidemics. Acute infections of
smallpox, measles, and influenza dominated initial encounters. The
reservation system led to the rise of chronic tuberculosis. Eventually
this was replaced by diabetes, heart disease, and substance abuse. As
recognized by both Indians and colonists since the sixteenth century,
disease was socially produced: Europeans brought new pathogens to
the Americas and triggered the conditions that made them so destructive.[5]

Understandings of disease changed just as dramatically as the diseases themselves. Everyone has an intuitive sense of what a disease is.
We all suffer from common colds, and we all know someone who has
died from cancer or heart disease. Medical researchers have described
the molecular mechanisms of many of these diseases. Historians have,
however, shown that these intuitive and scientific definitions fail to account for the historical diversity of the phenomena of disease. Cancer,
stigmatized in the 1950s, had become more accepted by the 1990s.
AIDS, a disease of social deviance in the United States in the 1980s, became a leading threat to economic development in the twenty-first
century. Other diagnoses, from neurasthenia and masturbation to alcoholism and chronic fatigue syndrome, challenged the very effort to define diseases. Although the tubercle bacillus that killed Capawack students at Harvard College in the 1650s likely resembled the bacillus that
afflicted the Navajo in the 1950s, understandings of that disease were
radically different in these two contexts.[6]

This malleability of disease meanings has many implications. Diseases exist as negotiated social phenomena that patients, doctors, and societies use to assign value and meaning to bodily phenomena. This negotiation once led historians to argue that diagnoses were arbitrary labels used to control social deviancy. The shock of HIV and AIDS in the 1980s pushed historians away from such relativism. As Charles Rosenberg noted, AIDS "has proved an occasion for labeling, but it is not simply an exercise in labeling." Instead, it led to the emergence of "a new consensus in regard to disease, one that finds a place for both biological and social factors and emphasizes their interaction."[7] Any historian studying disease must therefore manage a difficult challenge: balancing the desire to apply modern medical understanding to past experience and the need to acknowledge the historical specificity of disease meanings.

The complex processes that create disease and their meanings also influence the existence and interpretation of disparities in health status. Disparities have been reported since the earliest contact between Europeans and American Indians. Early explorers watched coastal tribes die while their own crews remained healthy. Fur traders and missionaries survived amidst epidemics of smallpox that devastated their hosts. As late as the mid-twentieth century, rates of tuberculosis and other infectious diseases among American Indians exceeded those among the general population by factors of ten, one hundred, or even one thousand. But these reports defy easy interpretation. Did colonists really know the prevalence of disease among Indians and Europeans? Did they lump many different eruptive fevers within the convenient label of smallpox? Would Walsh McDermott have agreed with diagnoses of consumption or scrofula given by his predecessors who cared for Indian patients?

Focusing explicitly on health disparities avoids some of these dangers. Regardless of the accuracy of past diagnoses, observers recognized disparities in disease experience. Regardless of the accuracy of the estimated magnitude of the disparity, belief in disparity triggered explanations that, in turn, motivated responses. Therefore the rationalization of disparities can be studied without attempting to establish the "true" diagnosis of a past epidemic. The focus is not on diseases themselves, but on beliefs about diseases and disparities.

An examination of the history of health disparities is aided by the vast literature on the causes of health disparities. Some modern epidemiologists emphasize behavior, believing that personal choices about such matters as tobacco, sexual behavior, diet, exercise, and alcohol consumption are crucial determinants of health. Others avoid this implicit victim-blaming and argue that behavior simply reflects the constraints of social environments. The issue of race has long been fiercely debated, with every assertion of racial distinction matched by an argument that racial disparities reflect underlying economic disadvantage. Abundant evidence also shows the dominant role played by socioeconomic status, both the amount of wealth in society and how equitably that wealth is distributed. Even such abstract concepts as civic participation, cooperation, and reciprocity can make crucial contributions to health status. While some see medical care as the solution to health disparities, others believe that the health care system simply drains resources from worthier investments.[8]

These debates about the causes of health disparity are part of a broader discourse about the causes of differential economic and political development. Since the nineteenth century, theorists have traced Euro-American success to the transformative power of capitalism, the nurturing stability of the English countryside, or the shape and orientation of the earth's continents. Clear links often exist between these narratives of global development and the disparities in health status between populations. Jared Diamond, for instance, has argued that the same cultural sharing that produced agriculture and technology in Eurasia also gave Eurasians resistance to the diseases that devastated indigenous populations worldwide. These attempts to find the fundamental mechanisms that underlie disparities have been balanced by an opposing project that situates disparities in the contingencies of local circumstances. Amartya Sen has shown how famines and disparities in health, wealth, and freedom have all resulted from specific forms of political (in)action. Anthropologists have documented countless cases in which specific (if inadvertent) political and economic decisions have aggravated the plight of impoverished populations. By tracing disparities to social agency, such analyses seek to obligate those at the healthy end of disparities to intervene.[9]

While these theorists seek to identify the causes of disparities of health and wealth, I am more interested in a parallel project: to uncover the meanings and functions of such theorizing. Every time that colonists, settlers, or medical researchers proposed an explanation for an observed disparity in health status, they made judgments that reflected their beliefs and their needs. Diseases and their disparities were never objective scientific facts. Instead, they were produced by social forces, interpreted through social biases, and used to perpetuate social advantage.

Peoples

When William Bradford reached the beaches of Cape Cod in 1620, he faced "a hideous and desolate wilderness, full of wild beasts and wild men."[10] His descendants established a radically different relationship with the land and its original inhabitants. By the end of the nineteenth century, the United States government had taken stewardship responsibility over those "wild men." When Sioux children died from malnutrition, government officials were embarrassed and outraged. When tuberculosis persisted among American Indians long after it had receded from the general population, physicians worked hard to overcome the problem. Any understanding of the responses by Europeans and Americans to American Indian health and disease requires an understanding of the changing relationships of the different populations in the Americas.

American Indians had created diverse and sophisticated societies before European colonization. When Europeans came to America in pursuit of land, freedom, furs, converts, and gold, they triggered a turbulent period of destruction and reconfiguration. European motivations and institutions shaped these encounters. Missionaries converted Indians; soldiers attacked them; and entrepreneurs traded with them, for furs and corn in the 1630s, and for uranium and natural gas in the 1950s. As colonies evolved into a nation, the federal government became increasingly involved. Responsibility for American Indians, instituted in the Bureau of Indian Affairs in 1824, moved from the War Department to the new Department of the Interior in 1849. Responsibility for American Indian health, assigned to the medical service of the Bureau of Indian Affairs in the 1870s, moved in 1955 to the Public Health Service. These changes occurred in parallel with growing faith in the power of government intervention.[11] However, despite centuries of effort to "civilize" and assimilate American Indians, many remained as exotic enclaves within the United States. As a consequence, intriguing parallels exist between Indian policy and international development.

These interactions had severe consequences for American Indians. Year after year settlers took Indian lands, government officials broke treaties, and diseases shattered Indian populations. Federal activism, even when well-intentioned, inevitably created barriers that constrained American Indian freedom. Paternalism knew few bounds: unfettered faith in Christian civilization inspired officials to impose their own values on Indians. Pursuit of health became a powerful justification of this process. Only recently has such paternalism been abandoned in favor of partially restored autonomy. Traditional histories portrayed Indians as stunned witnesses to these developments. For Frederick Jackson Turner, American Indians simply provided the frontier savagery that transformed European civilization into American freedom and opportunity.[12] Since the 1950s, however, historians and anthropologists have provided more nuanced models of these interactions, placing American Indians at the center of their analyses.

Historians now emphasize the many ways in which Indians participated in the evolution of Euro-American societies. American Indians reacted dynamically to colonists and settlers, recognizing them as economic opportunities, political allies, or misguided paternalists who tied tribes into webs of dependency. Notions of irresistibly advancing frontiers have given way to sophisticated analyses of the "middle ground" on which both groups interacted. This new American Indian history has uncovered the experiences of Indians during the transformations of encounter and national development.[13] My approach takes the lessons of this new historiography—the need for contextualized understandings of the interactions between American Indians and other groups— and applies them to those other groups. Just as encounter destabilized American Indian expectations and forced them to create new worlds, it challenged the preconceptions of colonists and settlers, who also struggled with the difficulties both groups faced during their turbulent interactions.

The ensuing creativity was decisively shaped by the demographic collapse of the American Indians. In 1614 John Smith found the islands of Massachusetts Bay inhabited by healthy people. When Philip Maximilian saw those same islands in 1832, he found no surviving Indians. The intervening centuries had seen the largest demographic catastrophe in world history. Although exact numbers remain contested, roughly 90 to 95 percent of the native population of the Americas lost their lives after European arrival, with epidemics taking a severe toll. This catastrophe shaped every aspect of the interaction between American Indians, colonists, and settlers. When nineteenth-century government officials established the reservation system, many assumed that they were simply providing palliative care for a dying race.[14] When American Indians defied the odds, when their populations grew throughout the twentieth century, they were left on reservations never meant to support them. The result has been a lingering burden of poverty and disease.

Ambiguous Responses

The recurring recognition of health disparities between American Indians and those who encountered them triggered exploitation and opportunism. Although such acts may have been the most dramatic responses to health disparities, efforts to alleviate disparities have been at least as persistent. As smallpox ravaged the Massachusett in 1633, Samuel Maverick and his family nursed its victims. On the verge of hostilities between the British and Delaware in 1763, Quaker trader James Kenny therapeutically bled ailing Indians. As early as 1760, Indians near Detroit petitioned the English to provide them with a doctor.[15] By 1888 the federal government employed 81 doctors to treat 200,000 American Indians. In 1966 there were 300 physicians and an elaborate system of clinics and hospitals on the reservations. While colonists feared that their efforts had little impact, by the late twentieth century the Indian Health Service claimed great success against American Indian health disparities. However, even these seemingly transparent episodes of medical humanitarianism were actions of surprising complexity.

Every therapeutic act must be understood with an appreciation of the elusiveness of medical efficacy. As European and American interventions evolved from haphazard efforts, by untrained individuals, to organized systems of medical care, the nature and meaning of efficacy changed significantly. Although Kenny and his Delaware patients likely had as much faith in bloodletting as Walsh McDermott had in antibiotics, the nature of their faith was quite different. Until the nineteenth century, treatment focused on control of symptoms. A purgative given to treat a disease was considered effective simply if it caused purging. By McDermott's time, the ambitions of medicine had changed. Symptoms had been recognized as reflections of underlying disease processes; efficacy could only be judged by decreased mortality and incidence of disease, proven by statistical demonstrations and controlled scientific investigation.[16] But beneath this mantle of scientific expertise, McDermott and his collaborators recognized the importance of less tangible aspects of medicine, especially its ability to reassure and comfort patients. These many meanings of efficacy have perplexed physicians and historians whenever they have tried to assess medical interventions.[17]

The ambiguity of efficacy is further complicated by the many challenges faced when deploying medical technologies. Some interventions have obvious power, such as the antibiotics that contributed to the twentieth century's "golden age" of medicine. The implementation of these technologies, however, has never been simple or obvious: social, economic, political, and technical obstacles have shaped the utilization, and thus the final efficacy, of all medical technologies.[18] Geographic isolation, socioeconomic conditions, and imperfect motivation have all limited the use of vaccination, antibiotics, and other treatments among American Indians. As a result, attention must be paid to both the potential and the actual impact of a treatment.

An appreciation of the imperfect power of medical technology and the complex determinants of medical efficacy is essential for understanding efforts by Europeans and Americans against Indian disease. Did tuberculosis persist because of unsuccessful treatments, overcrowded housing, overextended physicians, or indifferent bureaucrats? All of these factors likely contributed. Meanwhile, doctors and many of their patients trusted the efficacy of their remedies. This must be remembered when evaluating the decisions of physicians, traders, and bureaucrats. Whenever individuals failed to provide care, they failed to provide the same care they would have sought for themselves.

Every therapeutic act must also be understood with an appreciation of the complexity of therapeutic motivation. Many people certainly sought to relieve the suffering caused by Indian disease. This desire was motivated, in part, by the enduring suspicion that many of those diseases had been introduced by Europeans and Americans. By the late nineteenth century, however, American officials began to fear that the tide of disease had reversed direction, that the persistence of high levels of tuberculosis and other diseases on the reservations had become a dangerous "reservoir of infection" that threatened white settlers. Hand in hand with desire to treat American Indian disease came desire to use it as a substrate for medical experiment. Colonists, physicians, and even President Thomas Jefferson offered treatment to Indians in the spirit of experimentation. These experiments operated at multiple levels. They tested whether medical remedies could treat specific diseases, whether American Indians could be cured by European and American therapies, and whether systems of medical care would work in underdeveloped regions of the world. Such experiments are always ethically complex. Indians were harmed in some experiments, but benefited in others.[19]

The relationship between medical treatment and the "civilizing process" is similarly ambiguous. Missionaries and government officials long used medical arguments to justify their demands for behavioral change and social reform among American Indians. Physicians served as the front line in the government's efforts to "civilize" the Indians and took aggressive action to ensure that their instructions were followed. Knowing that they could not eradicate cultural difference, physicians tried to minimize its perceived health consequences by identifying and mitigating its most pathogenic aspects. This role appears in everything from explanations given for American Indian disease (such as religious practice or hygienic behavior) to medical interventions (such as health education and regulation of slaughterhouses) and faith that health disparities would vanish once Indians were incorporated into general society.[20] Every therapeutic act simultaneously served many needs. Medical care relieved suffering, tested new remedies, modified behaviors, purged reservoirs of infection, refined foreign aid programs, and demonstrated the virtues of Christian civilization.

Ambiguous Attitudes

The many meanings of epidemics and the many motivations of medical interventions arose from the diversity of relationships between Europeans, Americans, and American Indians. Some policies reflected con-

siderable moral distance between the populations. Before leaving England, John Winthrop celebrated the "miraculous plague" that
consumed the Indians. More than a century later, in 1763, General
Jeffrey Amherst conspired to disseminate smallpox among the Delaware and Shawnee. Such aggressive callousness contrasts with the experiences of those who shared the lived worlds of American Indians.
Plymouth colonists aided the Wampanoag in 1621, providing food
and shelter in the frigid winter. Francis Chardon believed that the
Christmas feast at Fort Clark, in which Mandan warriors, white traders, their Mandan wives, and mixed-blood children shared a dinner of
meat pies, pheasants, and coffee, would have "astonished" unaccus-
tomed observers.[21] American Indians were not simply savages facing
extinction. They were part of the daily lives of missionaries, traders,
soldiers, physicians, and bureaucrats. Indians were trading partners,
enemies, congregants, allies, and lovers.

The contrast between remote and direct experiences with American
Indians contributed to the contrasting responses of Europeans and
Americans. The experiences and resulting decisions were further shaped
by local interests. As Arthur Kleinman has shown, the "world is defined
by what is vitally at stake for groups and individuals. While preservation of life, aspiration, prestige, and the like may be shared structures of
relevance for *human conditions* across societies, that which is at stake in
daily situations differs (often dramatically) owing to cultural elaboration, personal idiosyncrasy, historical particularities, and the specifics
of the situation."[22] Any effort to understand the processes of rationalizing epidemics must recognize the needs and interests of the people
involved.

It is not possible to re-enter the minds of historical actors and see
the epidemics through their eyes. Anthropologists, however, have pio-
neered ethnographic techniques that allow acts of daily life to be understood as products of interactions between local needs, systems of
belief, and broader social forces. Social and cultural historians have
adapted these approaches with great success. Such analyses of American Indian history have been made difficult by limitations of surviving
sources, particularly the paucity of early materials written by American
Indians. Through creativity and perseverance, historians have begun
to overcome these limitations and produce impressively detailed
microhistories of the interactions of American Indians, Europeans, and

Americans.[23] They succeed because their micronarratives provide the detail, depth, and complexity needed to understand the multiple meanings of the events. They reveal what was at stake for the actors. Analyses of health disparities must be grounded at a similar level of analysis.

This requires a special historical approach, a history of meanings. Unlike an intellectual history of epidemic disease that takes place in the minds and writings of physicians and public health officials, or a social history of public health grounded in policies and the daily lives of victims, a history of the meanings of health disparities exists at the intersections of intellectual, social, and cultural history. The history of meaning shifts its emphasis "from raw historical experience (i.e., what happens to people) to what human beings have made out of that experience."[24] Any attempt at such a history is humbled by the ephemeral subtlety of meaning. Historians can neither know exactly why William Trent chose to infect the Delaware with smallpox in 1763 nor assess the authenticity of McDermott's desires to help American Indians. Historians can, however, document the nuances of responses and define many of the interests that shaped individuals' decisions. Reactions to health disparities have never been simple processes of observation, explanation, and action. Instead they demonstrate the coexistence of compassion, pragmatism, opportunism, and ideology. Such puzzling inconsistencies provide productive openings for historical analysis.

Exploring the motives behind responses to American Indian epidemics raises difficult problems. Is motivation an accessible category for historical analysis? Given the limitations of their sources, can historians fairly assess the intent behind actions? Can they recognize compassion, empathy, and authenticity? It is far easier to argue that a person acted out of self-interest than out of compassion. Even a single selfish motive undermines faith that a person ever acted altruistically. This sets too high a standard. A person may have acted with both compassion and self-interest. Many existing analyses have shown such mixed motivations in health care, from routine acts of blood donations to global campaigns of international health.[25]

My goal is not to answer these questions, only to consider them. Some things are clear. The political and economic stakes of local contexts drove specific decisions, from colonists' need for land to officials' desire to confine Indians on reservations. Such opportunistic acts reflected a specific moral relationship between Europeans, Americans, and American Indians, one of indifference to the plight of Indian populations. The concept of moral communities helps understand how this indifference may have worked. Every community defines the limits of its empathy and concern. If suffering occurs within the reach of this moral community, members feel an obligation to intervene and provide assistance. Suffering outside the moral community does not have the same impact. As David Morris has argued, suffering "is not a raw datum, a natural phenomenon we can identify and measure, but a social status that we extend or withhold."[26] Sometimes American Indians have been accepted into the moral community of the dominant groups of American culture, and at other times they have not. This acceptance or rejection has depended on war, treaties, missionary spirit, trade relations, or medical capacity.

These questions are part of the broader problem of social suffering. The structures of political and economic interaction inevitably create conditions in which certain (often marginalized) populations suffer. The appeal of these social structures to the dominant groups ensures the persistence of both the structures and the suffering. Human groups have long demonstrated remarkable tolerance of such suffering.[27] Observers of health disparities may seek almost any reason to erect emotional barriers between themselves and those who suffer. People with lung cancer suffer because of their bad habit of smoking. Uninsured populations remain uninsured because they choose not to pay for insurance. The human genome project promises to identify people for whom diseases will seem inevitable. Such mechanisms blame victims for their diseases and disguise the consequences of social inequality.

Many factors converge on the responses to disparities in health status. An empathic observer might desire to intervene, fail to do so, and then take solace in faith that the disparity is inevitable. A fur trader might vaccinate Indians to ensure access to a steady supply of furs, thereby saving a tribe from smallpox. Such actions cannot be easily judged.

Organization of the Book

The multitiered processes of rationalization arise from the subtle interplay between local interests and political economy. This interplay both generates the distribution of disease and shapes responses to it. These processes can be analyzed only through careful case studies. Since disparities in health status have existed in all cultures at all times, countless cases could be chosen. The history of American Indian populations provides a particularly valuable collection. Their burden of ill health has persisted over the five centuries since European contact. They continue to have the worst health outcomes of any ethnic group in the United States. The broad nexus of social and cultural forces reflected in their ill health connects this history to vital questions of race, class, medicine, colonialism, compassion, paternalism, and power.[28]

It is not possible to provide a detailed, contextualized history of all of American Indian health in a single project. I have chosen four specific cases: (1) responses to the decline of Indian populations in the first decades of colonization in New England; (2) efforts to spread and contain smallpox on the western frontier from the 1760s to the 1830s; (3) the emergence and management of tuberculosis on the Sioux reservation in the late nineteenth century; and (4) health research on the Navajo reservation in the 1950s and 1960s (Figure 1). Although my analyses make use of Indian perspectives, they focus on the responses by Europeans and Americans to the suffering of American Indians.[29] This is a limited perspective. Since these groups dominated economic and political power, however, their perspectives dictated health policy for American Indians.

My approach is unusual in that I compare four different cases widely separated in time and place, from seventeenth-century Massachusetts to twentieth-century Arizona. This approach risks incommensurability. Can decisions by people in such different contexts be placed into the same analysis? Does the search for connections across the cases do injustice to the unique details and meanings of each? The benefits outweigh the risks. First, each case has independent value, representing a period of particularly intense cultural interaction that produced crucial transitions in the relationship between Euro-Americans and American Indian disease. Second, the cases trace the evolution of smallpox and tuberculosis, the two diseases that dominated American Indian mortality from the sixteenth to the twentieth century. Third, the cases are tied together by their focus on a specific group, American Indians, and their focus on a single problem, responses to disparities in health status. This gives the coherence needed for any comparative study.

Each case is discussed over two chapters. The first chapter of each pair focuses on how the epidemics of smallpox or tuberculosis were un-

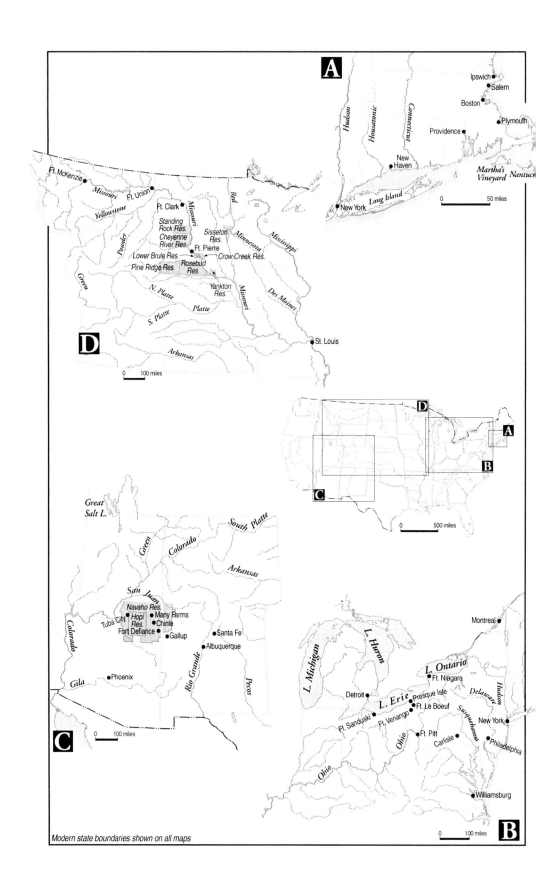

A

Ipswich
Salem
Boston
Plymouth
Providence
New Haven
Martha's Vineyard Nantuc
New York Long Island

Hudson
Housatonic
Connecticut

0   50 miles

D

Ft. McKenzie
Missouri
Ft. Union
Yellowstone
Ft. Clark
Missouri
Standing Rock Res.
Cheyenne River Res.
Lower Brule Res.
Pine Ridge Res.
Rosebud Res.
Powder
Green
N. Platte
S. Platte
Platte
Sisseton Res.
Ft. Pierre
Crow Creek Res.
Yankton Res.
Red
Minnesota
Mississippi
Des Moines
Missouri
St. Louis
Arkansas

0   100 miles

D
A
B
C

0   500 miles

C

Great Salt L.
Green
Colorado
South Platte
Arkansas
San Juan
Navaho Res.
Tuba City
Hopi Res.
Fort Defiance
Chinle
Many Farms
Gallup
Santa Fe
Albuquerque
Colorado
Gila
Phoenix
Rio Grande
Pecos

0   100 miles

B

L. Michigan
L. Huron
L. Ontario
Montreal
Ft. Niagara
Detroit
L. Erie
Presque Isle
Ft. Le Boeuf
Ft. Sanduski
Ft. Venango
Ft. Pitt
Carlisle
Ohio
Ohio
Delaware
Hudson
Susquehanna
New York
Philadelphia
Williamsburg

Modern state boundaries shown on all maps

0   100 miles

derstood at the time. The second chapter focuses on responses to the epidemics. Taken as a set, the first chapters of each case trace the history of explanations of epidemics and health disparities from the seventeenth to the twentieth century. The second chapters tell a history of Indian and health policy.

The story begins in England, on the eve of colonists' departure for America. Having heard sketchy reports from early explorers and colonists, members of the Plymouth and Massachusetts Bay Companies expected to find disease devastating American Indian populations. Epidemics seemed to be the means by which God prepared the way for the English. The exigencies of arrival and encounter destabilized this simple narrative. Acknowledging both their own vulnerability to disease and the common humanity of American Indians, colonists generated a rich diversity of potential explanations of Indian epidemics. Faced with this abundance, colonists assigned relevance to selected explanations. Their choices inevitably reflected the utility of different explanations during the turbulence of colonization.

As settlers moved beyond the Atlantic coast in the eighteenth and nineteenth centuries, smallpox followed them into the river valleys of the American interior and devastated previously isolated tribes. The spread of disease became a central issue in the moral and diplomatic discourse between colonists and American Indians on the western frontiers. While missionaries preached that health could come through

---

1. Map of regions discussed in the case studies (modern state boundaries included for reference). A: Southern New England, showing the location of the initial English settlements in the seventeenth century, many of which had previously been Indian villages. B: The Great Lakes region, showing the location of the forts involved in the Indian wars of 1763; Carlisle marked the western edge of English settlement on the Pennsylvania frontier. C: The Navajo Reservation, roughly the size of West Virginia, straddles the border of New Mexico and Arizona; Many Farms was chosen as a representative community in the middle of the reservation. D: The Upper Missouri Valley, with two different time periods superimposed. Forts Pierre, Clark, Union, and McKenzie, the fur trading posts involved in the smallpox epidemic of 1837, were far removed from St. Louis, then the limit of white settlement. The various Indian reservations in South Dakota, shown with their modern boundaries (stable since the 1890s), are the remnants of the Great Sioux Reservation, established in 1877 and including most of the Dakotas west of the Missouri River. (Map prepared by Philip Schwartzberg, Meridian Mapping, Minneapolis.)

Christian living, government agents offered gifts to reaffirm alliances strained by the disease. Into this devastation and negotiation came inoculation and vaccination, two new technologies that promised to harness the power of smallpox. Soldiers and traders hoped to take smallpox out of the hands of God and make it serve their own military and economic interests.

By the late nineteenth century, American Indians had been confined on isolated reservations. Government officials gained control over smallpox and other acute infections in this changed disease environment, only to face the emergence of tuberculosis. Thriving in the conditions of reservation life, tuberculosis attacked the Sioux and other tribes with a ferocity seen only in the darkest slums of eastern cities. It quickly replaced smallpox as the dominant cause of morbidity and mortality. Physicians and government officials began a critical debate. Did tuberculosis foretell the inevitable demise of the Indian race, or merely their passing struggles on the road to civilization? The government, eventually accepting the challenge to restore Indian health, sent a small group of agency physicians on an impossible quest against a threatening environment, unyielding poverty, and an inflexible bureaucracy.

Tuberculosis continued to assail American Indians through the middle of the twentieth century. Researchers increasingly understood the socioeconomic origins of tuberculosis, recognizing parallels between the plight of American Indian populations and that of developing populations worldwide. The suffering of the Navajo and other tribes eventually inspired the federal government to commit substantial resources to their rehabilitation. This new effort provided Walsh McDermott and a team of Cornell physicians with an opportunity to work with the Navajo to test promising new antibiotics against tuberculosis, and to test the power of modern medicine against the full disease burden of an impoverished society. Their work, the famous "Health Care Experiment at Many Farms," failed to alleviate Navajo health disparities and eventually inspired the Navajo to articulate a new vision of medical self-sufficiency.

By examining cases separated in time, I document enduring concerns and challenges. Century after century, colonists and their descendants tried to understand the etiology of epidemics, the vulnerability of American Indians, and the persistence of disparities in health status. Choosing salient explanations, they assessed their own responsibility for the epidemics, their obligation to intervene, and the role of medical and social approaches in improving health status. Because such questions persist across time and place, the specific case studies must be connected, even while respecting their contextual uniqueness. My long perspective also defines a series of striking trajectories. Medical practice evolved from individual efforts at alleviating symptoms to institutionalized programs to prevent and control disease. Policy toward the Indians grew from the efforts of isolated missionaries and traders to a formidable arm of the federal bureaucracy. All the while, health disparities persisted.

My analysis supports a number of important conclusions. First, whether the prevailing diseases were acute infections (such as smallpox and measles), chronic infections (such as tuberculosis), or the endemic ailments of modern society (such as diabetes and alcoholism), American Indians have always experienced higher rates of disease than their European and American contemporaries. The existence of disparities regardless of the underlying disease environment provides a powerful argument against the belief that each disparity reflected an inherent susceptibility of American Indian populations. Instead, the disparities in health status must actually reflect the disparities in wealth and power that have endured since colonization.

Second, striking patterns exist in the attempts to rationalize the distribution of health and disease. Explanations can emphasize intrinsic factors (such as racial difference), extrinsic factors (such as climate or socioeconomic status), or behavior (such as hygiene). Some explanations persisted (housing conditions, for instance); others did not. Invocations of providence, for example, gave way to genetic determinism as the most common argument for inevitable disparity. Crucial debates have also endured. While some observers assigned pathogenic agency to personal choices, others argued that Indian disease was the product of the disrupted social conditions produced by colonization. The continuities suggest that discrete modes of response exist when one population confronts the ill health of another. Responsibility must be assigned somewhere. It can fall on the sick (such as victims of genetic susceptibility); it can fall on the healthy (such as the misguided architects of the reservation system), or it can be transferred to an outside authority (such as God's providence). These assignments have crucial implications for health policy.

Third, the choice of explanation and the assignment of responsibility always reflect the specific needs and interests of local communities. No single explanation defines the phenomena of diseases so clearly that other explanations are precluded. Observers, faced with an abundance of theories, can then emphasize the most meaningful or useful understandings of disease. Needing land, colonists saw Massachusett depopulation as a gift of land. Wanting absolution for the destruction of Indian societies, federal officials saw Sioux tuberculosis as proof of their inevitable demise. As medical anthropologists have shown, the stakes and interests of local communities, within the context of national and international economic and political pressures, determine how disease is explained and managed.

Fourth, the existence of epidemics and their contested explanations allow and demand a range of responses. In some settings, health disparities are seen as proof of a natural order that can be exploited for the observer's benefit (such as purchase of abandoned furs). In others disparities stand as markers of social injustice that the observer must remedy (for instance, with financial assistance). Meanwhile, fear of expanding epidemics justifies invasive social practices (such as the imposition of "civilization"). Since disparities in health status parallel disparities in wealth and power, responses to health disparities necessarily involve decisions to deploy or withhold economic and political resources. A remarkable range of responses can be rationalized in the midst of an epidemic. Recognition of the patterns that link these cases provides insight into the many dilemmas of modern health policy in which desire and action stand alongside indifference and inaction.

This overview does not suggest that all loose ends will be woven seamlessly together. Each case on its own raises puzzles that cannot easily be solved. Each has aspects that do not fit into overarching trajectories. This is to be expected. Responses to health disparities are never simple processes of observation, explanation, and action. People act with inadequate information, with motivations they may not understand, and with interventions they cannot always control. They recognize the ways in which social forces generate disparities, yet they yearn to attribute them to irresistible forces of religion or race. They may accept responsibility for creating conditions that allow epidemics to exist, yet they are willing to exploit the ensuing opportunities for social, economic, and political gain. They may attempt to intervene, yet lack the motivation to follow their efforts through to efficacy. Suffering triggers complex processes by which epidemics and interventions are rationalized.

1

Expecting Providence

WHEN ENGLISH COLONISTS settled the coast of New England, they found themselves on a threatening, unknown shore. Their only solace came from faith that God had blessed their mission in America. The colonists' labors were eventually rewarded with thriving communities, but at tremendous cost. English settlement triggered devastating epidemics among the American Indians who had inhabited the forests and river valleys of America. Between 1616 and 1636, nearly 90 percent of the Massachusett, Wampanoag, and other tribes of New England died from smallpox and other diseases. The colonists, knowing little about these people, had to respond to the unprecedented tragedy of depopulation.

How could this catastrophe be understood? When colonists left Europe for America, they were guided by theological narratives that interpreted Indian mortality as the means by which God prepared the way for English settlement. These narratives, however, would prove inadequate for explaining the realities of encounter. If colonists were God's chosen people, then why did they suffer so greatly during their first winters in America? Could they ignore the suffering of American Indians, with whom they shared so many fears and vulnerabilities? Their lived experiences destabilized the simple narrative of providence. In its place arose a proliferation of disease narratives. Disease could be a product of divine punishment, or the result of freezing winters, murky swamps, and unhealthful diets. Colonists could blame (or thank) God, themselves, or the American Indians.

Much can be learned from the ways in which colonists responded to American Indian demographic collapse. Observers of disparities in health status never respond simply or mechanically to the suffering they witness. They respond actively and thoughtfully. Explanations are generated, organized, evaluated, and utilized. The process of expectation, destabilization, and proliferation of disease narratives occurred time and time again, whenever settlers encountered new groups of American Indians. As will be seen, subsequent Indian epidemics continued to trigger diverse explanations that emphasized environment, behavior, culture, or race. In the tentative wonderings of bewildered colonists can be seen the seeds of centuries of medical theorizing.

Expectation

On 11 November 1620, William Bradford and his fellow Separatists arrived on the gray and foreboding shores of Cape Cod. He described it as "a hideous and desolate wilderness, full of wild beasts and wild men—and what multitudes there might be of them they knew not." But this land was not completely unknown to the colonists. Decades of English fishing, exploration, and trade had provided glimpses of the land and the "savage barbarians" that English colonists would encounter.[1] These reports included the hints of dire epidemics striking down the American Indians that would fuel Puritan providential narratives.

Although American mythology traces English presence in America to the settlements at Jamestown and Plymouth in 1607 and 1620, these colonies came at the end of more than a century of sporadic encounters. Europeans reached the Atlantic coasts of northeastern America in the late fifteenth century and made intermittent appearances throughout the sixteenth century. During these early visits, they met a surprising variety of American Indian groups. They described many villages along the Massachusetts coast, from Agawam, Shawmut, and Wessagusset to Monomoy, Capawack and Nantucket. These settlements belonged to the varied tribes of southern New England: the Pawtucket, Massachusett, Wampanoag (or Pokanoket), Narragansett, Pequot, Niantic, Nipmuck, Mohegan, and Montauk. The people, who spoke dialects of a common Algonquian language, named themselves the Ninnimissinuok.[2]

Although exact numbers are unavailable, between 70,000 and 144,000 Ninnimissinuok lived in southern New England around 1600, with 17,600 to 37,600 in eastern Massachusetts. These people had been living in New England for over 10,000 years. Adapting to changing post-glacial environments, they created sophisticated systems of subsistence by hunting, gathering, fishing, and planting. Long-distance trade brought goods from as far as the Great Lakes. Although hereditary sachems governed the tribes, their authority depended on persuasion and consensus. Powwaws (shamans) oversaw their world of rituals, totems, and guardian spirits.

Increasing population density in the fifteenth and sixteenth centuries fueled increasing sociocultural complexity and intertribal strife. European arrival added new pressures. Bristol fishermen reached New England as early as 1480, exploring intermittently and taking several dozen Micmac captives. Sailing from Carolina to Maine in 1524, Giovanni de Verrazano found the Narragansett to be "kind and gentle," while the natives of Cape Cod were "rude and barbarous." Ten years later, Jacques Cartier found the Micmac already familiar with European traders' interests and expectations. Exploiting the riches of the Grand Banks fisheries, English, Basque, Portuguese, and Norman fishermen became an increasing presence over the sixteenth century, establishing drying stations from Labrador to Acadia. By 1580 between 350 and 700 ships, carrying 8,000 to 10,000 Europeans, plied the waters off Newfoundland each summer. Europeans and American Indians traded copper, jewelry, mirrors, bells, scissors, knives, axes, hooks, cloth, and beaver pelts.[3]

Sustained contact between Europeans and Indians in the northeast began with Samuel de Champlain's explorations of Quebec and New England in 1604 and 1606. The French base at Port Royal, established in 1610, soon became a center of Jesuit missionary activity. The Dutch arrived in 1609, with Henry Hudson's exploration of what he named the North (Hudson) River. By 1624 Dutch merchants had established agricultural outposts at Fort Orange (Albany), Manhattan, and the mouths of the Fresh (Connecticut) and South (Delaware) Rivers.[4]

English efforts evolved in parallel. Bartholomew Gosnold explored the coasts of Maine, Cape Cod, and Martha's Vineyard in 1602, found the natives already wearing European clothes, angered the Indians, and returned to England without attempting a settlement. Martin Pring, leading a trade mission in 1603, impressed the Indians with guitar music. But when the Indians turned hostile, he attacked with guns and fierce mastiffs, and then returned to England. In 1605 George Waymouth traded along the Maine coast and took five Indians captive, planning to train them as interpreters. Hoping to use these captives to facilitate relations with the natives, Ferdinando Gorges sent two voyages to Maine in 1606. The first was lost at sea. The other, after betrayal by the captives, bitter factionalism, and a fierce Maine winter, returned to England in 1607. Gorges tried again in 1611 and 1614, but both trips failed. John Smith explored the coast in 1614 and then attempted to establish a colony at Pemaquid in 1615. Richard Vines, an agent of Gorges, spent a winter on the Maine coast in 1616 and 1617. Thomas Dermer, another agent, led a series of voyages between 1617 and 1620, before dying after a Capawack attack.[5]

These early explorations encountered thriving Indian populations. Gosnold's expedition to Cape Cod met "manie Indians," who were "active, strong, healthfull, and very wittie," and, most important, eager for trade. In 1605, as Champlain sailed through the islands of Massachusetts Bay, he "observed many smokes along the shore, and many savages running up to see us." Receiving a hostile reception, he concluded that Massachusetts was too thickly settled for colonization (Figure 2). John Smith explored these same islands in 1614 and found them "planted with Gardens and Corne fields, and so well inhabited with a goodly, strong and well proportioned people." At Accomack (also Patuxet, later Plymouth), Smith fought with forty or fifty of the natives, but then befriended the survivors.[6]

New England, it seemed, was filled with healthy and aggressive people. The explorers feared that it would be dangerous land for colonists. This fear could only have been strengthened by knowledge of the struggles of English colonists in the south. Three attempts to settle the Outer Banks of the Carolinas failed in the 1580s. The first group ran afoul of the Roanoks, who taunted and threatened the starving colonists, forcing them to leave after a single winter. The second group was attacked within months of arrival; thirteen escaped, but were never heard from again. The third group, deposited in 1587, disappeared by 1590, leaving only three mysterious letters, "CRO," carved into the trunk of a tree.[7] English efforts at Jamestown had only slightly better success. Doomed by laziness and quarrels, only 38 of 108 colonists survived the first winter. During the second winter, starving colonists re-

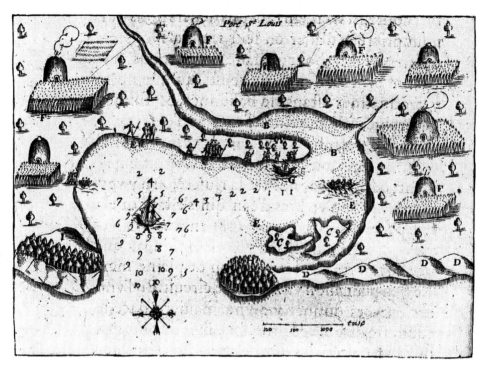

2. Port St. Louis (Plymouth Harbor). From Samuel de Champlain, *Les Voyages du Sieur de Champlain Xaintongeois* (Paris: 1613). The map shows the Wampanoag settlements at Accomack in 1605, before the devastating epidemic. Note the many dwellings, cleared forest, and bountiful crops, suggesting active, healthy precontact populations. (By permission of the Houghton Library, Harvard University.)

sorted to cannibalism, digging up graves to eat corpses. One man even murdered and salted his own wife. Of the 6,000 colonists sent between 1607 and 1624, only 1,200 were alive in 1625, victims of starvation, disease, and depression. When Dermer visited "James Citie" in 1619, he found "generall sicknesse over the Land." His crew barely escaped with their lives.[8]

News of such disasters surely discouraged would-be colonists. But the colonists also knew that the arrival of the Europeans had been dangerous for the American Indians. William Bradford had read Peter Martyr's accounts of Spanish America. Martyr provided abundant evidence of the "Black Legend" of Spanish brutality, describing, for instance, how the Spanish hunted the Caribs and Taino with dogs and abused them so badly in mines that the terrorized natives destroyed their crops and killed themselves and their children. He acknowledged, however, that much of the devastation came from disease. In 1518 "newe and straunge diseases . . . consumed theym lyke rotton sheepe." The combined impact of abuse and disease was devastating: "The number of the poore wretches is woonderfully extenuate. They were once rekened to bee above twelve hundreth thousande heades: But what they are nowe, I abhorre to rehearse."[9]

Martyr described a process that happened time and time again. Whenever Europeans encountered new populations, in Hispaniola and Mexico in the 1500s, in New England and Quebec in the 1600s, and even in Alaska and the Amazon in the 1900s, they witnessed terrible mortality. Epidemics of smallpox, measles, and influenza took the highest toll. These diseases, endemic in Europe, had not been present in the Americas before European arrival. Europeans, exposed as children, developed immunity that protected them as adults. American Indians, without this immunity from prior exposure, and stressed by the chaos of European colonization, were dangerously vulnerable. They died in great numbers.[10]

The English first encountered this mortality among the Indians at Roanoke. Over the winter of 1585 and 1586, Ralph Lane and Thomas Hariot observed epidemics among the local tribes. The disease was "so strange, that they neither knew what it was, nor how to cure it; the like by report of the oldest men in the countrey never happened before." This disease only struck villages that had been visited by the English: "within a few dayes after our departure from everie such towne, the people began to die very fast." When the English did not similarly succumb, Ensenore and other local elders reasonably concluded that the English controlled disease. They asked the English to unleash the disease against their enemies. The English declined, explaining that disease was in the hands of God: "our God would not subject him selfe to anie such praiers and requestes of men." While some English attributed these remarkable events to a recent comet or eclipse of the sun, Hariot believed that it was "the speciall woorke of God for our sakes."[11]

Early experiences in New England were strikingly similar. Vines spent the winter of 1616 and 1617 with the Pemaquid near Saco on the Maine coast. As Gorges described, the local tribes "were sore afflicted with the Plague, for that the Country was in a manner left void of inhabitants." Dermer, who sailed the coasts of Maine and Massachusetts in the summer of 1619, witnessed the end of this epidemic: "I passed alongst the Coast where I found some antient Plantations, not long since populous now utterly void; in other places a remnant remaines, but not free of sicknesse. Their disease was the Plague." Dermer had brought Squanto, a Wampanoag captured at Patuxet (Plymouth) in 1614, whom he hoped to use as an interpreter to establish peaceful relations with the Wampanoag. But on reaching Patuxet, "finding all dead," he abandoned this plan. As had happened at Roanoke, this plague left the English untouched. Although Vines and his crew had shared winter cabins with the dying Pemaquid, "(blessed be *GOD* for it) not one of them ever felt their heads to ake while they stayed there."[12]

By 1619, despite over ten years of effort, Gorges had failed to plant a colony on the New England coast. However, he had learned of the crucial weakness of the plague-stricken natives. The resistance met by Champlain and Smith was gone. Prospects for colonization seemed brighter. Such news may have shaped the hopes of Bradford and his fellow Separatists, who set their sights on "those vast and unpeopled countries of America, which are fruitful and fit for habitation." These reports clearly figured in the thoughts of King James I, who granted Gorges a patent for the Plymouth (Northern Virginia) Company on 3 November 1620: "within these late Yeares, there hath by God's Visitation, raigned a wonderfull Plague, together with many horrible Slaughters and Murthers, committed amongst the Savagees and brutish People there, heertofore inhabiting, in a Manner to the utter Destruction, Devastation and Depopulacion of that whole Territorye." The message seemed clear: "We in our Judgment are persuaded and satisfied that the appointed Time is come in which Almighty God in his great Goodness and Bountie towards Us and our People hath thought fitt and determined, that those large and goodly Territoryes, deserted as it were by their naturall Inhabitants, should be possessed and enjoyed by such of our Subjects and People."[13]

Similar thoughts filled the minds of John Winthrop and the leaders of the Massachusetts Bay Company in 1629 as they planned the Puritan migration. Winthrop wrote his "General Observations" as an argument in support of emigration, addressing a series of specific concerns. Asked "what warrant have we to take that lande which is and hathe been of longe tyme possessed by other sonnes of Adam," Winthrop replied that "God hathe consumed the natives with a miraculous plague, wherby a great parte of the Country is left voyde of Inhabitantes."[14]

As these explorers and colonists attempted to settle the foreboding shores of America, they witnessed epidemics that devastated the American Indian populations. Their brief accounts were quickly written into narratives of divine providence. While England overflowed with populations and religious strife, the original inhabitants of New England had been consumed by war and plague, leaving the land void. None could doubt that God had prepared this land for English colonization. Bradford's Separatists and Winthrop's Puritans could not have asked for a clearer sign of their destiny. On 6 September 1620 Bradford and 101 others set sail "with a prosperous wind" filling the *Mayflower's* sails. Ten years later, leading 1,000 colonists, Winthrop set sail on the *Arbella* with "faire weather" on 8 April 1630.[15]

Destabilization

As soon as they arrived at Cape Cod, the Separatists set out to explore their "desolate wilderness." Their initial forays found the area densely settled. On 15 November they saw "five or six persons with a dog coming towards them, who were savages; but they fled." The next day they found an Indian settlement and helped themselves to "divers fair Indian baskets filled with corn." Further searching revealed more villages with Indians who hid, leaving corn and beans for the taking. On 7 December Indians attacked Bradford's exploring party, but retreated from the English muskets.[16]

However, the colonists soon began to encounter the expected signs of epidemic devastation. On 11 December the *Mayflower's* shallop sailed into a harbor and found an abandoned village with "divers cornfields and little running brooks, a place (as they supposed) fit for situation." They summoned the *Mayflower* from Cape Cod and, on Christmas Day, began to erect the first houses of Plymouth. Three months later they learned the source of their good fortune. In March 1621 Samoset, a Pemaquid chief who had long traded with the English in Maine, walked into Plymouth village. As he described, the site had once been Patuxet, but "about foure yeares agoe, all the Inhabitants dyed of an extraordinary plague, and there is neither man, woman, nor childe remaining . . . to hinder our possession."[17]

Wherever the colonists looked, they saw more evidence of depopulation. Samoset soon returned with Squanto (the sole survivor of Patuxet), who proved a valuable interpreter. When Squanto led Edward Winslow to the village of Massasoit, the Wampanoag chief, they found many fields that had been cleared, but lay empty: "Thousands of men have lived there, which dyed in a great plague not long since." As Bradford described, the victims "not being able to bury one another, their skulls and bones were found in many places lying still above the ground where their houses and dwelling had been, a very sad spectacle to behold." When Winslow explored Massachusetts Bay, he did not find islands full of Indians. Instead, "most of the Ilands have beene inhabited . . . but the people are all dead, or removed." Robert Cushman, who visited Plymouth in the summer of 1621, estimated that "the twentieth person is scarce left alive."[18]

Winslow, Bradford, and Cushman witnessed the impact of a catastrophic epidemic that struck the New England coast in 1616. Although historians still debate the point, European diseases do not seem to have had a significant presence in the Northeast until after 1600. This changed quickly. The French established themselves at Port Royal in 1610. Within a year 75 percent of the nearby Micmac were dead from epidemics. An epidemic might have struck the Wampanoag in 1612 and 1613. In 1616 disease broke out in New England and raged until 1619. Although the nature of the "plague" remains unclear (smallpox? chicken pox? hepatitis?), it extended from the Penobscot River, south along the coast of Maine and Massachusetts Bay, to the eastern shore of Narragansett Bay. Thousands of Eastern Abneki, Massachusett, and Wampanoag died. Whole villages disappeared.[19]

The Plymouth colonists also found ongoing epidemics. In 1622 Squanto "fell sick of an Indian fever" and died within days. When Winslow led a trading mission to the Massachusett in 1623, "they found a great sickness to be amongst the Indians, not unlike the plague, if not the same." Trading at Nemasket, they found "a great sickness arising amongst them" as well. Other settlers who arrived in the 1620s found similar desolation. Thomas Morton, who spent several years near Massachusetts Bay, described how the Indians had "died on heapes." Survivors fled without burying the corpses, leaving them "for Crowes, Kites, and vermin to pray upon." Skulls and bones littered the forest. For Morton, it seemed "a new found Golgatha."[20] It is difficult to imagine the impact of such desolation on the English observers, let alone on the Indian survivors.

The arrival of Winthrop and the Massachusetts Bay Company in 1630 greatly expanded the scale of encounter between the peoples of England and America. The creative potential of the interaction between these groups was almost immediately devastated by epidemic disease. The Great Migration began hesitantly in 1623, when Puritans from Dorchester established a fishing settlement on Cape Ann. They abandoned the site in 1626; thirty remained, but moved their settlement to Naumkeag. In 1628 the Massachusetts Bay Company received a charter for lands between the Charles and Merrimac Rivers. Forty settlers were sent to reinforce the small remnant at Naumkeag. Another 200 arrived in 1629 and renamed the settlement Salem. Motivated by economic recession and religious intolerance in England, one thousand colonists, led by John Winthrop, sailed for Massachusetts Bay in 1630. They quickly settled Charlestown, Boston, Newtown (Cambridge), Medford, Watertown, Rocksbury, Saugus, and Dorchester. Aided by a continuing flood of immigrants—20,000 between 1630 and 1660—the settlers filled the lowlands surrounding Massachusetts Bay and spread along the river valleys and coastlines into Connecticut. Dissidents settled in Rhode Island, New Hampshire, and Nantucket.[21]

Winthrop and his companions had been confident, before their departure, that God had sent epidemics to clear the way for their settlement. Like their predecessors at Plymouth, they found much evidence of this recent mortality. John White marveled that the English could settle land that was already cleared, "which comes to passe by the desolatio hapning through a three yeere Plague, about twelve or sixteene yeeres past, which swept away most of the Inhabitants all along the Sea coast, and in some places utterly consumed man, woman & childe, so that there is no person left to lay claime to the soyle which they possessed." William Wood found other places, once cleared of underbrush, now overgrown. Francis Higginson heard of sagamores (chieftains) who had as few as two Indians left in their tribes, all others having been "swept away by a great and grievous Plague."[22]

The suffering of the Massachusett continued after the colonists arrived. An epidemic may have struck in 1628. John Pond described an outbreak during the winter of 1630 and 1631: "her ar but fewoe eingeines and a gret sorte of them deyeid theis winture it wase thought it wase of the plage."[23] The next two years appear to have been healthy ones, but when cicadas emerged in May 1633, the Wampanoag predicted that "sickness would follow." That summer "pestilent feavers," likely smallpox, struck Plymouth. Although several colonists died, the epidemic among them soon died out. The American Indians, who had forecast the epidemic, did not get off so easily. Bradford described how it soon "swept away many of the Indians from all the places near adjoining." Others told how this epidemic "swept away multitudes of them, young and old. They could not bury their dead." This time, in contrast to the epidemic of 1616, the outbreak did not remain confined to the coast. Instead, it spread quickly throughout New England and into New York and Quebec. The epidemic, apparently the northeast Algonquin's first experience with smallpox, became the greatest epidemic ever to strike the New England Indians. Overall mortality approached 86 percent.[24]

The impact of the epidemic was immediately clear to Winthrop and Bradford. Smallpox killed many of the leaders of the Massachusetts Bay tribes who had met Winthrop on his arrival. Plymouth traders at their post at Windsor on the Connecticut River watched as Indians "died most miserably." Traders from Massachusetts Bay "could have no trade" because the epidemic had spread "as farr as any Indian plantation was knowne to the west." Bradford left the most graphic account, describing how their skin, covered with matted sores and scabs, sloughed off, leaving them "all of a gore blood, most fearful to behold. And then being very sore, what with cold and other distempers, they die like rotten sheep." Unable to care for each other, "some would crawl out on all fours to get a little water, and sometimes die by the way and not be able to get in again."[25] As will be seen, such misery would recur time and time again.

After 1634, less serious outbreaks of various diseases continued amongst the Indians. Thomas Mayhew described a "very strange disease" among the Capawack of Martha's Vineyard in 1643: "they did run up and down till they could run no longer, they made their faces as black as a coale, snatched up any weapon, spake great words, but did no hurt." In later years, Mayhew and his fellow missionaries watched their converts die of "a consuming disease," of smallpox, and of "that grievous disease of the Bloody-Flux, whereof some with great torments in their bowels died." In June 1647 an "Epidemicall sickness" struck Indian, English, French, and Dutch; "it tooke them like a Colde, & a high feaver with it: suche as bledd or used Coolinge drinkes dyed: those who took comfortable things, for most parte recovered." John Josselyn encountered a host of ailments during his travels among the Indians and English: bloody flux, old aches, shrunk sinews, "wind in the stomach," overflowing courses, scalds and burns, mother fits, frozen limbs, "shortness of Wind," ptisick, scurvy, dropsie, worms, fevers, and *"Plague of the Back."*[26]

None of these outbreaks approached the devastation of 1633. Nonetheless, they all contributed to the decimation of the New England Indians over the seventeenth century. A number of contemporary observers tried to estimate the impact of these diseases. John Smith and Robert Cushman both estimated that the epidemic of 1616 to 1619 killed up to 95 percent of the coastal population. White suggested an even more severe estimate: "the Contagion hath scarce left alive one person of an hundred." Bradford made similar estimates for the epidemic of 1633 and 1634: "of a thousand, above nine and a half hundred of them died."[27] While exact numbers are not known, modern estimates suggest that populations fell from at least 70,000 in 1600 to no more than 12,000 in 1700. This is only an average: mortality for specific groups varied between 75 and 100 percent. Similar mortality rates were seen throughout the hemisphere: estimates of total mortality range from 7 to 100 million, out of a total pre-contact population of 8 to 112 million. Die-off ratios—the ratio of pre-contact to post-contact population size—varied between 2:1 and 50:1.[28]

The initial devastation and ongoing depopulation of the New England Indians seemed to fulfill the colonists' expectations of providence, but God did not leave unambiguous messages for his servants. The first years of settlement brought similar devastation to the English. Like their predecessors at Roanoke and Jamestown, the Plymouth colonists faced disaster their first winter. Bradford described how "it pleased God to visit us then with death daily, and with so general a disease that the living were scarce able to bury the dead." Two or three of the colonists died each day, victims of exposure, scurvy, or other diseases brought on by their "inaccommodate condition." By the end of winter, "of 100 odd persons, scarce fifty remained." Cushman lamented this "cruel mortality." In 1623 new colonists arrived in Plymouth. Seeing the miserable condition, they were "daunted and dismayed . . . Some wished themselves in England again; others fell a-weeping . . . In a word, all were full of sadness." If the colonists really believed that God had blessed the English, then they had to admit that God worked in mysterious ways. Only slowly did the colony learn to provide for its own subsistence.[29]

Other groups fared just as poorly. In 1622 sixty men (including Thomas Morton) established a colony at Wessagusset, at the mouth of the Neponset River on Massachusetts Bay. As had happened at Jamestown, they worried more about building forts than planting corn or catching fish. Winter made them regret these decisions: "their forts would not keep out hunger . . . many were starved to death." The suffering men died easily: "one in gathering Shell-fish was so weak, as he stuck fast in the mud, and was found dead in the place." After colonists stole corn from the Massachusett, the Indians plotted to destroy both Wessagusset and Plymouth. Although the plot was broken by colonists from Plymouth, Wessagusset was abandoned in 1623. Gorges sent a group in 1624 to reoccupy the site at Wessagusset, but most left after the first winter. Some remained, including Samuel Maverick, who built himself a fortified house at Winnesimet (now Chelsea). In 1625 four trading partners established a trading post near Wessagusset, named Mt. Woolaston. In 1627 two of the partners left for Virginia. The third partner, Morton, staged a coup, re-established the settlement as "Mare Mount," and attracted the wrath of the Separatists for his irreligious ways. The Plymouth colonists disbanded Ma-Re Mount and shipped Morton back to England in chains.[30]

Although larger and better funded, the Massachusetts Bay Company initially met similar misfortune. Smallpox assailed the colonists as they sailed from England. On one ship it killed fourteen, "we are wondurfule seick." Smallpox, scurvy, and "an infectious fever" followed John Endecott's group ashore at Salem in 1629. Consumption seized Higginson during the winter of 1629 and 1630; he died the following August. Eighty of these 200 settlers perished that winter. When Winthrop and the main Puritan migration arrived in the summer of 1630, they expected to find Endecott and Higginson well established. Instead, as described by Thomas Dudley, they found "the Colony in a sad and unexpected condition": many had died, the survivors were sick and weak. Meanwhile, many of the new arrivals, "being sick of fevers and the scurvy," were too weak to unload their own provisions. Starvation and disease took hold. By December, "there died by estimation about two hundred at the least: so low hath the Lord brought us!" Dudley compared this suffering to that unleashed by Moses on Egypt: "there is not a house where there is not one dead, and in some houses many." John Pond told how settlers at Sudbury suffered severely from scurvy and a burning fever, "all sudberey men ar ded but three and thee woomen and sume cheilldren."[31]

News of this suffering reached Plymouth. Winslow and Samuel Fuller, Plymouth's physician, found "the hand of God to be upon them and against them at Charlestown . . . not sparing the righteous but partaking with the wicked in these bodily judgments." Winthrop saw God's judgment in the mortality, but had faith that it would pass once their faith had been purified: "the Lord is pleased to humble us . . . but in his due tyme, will doe us good, according to the measure of our Afflictions." The health of the colonists did improve after the first winter, the result of assistance from the established colony at Plymouth, and their ability to summon substantial resources from England. For instance, when the *Lyon* arrived in February 1631, it brought a "store of Juice of Lemons"; many who suffered from scurvy "recovered speedyle." But even after surviving the challenges of their first winters, the colonists remained vulnerable to many diseases. The great epidemic of 1633, as noted above, started at Plymouth, "many fell very sick." Over twenty colonists died, including Fuller. Smallpox "caused them to humble themselves and seek the Lord; and towards winter it pleased the Lord the sickness ceased."[32] Disease was never far from their minds.

These early years of English settlement had not fulfilled English expectations. The sorry fate of most of the early colonies produced little evidence of divine blessing. Meanwhile, the colonists saw only conflicting evidence of God's wrath towards the Indians. The epidemic of 1616 to 1619 had laid waste to many coastal tribes, but many groups remained. Enough Wampanoag survived to become crucial suppliers of corn to Plymouth. Enough of the Massachusett survived to threaten the first colony at Wessagusset. The Narragansett "had not been at all touched with this wasting plague." With his "great people" estimated "to be many thousands strong," the Narragansett chief Canonicus could "breathe forth many threats against us" and harass the Plymouth colonists for several years. The survival of western tribes disrupted plans for an English plantation along the Connecticut River in 1633: "the place was not fitt for plantation, there beinge 3: or 4000: warlike Indians." Nantucket in 1634 remained "full of Indians."[33]

Winthrop and the Massachusetts Bay Company also encountered an initial abundance of Indians. Their populations might have been thinned, but they remained "exceeding numerous about us." The *Arbella* sighted land on 6 June 1630; it anchored off Cape Ann on 12 June. That first day, an "Indian came abord us, & laye there all night." The next morning, Masconomo, the Pawtucket sagamore at Agawam, visited with one of his men. Local leaders made frequent visits to Winthrop in Boston. On 23 March 1631, Chickatabot, sagamore of the Massachusett south of Boston, presented Winthrop with a hogshead of corn. On 26 March Winthrop hosted brothers John and James Sagamore, who led the Pawtucket of the Mystic and Saugus rivers north of Boston. On 4 April Wahginnacut, a sagamore from the Quoanehtacut (Connecticut) river, arrived. On 13 July Winthrop received Miantonomi, nephew of Canonicus. Indians were such a presence in the colonists' lives that by 6 September John Dawe, an English servant, had been whipped "for solicitinge an indian Sqa to incontinencye."[34] Had God really intended to clear the Indians to make way for the English? Enough Indians remained to help or to hinder the colonists.

As initial events clouded providential visions, the colonists were moved less by faith in providential destruction of the American Indians than by faith in their common humanity. They recognized that both groups shared common struggles. Colonists at Plymouth and Wessagusset starved to death, fell sick after gorging on certain foods, and suffered from frigid winter snows and seas. The Wampanoag and Massachusett suffered from these same susceptibilities. After the colonists routed the conspiracy at Wessagusset in 1623, many terrified Massachusett "forsook their houses, running to and fro like men distracted, living in swamps and other desert places, and so brought manifold diseases amongst themselves, whereof very many are dead." The Plymouth colonists, moved by shared suffering, also tried to help ailing Indians. Cushman, writing in December 1621, claimed that "when any of them are in want, as often they are in the winter, when their corn is done, we supply them to our power, and have them in our houses eating and drinking, and warming themselves." In 1623 Winslow was called to pay respects to Massasoit, who supposedly lay dying. Finding him suffering only from constipation, Winslow cured him with "a confection of many comfortable conserves" and a broth of strawberry and sassafras. Massasoit long remained grateful to the colonists.[35]

Similar stories emerged during the early years of the Massachusetts Bay Colony. When smallpox struck the Massachusett in November 1633, the English tried to help. According to Winthrop, "some of them were cured." As the epidemic intensified in December, healthy Indians fled, leaving the English to care for the languishing victims: "It wrought muche with them, that when their owne people forsooke them, yet the Englishe came dayly & ministered to them." Winthrop singled out one family in particular, the Mavericks at Winnesimet, who "ministerd to their necessityes, & buried their dead, & took home many of their Children." Plymouth traders at Windsor also nursed the dying Indians: "though at first they were afraid of the infection, yet seeing their woeful and sad condition and hearing their pitiful cries and lamentations, they had compassion of them, and daily fetched them wood and water and made them fires, got them victuals whilst they lived; and buried them when they died."[36] Although it is unclear how often such assistance was given, the efforts do show that colonists did not simply rejoice at the providential destruction of Indian populations. Motivated by sympathy for the dying Indians, the English were "constrained to help."[37]

When colonists had imagined America from the comforts of England, news of American Indian depopulation had easily been placed into narratives of providence. Indians could be dismissed as savages casually eradicated by an obliging God. Colonists' early experiences in America challenged this simple vision. While the Wampanoag and Massachusett had been wasted by epidemics, the colonists experienced extraordinary mortality as well. Although Bradford had expected to find "wild beasts and wild men" in America, the colonists quickly recognized the common humanity of the American Indians. Sharing vulnerabilities to famine, frostbite, and constipation, the colonists acted out of compassion to relieve Indian suffering.

Proliferation

As the events of colonization unfolded in unexpected ways, colonists' explanations of Indian epidemics evolved a complexity that historians have not fully appreciated. Evocations of providential decline did continue to appear despite colonists' own mortality. However, these voices were but one of many in the wilderness of New England.

Well aware of their own sufferings, the Plymouth colonists seldom attributed Indian disease to acts of God. Neither Bradford nor Winslow described the epidemic of 1616 to 1619 as an act of God. Winslow's only mention of God and disease came when God "struck Tisquantum with sickness, insomuch as he there died." For Cushman, the real miracle was that the Wampanoag had not eradicated the colonists during their first winter: "when there was not six able persons among us, and that they came daily to us by hundreds, with their sachems or kings, and might in one hour have made a dispatch of us." Others were more willing to read the will of God. Despite his own failures in the 1620s, Thomas Morton did not doubt the cause of American Indian epidemics: "the hand of God fell heavily upon them." John Smith, who had once seen the thriving populations of Massachusetts Bay, heard of their demise and believed that "God had laid this Country open for us, and slaine the most part of the inhabitants by cruell warres and a mortall disease."[38]

Providence made a stronger showing in the aftermath of 1633. Bradford described how "it pleased God to visit these Indians with a great sickness." Winthrop noted that "Gods hand hath so pursued them, as for 300 miles space, the greatest parte of them are swept awaye by the small poxe." He concluded that "God hathe hereby cleered our title to this place." After all, "if God were not pleased with our inheriting these parts, why did he drive out the natives before us? and why dothe he still make roome for us, by deminishinge them as we increace?" The anonymous chronicler of Charlestown and John Cotton, the leading Puritan theologian in Massachusetts, both used the epidemic to defend the legitimacy of Puritan land claims. Without "this remarkable and terrible stroke of God," the colonists "would with much more difficulty have found room, and at far greater charge have obtained and purchased land." Thomas Gorges, who spent two frustrating years in Maine as the deputy of his cousin Ferdinando Gorges, found that "The Indians are tractable. The Lord sent his avenging Angel & swept the most part away." An anonymous 1642 tract provided a list of things for which the colonists should give thanks. God's gift of epidemics led the list: "1. In sweeping away great multitudes of the Natives by the small Pox."[39]

Historians have long been impressed by these providential explanations of Indian epidemics. Defining the standard interpretation in 1909, Herbert Williams concluded that the English regarded the epidemics "as the method by which Providence removed the savages to make room for Englishmen." John Heagerty commented wryly that Puritan "faith had the virtue of simplicity and directness." According to Alden Vaughan, the disparity between Indian demise and English health "was proof positive of the Lord's intention of making New England a haven for His true church." Such assertions have been reiterated by historian after historian.[40] This common account of English responses equates providential interpretation with utter callousness. According to historians, the colonists saw the Indian mortality "as the destruction of devils." They considered the depopulation "a blessed event." The devastation "was a Golgotha the Puritans delighted in discovering."[41]

However, historians' focus on this one aspect of response obscures a more interesting narrative. Karen Kupperman has shown that colonists' responses to American Indians were more complex than past analyses have allowed: "within a single brief book writers could be contemptuous and admiring, hostile and friendly, self-confident and terrified."[42] The complexity of English responses to Indian disease demonstrates this particularly well. Although providential celebrations of American Indian mortality did occur, they were but one mode of explanation.

During the early years of colonization, English and Indians encountered each other with mutual curiosity. Neither side initially believed the other to be intrinsically different at a physical level. Philip Vincent, a leader of the English forces in the Pequot War, saw Indian bodies as indistinguishable from the English: "Their outsides say they are men . . . Their correspondency of disposition with us, argueth all to be of the same constitution, and the sons of Adam, and that we had the same matter, the same mould. Only art and grace have given us that perfection which yet they want, but may perhaps be as capable thereof as we." Roger Williams agreed: "Nature knows no difference between *Europe* and *Americans* in blood, birth, bodies, &c. God having of one blood made all mankind." Williams even wrote a poem on the subject: "Boast not proud English, of thy birth & blood, / Thy brother Indian is by birth as Good. / Of one blood God made Him, and Thee & All, / As wise, as faire, as strong, as personall."[43]

Even skin color was misleading. As Morton described, Massachusett infants "are of complexion white as our nation, but their mothers in their infancy make a bath of Wallnut leaves, huskes of Walnuts, and such things as will staine their skinne for ever, wherein they dip and washe them to make them tawny." Wood held a similar belief, but with a different mechanism: "Their swarthiness is the sun's livery, for they are born fair." Kupperman has shown that this faith in the artificial origins of Indian complexion reassured the English that the Indians were not a different race. Only later in the century would colonists begin to suspect that Indian disease reflected some sort of inherent constitutional susceptibility. Joyce Chaplin has argued that this attribution of disease to "innate weakness" was crucial to the gradual articulation of "a racial definition of humanity in America." Racial definitions, however, did not consolidate until the nineteenth century, and even then (as will be seen) observers continued to downplay ideas of inherent difference and instead emphasize the pathogenic power of behavior and environment.[44]

Until the racial definition emerged, colonists believed that their bodies and Indian bodies shared the same vulnerabilities. As a result, colonists often explained Indian epidemics in the same ways that they explained their own diseases. Although some historians ignore the complexity of colonists' medical thought, the English brought elaborate theories of disease etiology to America. Theology certainly remained central to their thoughts, but the colonists were practical people dealing with practical problems: disease and its causes could be familiar and mundane. Moreover, leading colonists, educated at Cambridge University, were well versed in Aristotelian natural philosophy. As a result of these practical and academic experiences, they entertained a wide range of natural explanations of disease.[45]

Colonial environments could bring health or disease. William Wood found that New England had a "medicinable climate" for English constitutions. Higginson and many others agreed: "there is hardly a more healthfull place to be found in the World that agreeth better with our English Bodyes." The clear and dry air cured disease by "altering, digesting, and drying up the cold and crude humors of the Body." The water kept the body "temperately soluble." Native crops, particularly corn, kept "the body in a constant moderate loosenesse."[46] This same environment, however, could also turn deadly. Wet lodgings and cold weather "so taynted" the Plymouth colonists that Bradford feared they would "breed diseases and infection amongst us." Colonists' bodies, corrupted by rotten provisions during their long Atlantic voyages, were particularly vulnerable when they first arrived in New England: "the searching sharpness of that purer climate creeping in at the crannies of their crazed bodies, caused death and sickness." Damp lodgings caused scurvy among the Massachusetts Bay colonists. As always, "The poorer sorte of people (who laye longe in tentes &c:)" suffered the most.[47] Similar "natural causes" produced fevers in colonists during hot weather. The heat of even Connecticut could be a threat: "All that southerly part of the seacoast having, as more propinquity to Virginia in situation, so a participation with it in its climatical diseases."[48]

Other causes of disease abounded. Colonists died, or lost fingers and feet, to frostbite. Many starved. Others suffered from exhaustion: lacking horses, "many an honest Gentleman travell a foot for a long time, and some have even perished with extreame heate in their travells." Certain foods, such as fresh mussels which the Plymouth colonists found on Cape Cod, "made use all sicke that did eat." John Winthrop Jr. had heard that leprosy might be caused by consuming too many fish. Specific foods could also heal. Winthrop described how "Oranges and Limons," shipped from Bermuda in 1636, brought "a great reliefe to our people." Josselyn praised native cranberries as "excellent against the Scurvy." Some diseases were contagious and could spread from person to person. Women were vulnerable to a unique set of problems, including unskilled midwives, excessive reading, and promiscuous suckling. Winthrop also knew that pessimism and depression could kill: "It hathe been always observed heere, that such as fell into discontente & lingered after their former Conditions in Englande, fell into the skirvye, & dyed." Writing in 1643, Bradford saw clear lessons from their experiences: "change of air, famine or unwholesome food, much drinking of water, sorrows and troubles, etc., all of them are enemies to health, causes of many diseases, consumers of natural vigour and the bodies of men, and shorteners of life."[49]

Believing that Indian bodies resembled European bodies, the colonists attributed Indian diseases to the same exposure and deprivation that caused English disease. Gorges traced the epidemic that devastated the Maine coast in 1616 to unrest that followed the death of the local chief: competing groups "fell at variance among themselves, spoiled and destroyed each others people and provision, and famine took hould of many; which was seconded by a great and generall plague." After the Plymouth colonists routed the Massachusett conspiracy at Wessagusset, the terrified Indians abandoned their houses and corn, fled into swamps, and died in great numbers. Roger Williams argued that the Narragansett suffered from lack of "a raisin or currant or any physick, Fruit or spice, or any Comfort more than their Corne and Water." Excessive food could also be a culprit. After Winslow cured Massasoit of his nearly fatal constipation, the relieved sachem gorged himself on fatty duck and nearly died again.[50]

The colonists also described a series of American Indian behaviors that they considered dangerous. Winslow noted that the Wampanoag exposed themselves by visiting people who were "dangerously sick" in their homes. Williams, however, noted that such visits were not made if "it be an infectious disease." Colonists described the offensive, supposedly harmful, antics of Indian healers. Winslow criticized Massasoit's powwaws, who made "such a hellish noice, as it distempered us that were well, and therefore unlike to ease him that was sick." Mayhew accepted that the powwaws might once have been effective, but "since the Word of God hath been taught unto them in this place, the *Pawwaws* have been much foiled in their devillish tasks, and that instead of curing have rather killed many." Josselyn attributed syphilis to Indian cannibalism. Such victim blaming has always remained popular among observers of American Indian epidemics.[51]

Some colonists also took seriously the Indians' own explanations of the epidemics. Thomas Gorges described how the natives near Accomenticus believed in a link between a lunar eclipse and Indian mortality: there "hapned an ecclipse of the moon such as was never heer seen by Inglish or Indians, for she was totally ecclipsed for the space of 2 hours. The Indians suppose because the moon dyed (as they terme it). This will be a fatal year to them." Roger Williams described a similar belief about earthquakes. After the earthquake in June 1638, Narragansett elders told Williams that this was the fifth earthquake in eighty years, and that "they allwayes observed either Plauge or Pox or some other Epidemicall disease followed: 3, 4 or 5 yeare after the Earthquake (or Naunaumemoauke, as they speake)." The English and American Indians could participate in a mutual discourse on disease etiology, one based wholly on natural mechanisms.[52]

At times the colonists even admitted a sense of responsibility for

American Indian mortality, attributing it to the changes in traditional customs that followed contact with the Europeans. William Wood observed that when the Indians changed "their bare Indian commons for the plenty of England's fuller diet, it is so contrary to their stomachs that death or a desperate sickness immediately accrues, which makes so few of them desirous to see England." When epidemics struck converts on Martha's Vineyard in 1643, Mayhew described how the Wampanoag "laid the cause of all their wants, sicknesses, and death, upon their departing from their old heathenish ways." When promising Indian scholars died at Harvard College, some observers "attributed it unto the great change upon their bodies, in respect of their diet, lodging, apparel, studies; so much different from what they were inured to among their own countrymen." Alcohol was often singled out. Williams blamed the liquor trade for the "many sudden deaths, what by *Consumptions* and *Dropsies*, the *Barbarians* have been murthered, *hundreds*, if not *thousands* in the whole Countrey." Daniel Gookin blamed this "beastly sin of drunkenness" among the Indians on "the English and other Christian nations."[53] Such attributions of morbidity and mortality to the process of cultural transition would become a dominant theme in the ensuing centuries of encounter.

The English were not alone in generating diverse explanations for American Indian epidemics. Spanish, French, Dutch, and Swedish colonists also observed the initial depopulation of the Atlantic coast of the Americas. All of the groups described similar processes of divine providence and natural mechanism. Consider the epidemic that struck the Indians of Guatemala in 1576 and 1577. Spanish officials initially described the disease as a contagion that had spread from Mexico. A formal investigation disagreed, citing abuses perpetrated by the local Spaniards. A second investigation, hoping to exonerate the colonists, blamed divine mechanisms: "What causes the Indians to die and to diminish in number are secret judgments of God beyond the reach of man."[54]

The French experience is most useful here. While the English settled New England in the early seventeenth century, the French worked to convert and colonize Acadia and Quebec. Jesuit missionaries left a detailed and angst-ridden record of the ensuing Indian mortality. When the French arrived, they found healthy populations in Acadia (1610) and Quebec (1625). This quickly changed. By 1637 50 percent of the Huron had died from epidemics of smallpox and ill-defined fevers. The Huron "asked why so many of them died, saying that since the coming of the French their nation was going to destruction." The Jesuits accepted this challenge and proposed a wide range of explanations.[55]

Like their predecessors at Roanoke and Plymouth, the Jesuits were quick to see the hand of God behind daily events. Just as God rewarded drought-stricken converts with bountiful rains and restored health to missionaries afflicted with pestilence, God struck down blasphemers, whether French or Indian. When a Montagnais sorcerer ignored warnings that he would land himself in hell, "God did not fail to strike him; for the year had not yet expired, when his cabin took fire, I know not how, and he was dreadfully scorched, roasted and burned."[56] Few examples of God's judgment, however, involved Indian disease.

Instead, the French had many natural explanations for differential susceptibility to epidemics. Like the English, the French emphasized exposure and privation. Paul Le Jeune and Pierre Biard both attributed Indian deaths to the hardship of their "wretched" lives: "only the most robust can endure." Le Jeune also blamed "their filthy habits." Echoing Winslow's opinion of Wampanoag shamans, he criticized Huron sorcerers. One such "charlatan," trying to cure a sick child, "was beating upon and whirling around an instrument full of little stones, made exactly like a tambourine. With all this he howled immoderately. In a word, he and his companion, in order to cure this little boy of a fever, made enough noise to give one to a healthy man." The Jesuits also recognized that many diseases could be contagious. In a smallpox outbreak in 1640, "the evil spread from house to house, from village to village, and finally became scattered throughout the country." Hierosme Lalemant blamed the rapid spread on carelessness: "the Hurons—no matter what plague or contagion they may have—live in the midst of their sick."[57]

Le Jeune admitted that such explanations did not account for the increase in mortality since French arrival: "I would have considerable trouble to assign a natural cause for their dying so much more frequently than they did in the past." Biard had attributed worsening Micmac mortality to changed diets. Le Jeune singled out brandy and wine, "which they love with an utterly unrestrained passion." The alcohol trade, of course, he blamed on the English.[58] The Indians had other

ideas. As early as 1616, the Micmac had recognized a correlation between French contact and Indian mortality. They concluded that the
French poisoned them or sold them spoiled goods. When missionaries
remained healthy while their subjects died, the Huron concluded that
the French "had a secret understanding with the disease." Some
believed that the French spread pestilence with a "bewitched" cloak.
Some claimed that they kept a "crafty demon" concealed in a musket
and sent it wherever they wanted. Others accused the French of poi-
soning their water, of defiling pictures of their children, or of destroying them with the magical power of writing. Only when missionaries
fell sick did the Huron concede that the French might not be "undying
demons, and masters of maladies."[59]

Although the French denied Huron allegations of deliberate infection, they increasingly admitted their own culpability as they observed
the continuing epidemics. Lalemant conceded that "since our arrival in
these lands, those who had been the nearest to us, had happened to be
the most ruined by the diseases." The implication was unavoidable: "no
doubt we carried the trouble with us, since, wherever we set foot, either
death or disease followed us . . . where we were most welcome, where
we baptized most people, there it was in fact where they died the
most." Shaken by this, Lalemant sought solace in faith: "We shall see in
heaven the secret, but ever adorable, judgments of God therein."[60]
Guilt-stricken and fearing that they were the cause of depopulation,
the ever-inquisitive Jesuits set aside their curiosity.

Suspicion that the French brought death to Quebec threatened the
Jesuit mission. By the 1630s, however, severe mortality (from French-
acquired epidemics) left the Huron dependent on continuing French
assistance: they had become trapped in a deadly relationship. The Jesuits faced a different problem. Believing that their work depended on
the survival and conversion of the Huron, they could take no solace in
providential depopulation. Instead, they emphasized natural mechanisms of disease, especially ideas of contagion and contaminated goods
that reflected the central role played by commerce in French-Indian
relations.[61]

Taken together, the French and English experiences demonstrate
the appeal of providential interpretations across a range of European
cultures and religions. However, neither group saw the epidemics simply in moral terms. As Joyce Chaplin has argued, epidemics were both

"moral *and* material events."[62] The English and French understood that natural mechanisms of disease afflicted both colonists and Indians: the many hazards of the colonial environment undermined health, whereas specific behaviors increased the risk of disease. Some colonists, even in this early period, suspected that the process of encounter and ensuing cultural change created the vulnerabilities that devastated American Indians. As a result, theology had to accommodate pragmatism, which recognized disease as the proximate outcome of physical risks; sympathy, which acknowledged the shared suffering of the American Indians; and responsibility, which conceded European culpability for the mortality.

If God truly loved the English above all others, for the moment it was not clear. American Indians had suffered the tremendous mortality that the colonists had expected, but any obvious disparity in health status had been confounded by the colonists' own suffering during their first decade in New England. No simple messages lent themselves to providential interpretation. Instead, the destabilizing processes of colonization fueled diverse explanatory narratives. Everyone—colonist and Indian—was flawed, and thus vulnerable to divine judgment. Everyone had a mortal body, subject to hostile weather, inadequate food, and lurking disease. Colonists could rejoice when God favored them by removing American Indians, but they could also empathize with Indian suffering and regret their own responsibility for the calamity. The world was a complicated and dangerous place.

2

Meanings of Depopulation

AS THEY PLANNED their voyages of colonization, William Bradford, John Winthrop, and other English adventurers had optimistic visions of America. Although they had long been persecuted in Europe, they expected to find religious freedom and economic opportunity in America. They had faith that God blessed their mission, going so far as to send epidemics among the American Indians: by the "awful and admirable dispensation" of smallpox, "it pleased God to make room for his people of the English nation."[1] The first decade of colonization challenged such providential narratives. While the colonists did witness shocking mortality among the Pemaquid, Massachusett, and Wampanoag of coastal New England, they struggled with devastating problems of their own. Half the Plymouth colonists died in their first winter. Colonies planted throughout the 1620s failed. The colonists at Massachusetts Bay, who would eventually prevail through force of numbers, had to overcome smallpox, consumption, starvation, and depression before establishing themselves firmly on those dangerous shores.

These struggles of early colonization destabilized the clear narratives that had led the colonists to America. God did seem to strike down American Indians, but Europeans were similarly vulnerable to God's judgments. The practical concerns of daily life also fueled a parallel series of explanations, attributing diseases of colonists and Indians to much more tangible causes, including food, environment, behavior, and specific natural phenomena. With these understandings, the colonists struggled to overcome the diseases, holding days of prayer, acquiring lemons from Bermuda, and providing food and nursing care to afflicted Massachusett and Wampanoag. Such sympathy, however, was constrained by the realization that the colonists could often do little to overcome smallpox and other epidemics. Even as the colonists welcomed some American Indians into their moral communities, they set low expectations for their own interventions.

Despite this initial diversity of explanation and response, however, the colonists did not face insoluble confusion about the meanings of depopulation. Instead, their concept of providence provided a framework for integrating natural and theological mechanisms into a unified account of the horror of Indian demise. When the integration worked, it provided a powerful and reassuring understanding of the catastrophe that the colonists observed. This framework, however, proved imperfect. Many examples show how colonists contested the relevance of theological and natural explanations. These tensions enable an analysis of how colonists and Indians, filtering their perceptions of Indian epidemics through the needs and concerns of their local worlds, favored explanations that were the most meaningful and useful. Meaning can also be found in the way that the initial diversity of explanation was distilled over the seventeenth century. If the initial turbulence of colonization fueled instability of explanation, then the expansion of the English colonies allowed consolidation. As English populations grew while Indian populations declined, the colonists found new meaning in their initial expectations of providence. These re-emerged as the essential memory of American Indian epidemics.

Subtleties

During the initial encounter between colonists and American Indians, providential and natural explanations often appeared side by side. This diversity challenges our modern imagination. In defiance of our desire to assign effects to a single cause, early modern writers inhabited an intellectual world in which multiple causes operated simultaneously. Any attempt to understand the meanings of their explanations must acknowledge this difference. As Karen Kupperman warns, we cannot easily understand colonists' thoughts: "Their purposes and meanings are alien and require imaginative reconstruction."[2] Because of the difficulty of adopting their world view, it is only possible to make guarded progress in pursuit of meanings. This progress, however, is extremely useful.

The work of the many historians who have studied Puritan theories of providence offers a valuable starting point. Perry Miller provided the classic interpretation of the Puritan world view. He centered Puritan lives on the anguish that resulted from their inability to attain true harmony with God: "The ultimate reason of all things they called God, the dream of a possible harmony between man and his environment they named Eden, the actual fact of disharmony they denominated sin, the moment of illumination was to them divine grace, the effort to live in the strength of that illumination was faith, and the failure to abide by it was reprobation." More recent work has examined subtleties that Miller overlooked. Miller treated the first three generations of Puritans in New England as a homogenous group, their writings as "the product of a single intelligence." Historians have since emphasized the many inconsistencies and subtleties of Puritan thought. David Hall has shown that the "mental world of the colonists was far richer than we have supposed": they could "select among a range of meanings." As a result, interpreting their thoughts and contradictions, the "flows of meaning and how people acted on them," remains "more of an art than a science."[3]

Several aspects of Puritan thought are clear. Most Calvinists shared the belief of Thomas Beard, who wrote that "God was immediately and actively present in the world, the ultimate force behind everything that happened." As a consequence, Puritan minds did not draw our modern dichotomy between physical and spiritual. Instead, Puritans sought a seamless view of causation, in which natural and theological explanations operated in concert. God had once intervened directly, without acting through the laws of nature. Such miracles had ceased in biblical times, as soon as God completed the revelation. During the lives of the Puritans, God resorted only to special providences. Cotton Mather explained how these worked. All events had a teleology: by "the foreknowledge and decree of God, the first cause, all things come to pass immutably and infallibly." But God did not act directly: God did not make Indians vanish in a puff of smoke. Instead, providence was manifested through natural processes, "according to the nature of second causes, either necessarily, freely, or contingently."[4]

In this world, all events had natural and spiritual causes, simultaneously. As Perry Miller has described, God, "assuming for the moment the role of a natural agent and binding Himself by natural law," acted "by natural instruments, by arranging the causes or influencing the agents, rather than by forcible interposition and direct compulsion." Half of the Plymouth colonists died the first winter, clearly from exposure and disease. But as Mather explained, if such diseases had not "fetcht so many of this number away to Heaven," the whole group would have starved the following summer. When an earthquake rattled Boston in 1662, Nathaniel Morton noted that the "Efficient Cause is Supernatural, as either principally *God*, or instrumentally the *Angels*," but the formal cause was "naturally the Wind shut up within the Pores and Bowels of the Earth."[5] Although providential events might seem local and contingent, they could just as easily reflect plans laid by God at the origins of the cosmos.

Such special providences had many functions in Puritan life. Strict Calvinists believed that all events had been foreordained by God, even those that seemed to be remarkable coincidences conducted by people acting independently. God, extending grace, had already chosen whom to save. But this did not absolve Puritans of the responsibility to lead devout lives. As Charles Cohen has explained, grace was a dynamic interaction between God and humans: "Grace does not operate without human participation." Although individual action could not bring about salvation, individuals' choices reflected the status of their salvation. Individuals who did good works could suspect that they were good people who had been chosen. Perception of divine intent behind daily events oriented the Puritans to their status. It revealed God's love or anger, motivating them to good works whether to demonstrate their salvation or to regain God's love.[6] Providential interpretation restored aspects of agency and responsibility to a predestined world.

Providence also provided crucial reassurance in a bewildering world. Early modern life overflowed with danger, powerlessness, and death. As suggested by historian Michael Winship, faith in the purpose of events replaced anxiety with serenity, offering "consolation by assuring believers that all that befell them came from a loving, if often angry, God." In this way providence provided an "organizing and explanatory principle" for all aspects of Puritan lives and history. Thomas Shepard, who became the minister at Cambridge in 1636, could endure shipwreck, illness, and the death of his wife and son, confident that each had a role. For instance, when his son died, he recognized that "the Lord now showed me my weak faith, want of fear, pride, carnal content, immoderate love of creatures and of my child especially."[7] Such providential reassurance was not confined to the Puritans. English Anglicans and French Catholics just as easily found solace in faith that all occurred by the will of God.

With natural mechanisms energized by divine will, the world (in theory) could be both "unpredictable and communicative." As Winship described, it "bubbled forth a rich semiotic stew of intentions, which all could freely taste." Pursuit of such meanings motivated Puritan natural philosophy: "they took particular comfort in moralizing over oddities which seemed to be produced by natural causes, but in which the pious investigator could perceive the finger of God."[8] Snow might freeze feet; cranberries might cure scurvy; Indians might die from consuming English foods. God was behind it all: God's will motivated the weather; God graced humans with knowledge of medical therapeutics; and God willed that the Indians should die to make way for the English mission in America. When the system functioned smoothly, there was no choice between spiritual and natural explanations of disease. Both occurred, simultaneously. The synergy of meaning and mechanism aided Puritans in their pursuit of grace. Every event, of both health and disease, became a tool in their quest for salvation.

Even when this union of theology and natural process operated seamlessly, the faith was difficult to follow. Devout colonists lived a continuous struggle to accept their many calamities with faith. Why did God keep Plymouth without a minister, striking down their recruit with a fatal fever? Why did God strike down even the most godly and dedicated colonists? Thomas Shepard might have been willing to accept providential reassurance for every misfortune, seeing his illness in 1642 as a reminder that his life was "a vapor and bubble, a vanity . . . I was sinning and provoking God in every action."[9] But such feats of finding solace in misery were likely ones that few could accomplish.

Furthermore, colonists struggled to understand events in which theology and natural philosophy existed in tension. In some cases, events occurred in ways that defied Puritan understanding of the natural world. In others, events were assigned firmly to the natural or theological domains, but not to both. These discrepancies opened space for creative interpretation.

First, English colonists could not always find natural explanations for the phenomena they observed. During his missionary efforts, John Eliot was besieged by questions from the Massachusett about the causes of winds, tides, and thunder. When asked why "the Sea water was salt, and the Land water fresh," Eliot threw up his hands in frustration: "Tis so from the wonderfull worke of God, as why berries sweet and Cranberries sowre, there is no reason but the wonderfull worke of God that made them so." When no natural mechanism could be found to explain the disappearance of a plague of rats from Bermuda, John Smith pronounced it a miracle, "a more mediate and secret worke of God": "God doth sometimes effect his will without subordinate and secondary causes."[10] Where natural causes could not be found, colonists' dual-causal system collapsed simply to attribution of cause to divine will.

Second, some events defied known natural mechanisms. Having suffered so many hardships, the Plymouth colonists reasonably expected that they would live only short lives. To Bradford's surprise and amazement, the opposite occurred: "I cannot but here take occasion not only to mention but greatly to admire the marvelous providence of God! That notwithstanding the many changes and hardships that these people went through, and the many enemies they had and difficulties they met withal, that so many of them should live to very old age!" William Hubbard struggled to explain the vagaries of fevers in Connecticut in the 1630s: sometimes mild, sometimes fatal, sometimes general, sometimes afflicting a single plantation. This variability could only mean one thing: "though there might be something in the climate, yet a Divine Hand hath overruled." Other surprises occurred frequently, if on smaller scales. John Winthrop described the arrival of two ships in Boston in 1636: although they endured a month of "stinking water" and "very short and bad" provisions, "through the great providence of the Lord, they came all safe on shore, and most of them sound." In 1637 smallpox struck a ship but, according to Edmund Browne, few suffered: it was "ordered by the Lord's power, as if it had not been infectious."[11] God, apparently, could guide events away from their natural course.

Third, colonists could take questions that had both theological and natural aspects and assign them to one domain. When fleeing Massachusett conspirators died in swamps in 1623, Ianough, their sachem, feared that "the God of the English was offended with them, and would destroy them in his anger." Edward Winslow saw a more practical explanation: "through fear they set little or no corn, which is the staff of life, and without which they cannot long preserve health and strength." William Bradford attributed earthquakes to God, but whether the earthquake of 1638 caused the ensuing cold summer and poor corn harvest, "I leave it to naturalists to judge." In 1646 the "loathsome disease" of syphilis struck Boston, infecting a woman and sixteen children. Magistrates could "find no dishonesty" in the woman or her husband. They theorized that the disease began because many children had suckled her breasts. Winthrop, in a rare move, deferred judgment and concluded that "this is a question to be decided by Phisitians." When relief came "by the good providence of God," it took the form of a young surgeon from the West Indies "who had had experience of the right waye of the Cure of that disease."[12] Even the morality-laden disease of syphilis was better left to a surgeon's hands than to theological inquiry.

Finally, natural and providential explanations could compete in open debate. Thomas Dudley described a dispute he had with a minister, Mr. Wilson, about whether the early mortality of the Plymouth colonists arose from "natural causes" or from "Other causes God may have." Although Dudley did "forbear to mention" God's causes, he had no trouble listing potential natural causes: "the want of warm lodging and good diet . . . the sudden increase of heat which they endure that are landed here in summer, the salt meats at sea." Those who landed in winter "died of the scurvy, as did our poorer sort, whose houses and bedding kept them not sufficiently warm, nor their diet sufficiently in heart." Although he favored natural causes, Dudley, in the end, left "this matter to the further dispute of physicians and divines." Daniel Gookin described similar debates about why so many Indian students at Harvard College died from consumption. Some "have attributed it unto the great change upon their bodies, in respect of their diet, lodging, apparel, studies; so much different from what they were inured to among their own countrymen." Others saw the deaths as "severe dispensations of God," either because "God was not pleased yet to make use of any of the Indians to preach the gospel," or because Satan "did use all his strategems and endeavours to impede the spreading of the christian faith." Still others "did conclude that there was nothing more in these providences and remoras, than did usually attend and accompany all good designs, tending to the glory of God and salvation of souls."[13] In these cases, the colonists did not find integrated synergy of providence and mechanism. Instead, they struggled to choose between them.

Motivations

As these examples show, providential explanations were not simply the reflexive response of devout colonists. Instead, providence could be emphasized or de-emphasized, presumably where it suited the purposes of the colonists. Such choices, grounded in the local political or economic needs of their worlds, recurred whenever and wherever Europeans responded to American Indian epidemics. In these early colonial cases, it is possible to understand the cultural work performed by providence by examining cases in which providential explanations were most forceful. It is also possible to see how American Indians attempted to put their own understandings of the epidemics to good use.

The efforts of Massachusetts Bay Company officials to justify English settlement in New England provide the clearest demonstration of providence serving local needs. As they planned the Great Migration in 1629, Winthrop, White, and Higginson all defended their right "to take that lande which is and hathe been of longe tyme possessed by other sonnes of Adam." Not only was there more than enough room for everyone, but also "God hathe consumed the natives with a miraculous plague," leaving the land void. In 1634, after witnessing the great smallpox epidemic of 1633 and 1634, Winthrop continued this justification. In letters to Simonds D'Ewes and Nathaniel Rich he argued that God, using smallpox, had "cleared our title" to New England. John Cotton, Thomas Gorges, and the chronicler of Charlestown all made similar claims.[14] In this context, every Massachusett death simply strengthened English claims to New England. At a time when acquisition of land was the primary concern of the colonists' state-building process, providential depopulation provided the primary justification. As will be seen, as the needs of the state evolved from land, to trade, to international politics, American Indian disease always played a valuable role.

As early settlers made explicit linkages between Indian mortality and

English land rights, they also used Indian epidemics as proof that God favored the English over the American Indians. For instance, they believed that God often protected them when they were exposed to dying Indians. Richard Vines and his crew wintered with the dying Pemaquid in 1616 and 1617 but "(blessed be *GOD* for it) not one of them ever felt their heads to ake." John White and John Smith both celebrated this remarkable occurrence. When English colonists nursed Indians suffering from smallpox in 1633 and 1634, "by the marvelous goodness and providence of God, not one of the English was so much as sick."[15] The English deployed these precise examples of disparity in disease vulnerability to document their privileged status.

Even as they argued that epidemics demonstrated God's love of the colonists, they told how epidemics punished treacherous natives. One popular story told the fate of French fishermen shipwrecked on Cape Cod shortly before 1616. The Indians harassed and captured the survivors. According to Bradford, the captives were "sent from one sachem to another to make sport with, and used them worse than slaves." One Massachusett told Phineas Pratt that "we gave ym such meat as our dogs eate." In these early versions, providence is only a threat. When the Indians, fascinated by the French obsession with a book (presumably the Bible), asked what the book said, the French answered: "It saith, ther will a people, lick French men, com into this Cuntry and drive you all a way."[16] But as this story was told and retold, it accumulated substantial elaboration. According to John Smith, one of the French sailors learned some of the Massachusett language and attempted to convert them. They derided him. When he said that his God would destroy the Indians, they dismissed his claims: "so long they mocked him and his God, that not long after such a sicknesse came, that of five or six hundred about the Massachusetts there remained but thirty." Thomas Morton told a similar story. In these versions, and the many variations that followed, disease was the deserved punishment of heathen Indians.[17]

The colonists also deployed providential explanations of disease in their efforts to convert Indians to Christianity. Missionaries used the suffering caused by epidemics to encourage many Indians to accept God as their savior. When John Sagamore, the Massachusett leader at Winnesimet, suffered from smallpox he told the English that he "desired to be brought amonge the Englishe (so he was) & promised (if he recovered) to live with the Englishe, & serve their God. he lefte one sonne, which he disposed to mr willson the paster of Boston, to be brought up by him . . . he died in a perswasion that he should goe to the English mens God." Many of his people followed his lead: "diverse of them in their sicknesse, confessed that the English mens God was a good God, & that, if they recovered they would serve him." This story long remained popular among Puritan authors.[18]

Thomas Mayhew, working as a missionary on Martha's Vineyard, recorded many similar tales. Would-be Capawack converts had to describe the processes by which they had come to know God. These conversion narratives contain many accounts of disease inspiring the Capawack to pay closer attention to God. Nookau, for instance, went through several cycles of illness-inspired recognition of his sinning ways before finally promising to dedicate his life to God and prayer. He quickly recovered: "God gave me health and then I thought, truly, God in Heaven is merciful; then I much grieved, that I knew so little of Gods Word." Even a two-year old toddler, dying of the bloody flux, learned to accept Christ, "in this manner it lay calling upon God and Jesus Christ untill it died."[19]

The colonists also told how Indians, when they converted, became recipients of the benefits of providence. In the winter of 1649 and 1650, smallpox stalked the English. John Eliot reported that his Christian Indians were spared: "The Lord had shewed them a very great testimony of his mercy this winter, in that when formerly the English had the Pox much, they also had the same; but now though it was scattered in all or most of the Townes about them, yet the Lord hath preserved them from it." A group of "profane Indians," who lived nearby, were not similarly spared, "those which were cut off, were of the worst and mischievous of them all." This blessing was noted by everyone: "which Providences, all the good Indians do take a great notice of, and doth say that the Lord hath wrought a wonder for them; and it seemeth to me that the Lord hath blest this good Providence of his to be a strong ingagement of their hearts to the Lord."[20] In these narratives, the authors used disease status as evidence of the blessings gained by those who accepted Christianity. Just as epidemics had been made to serve the needs of the state, they could be made to serve the needs of the Church.

The colonists deployed providential narratives to serve the needs of their state-building and church-building enterprises: the English needed land, so God sent smallpox to clear the land; the English needed converts, so God sent smallpox to win over Indian hearts. But the English also felt anxiety about these justifications. Could they really take land that had been so long inhabited? Why did God not always protect converted Indians from disease? The English felt other anxieties as well. At times they felt motivated to intervene to help the suffering Indians, but these efforts to provide care produced few results. Bradford described how the efforts of Plymouth traders to nurse the Indians on the Connecticut River brought little benefit: "very few of them escaped, notwithstanding they did what they could for them themselves." Winthrop noted that although the English adopted Massachusett children orphaned by smallpox, "most of them died soone after." Cotton Mather later noted that "although the English gave them all the assistances of humanity in their calamities," most of the Massachusett died.[21]

This suggests another possible role for providential narratives. The colonists were surrounded by horrific mortality that they were powerless to stop. They could do little more than pray and provide nursing care. Indians for whom they cared died despite their care. Powerless to intervene, the colonists must have found solace in seeing the deaths as the will of God, as somehow fulfilling God's purposes. Faith that all things happened in accordance with the will of a loving, but often angry, God, provided comfort and serenity in this bewildering world of observed suffering.[22] Providence also naturalized the epidemics, making them expected and tolerable. It absolved the colonists of any responsibility and agency that they might have felt. There was little the colonists could do; perhaps it helped to believe that there was little they should do.

A potential parallel exists in modern histories of American Indian depopulation. Now, even more than the Puritans, modern historians emphasize the natural inevitability of the epidemics of encounter. As Alfred Crosby has described, the "initial appearance of these diseases is as certain to have set off deadly epidemics as dropping lighted matches into tinder is certain to cause fires." This is not simply a rhetorical flourish. Historians and scientists have long argued that American Indians, "genetically virgin peoples," were "immunologically defenseless." Such immunological determinism, embodied in the theory of virgin soil epidemics, has been hugely popular, from William McNeill's *Plagues and Peoples* to Jared Diamond's Pulitzer Prize–winning *Guns, Germs, and Steel*, persisting despite considerable evidence that demonstrates the social contingency of depopulation.[23] Why is immunologic vulnerability singled out as the most relevant explanation, amidst a wealth of sophisticated alternatives? Perhaps it has appeal, like Puritan providentialism, because it provides meaning and reassurance to historians and their audiences. Depopulation is represented as the product of a unique historical-immunological moment: the convergence of two long-isolated populations, one familiar with disease, the other immunologically naïve. The inevitable outcome cannot be blamed on colonists or their descendants, for if they had not introduced smallpox, someone else surely would have. This argument replaces Puritan theology with modern biology. Like Puritan providentialism, genetic determinism blames the inherent inferiority of disease victims, absolving observers of responsibility for the disparity, and of responsibility to intervene.

The colonists (and their historians) were not alone in assigning meanings to epidemics to make them serve specific purposes. Far from remaining passive victims of differential mortality, the Massachusett and Wampanoag responded opportunistically to the depopulation they suffered. Massasoit, for instance, tried to use the mortality as an excuse to further his political aims. After the epidemic of 1616, Massasoit and his weakened Wampanoag tribe had been forced to swear fealty to the Narragansett, who had not been touched by the plague. The Narragansett subsequently granted some of the Wampanoag land to Roger Williams, who founded Providence. Decades later Massasoit tried to reclaim this land from the English. He "acknowledged it to be true that he had so subjected as the Narragansett Sachems affirmed," but he argued that this subjugation was invalid: "he affirmed that he was not subdued by war, which himself and his father maintained against the Narragansetts, but God, he said, subdued me by a plague, which swept away my people, and forced me to yield."[24] Since the land had not been taken from him rightfully, he wanted it back.

Squanto, the sole survivor of Patuxet, also tried to use the epidemics to serve his political needs. Winslow provided the earliest account of his "notable, though wicked practice." Squanto had achieved prominence as the translator between the Plymouth colonists and the

Wampanoags. He realized that the more the Wampanoag feared the colonists, the more power he would have as the mediator between the two groups. Recognizing an opportunity, he manipulated the tribe's fear of disease. As Winslow described, Squanto told the Wampanoag that the colonists had "the plague buried in our store-house; which, at our pleasure, we could send forth to what place or people we would, and destroy them therewith, though we stirred not from home." When Hobbamock, one of Massasoit's counselors, visited Plymouth, Squanto pointed to some barrels of gun powder and told Hobbamock that they contained the plague. This ruse was uncovered when Hobbamock asked the English "whether such a thing were, and whether we had such a command of it." The English denied such power, but noted that "the God of the English had it in store, and could send it as his pleasure to the destruction of his and our enemies." For this, and other misbehavior, Massasoit nearly had Squanto executed.[25]

Thomas Morton told this story with an interesting twist. When Hobbamock heard from Squanto that the colonists had a store of plague, he became frightened. Squanto "more to encrease his feare told the Sachem if he should give offence to the English party, they would let out the plague to destroy them all, which kept him in great awe." Hobbamock quickly recovered from his fear and recognized that the colonists' supposed control over disease could become a great tool for the Wampanoag. Like his predecessors at Roanoke, he asked the colonists to use this disease against his enemies: "being at varience with another Sachem borderinge upon his Territories, he came in solemne manner and intreated the Governour, that he would let out the plague to destroy the Sachem, and his men who were his enemies, promising that he himselfe, and all his posterity would be their everlasting freindes, so great an opinion he had of the English."[26] Hobbamock had realized that if the English really did control disease, then they would be powerful allies.

Squanto and Hobbamock were not alone in their belief that the English had control over disease. Many others had noted that the epidemics began around the time of English arrival and that the English often did not suffer as severely. The conclusion seemed obvious. As Roger Williams described, Canonicus, the Narragansett sachem, was extremely suspicious of the English connection to disease: "At my first coming to them, Caunounicus (morosus aeque ac barbarus senex) was very sour, and accused the English and myself for sending the plague amongst them, and threatening to kill him especially." Williams had to remind Canonicus that the English also suffered from God's judgments to dissuade him from his suspicion: "the plague and other sicknesses were alone in the hand of the one God, who made him and us, who being displeased with the English for lying, stealing, idleness and uncleanness, (the natives' epidemical sins,) smote many thousands of us ourselves with general and late mortalities."[27]

The recurrent fears among the Wampanoag and Narragansett that the English sent disease among them suggest an interesting possibility. Did the colonists ever attempt to infect the American Indians with smallpox or other diseases? Did they ever bluff that they could do so? There is no evidence that the colonists at this time ever made such an attempt. Instead, in their writings Winslow and Williams both described telling American Indians that God, not the English, controlled disease. In the absence of threats, Indian fears of English control over disease could simply have been an obvious conclusion based on the apparent disparities in the groups' susceptibility to disease. But it is also imaginable that desperate colonists, isolated in the hostile wilderness of New England, attempted to frighten the Massachusett and Wampanoag into submission with claims of dominion over disease. Such bluffs certainly occurred in later encounters between Europeans and American Indians. If they occurred among the early colonists of Massachusetts, then they would represent remarkable early cases of instrumentalization, if not of disease itself, then of disease theories.

Histories

In the early years of colonization, the events of the encounter between Europeans and American Indians had destabilized English expectations of providential decline. Indian epidemics triggered a wide range of explanations. Colonists could pick among this range and emphasize the explanations that had the most meaning or value for their purposes. With the passage of time, however, the destabilization and proliferation of narratives produced by encounter slowly resolved, replaced by a resurgence of providence.

Although never as severe as in 1616 and 1633, disease continued to afflict New England Indians, steadily eroding their populations. When

Europeans had first arrived in New England in the early seventeenth century, they found a land full of Indians. By the late 1630s, they found the land increasingly vacated and empty. Edmund Browne described how, within a few years of arrival, the mains threats to the colony—Indians and wolves (he also mentioned mosquitoes)—had been eliminated: "The Indians are wholly subjected, and we more secure from land enemies and annoyances by thieves than in O[ld] England. I tell you no untruth: our outward door hath stood by a quarter of a year unlocked, and men ride and travel abroad ten or twenty miles without sword or offensive staff, for both wolves and Indians are afraid of us. (The Lord be praised.) There be very few Indians." Such devastation even occurred in places where the Indians and colonists maintained amiable relations. Cotton Mather described how in towns like New Haven, despite "kindnesses passed between them," "nevertheless there are few of those towns but what have seen their body of Indians utterly extirpated by nothing but *mortality* wasting them."[28]

As writers began compiling histories of the early years of settlement, the great epidemics became favorite topics. Most authors writing in the 1670s and 1680s drew heavily from existing accounts. Samuel Clarke simply reprinted William Wood's descriptions, with occasional modifications. William Hubbard used Winthrop's *History*, while Increase Mather used Bradford's. Some, like Daniel Gookin, sought to improve on existing histories. Hoping to identify the nature of the 1616 to 1619 epidemic, he "discoursed with some old Indians, that were then youths," who described how the disease turned victims' skin yellow. Others simply adapted existing material into more colorful prose. Edward Johnson's 1654 *History of New England* described how colonists entered a village stricken by smallpox in 1633 and "beheld a most sad spectacle, death having smitten them all save one poore Infant, which lay on the ground sucking the Breast of its dead Mother, seeking to draw living nourishment from her dead breast." Cotton Mather, writing nearly fifty years later, famously described how "those pernicious creatures" had given way to "a *better growth*."[29]

Natural explanations of disease did persist in these histories. Hubbard explained how the Plymouth colonists suffered "sicknesses and diseases" because of the "hard weather and many uncomfortable voyages." The first Massachusetts Bay Company colonists, arriving in 1628, were "seized with the scurvy and other distempers" because of the "want of wholesome diet and convenient lodgings" in the "uncultivated desert" of Cape Ann. Even Cotton Mather, the devotee of God's providence, included natural mechanisms for the spread of smallpox among the Indians in 1633: "This distemper getting in, I know not how, among them, swept them away with a most prodigious desolation." Mather later produced what is considered to be the first medical text written in the colonies, *The Angel of Bethesda*, in which he speculated about the role of animalculae (tiny animals) in causing smallpox.[30]

Providence, however, abounded. God eased the trials of the colonists by "changing the very nature of the seasons, moderating the Winters cold of late very much." The epidemic of 1616 to 1619 "not onely made roome for his people to plant; but also tamed the hard and cruell hearts of these barbarous Indians." The 50 percent mortality suffered by Plymouth colonists was a blessing in disguise: "if a *disease* had not more easily fetcht so many of this number away to Heaven, a *famine* would probably have destroyed them all, before their expected supplies from England were arrived." When the Massachusett began to quarrel about lands with Winthrop's newly arrived colonists, "the Lord put an end to this quarrell also, by smiting the Indians with a sore Disease, even the small Pox; of the which great numbers of them died." Similar statements appear in the writings of Nathaniel Morton, Increase Mather, William Hubbard, and even Daniel Gookin, the sympathetic superintendent of Indian affairs. Cotton Mather yearned for the days of the Puritan saints, when the hand of God swept the natives away, "We have heard with our ears, O God, our fathers have told us, what work thou didst in their days, in the times of old; how thou dravest out the heathen with thy hand, and plantedst them; how thou did'st afflict the people, and cast them out!"[31]

Certain stories received particular emphasis. The story of the French shipwreck, with disease striking down the abusive Indian captors, was retold many times. Many historians praised the colonists who nursed the Massachusett in 1633 and 1634. While Edward Johnson praised colonists for tending to both the bodies and souls of the dying Indians, Cotton Mather believed that these efforts were futile: "although the English gave them all the assistances of humanity in their calamities, yet there was, it may be, not *one* in *ten* among them left alive." The story of John Sagamore's smallpox-inspired conversion was also popular. Cotton Mather told how the "great plague" struck down "one of the Princes in the Massachusett-Bay, who yet seemed hopefully *christianized.*" Hubbard added substantial embellishment, noting that John had long wanted to convert but, "kept down by fear of the scoffs of the Indians," delayed until it was too late. Cotton Mather also told of the successful prayers of Christian Indians, as well as the limits of these prayers against disease.[32]

Providence dominated these narratives with a thoroughness not seen since before the colonists left England. Several developments help explain the increased prevalence of providence. First, the re-emergence of providence reflected a hardening of English attitudes towards American Indians, traces of which can be seen quite early. For instance, in the 1622 edition of his *New England Trials*, John Smith made his oft-cited comment: "God had laid this Country open for us, and slaine the most part of the inhabitants by cruell warres and a mortall disease." Neither of the prior versions of this document—a 1618 letter to Francis Bacon, and the 1620 edition of *New England's Trials*—mentioned either epidemics or divine vengeance.[33] What might have changed Smith's attitudes? Between the 1620 and 1622 editions, Powhatan and his forces had attacked the English settlements in Virginia. Perhaps Smith, outraged by this betrayal of the English by Indians he had once known, became more willing to see the death of the New England Indians as evidence of divine punishment.

Bradford's attitudes demonstrate a similar shift over time. His descriptions of the epidemic of 1616 to 1619 contained no providential interpretation. God, however, did appear in the epidemic of 1633 and 1634. What had changed? In the initial years of the colony, Bradford and the Plymouth colonists knew that their fate was tied to that of Massasoit and the Wampanoag. Whether motivated by sympathy or political interest, both groups assisted the other. Over time, however, the colonists became less dependent on the Wampanoag. With the arrival of the Massachusetts Bay colonists, the Plymouth colonists refocused their attention on the other English colonists, away from American Indians. Perhaps an emotional wall had developed by 1634 that left the Indians outside the moral community of the colonists. Such a wall was certainly in place by the Pequot War of 1637, when Bradford praised God for giving the English victory over several hundred Pequot women and children at Mystick: "It was a fearful sight to see them thus frying in the fire and the streams of blood quenching the same, and horrible was the stink and scent thereof; but the victory seemed a sweet sacrifice, and they have the praise thereof to God, who had wrought so wonderfully for them, thus to enclose their enemies in their hands and give them so speedy a victory over so proud and insulting an enemy." The war, born of perceptions of Indians as savages and exacerbated by misinterpretation of Pequot actions, brought new savagery into relations between English and Indians.[34]

Second, the emphasis on providence in narratives of American Indian epidemics was part of a broader discourse that emphasized providence in all parts of Puritan lives. As the seventeenth century wore on, concern over the increasingly secular culture of Massachusetts and the decline of religious spirit became a dominant preoccupation of Puritan theologians. With each passing generation, the colonists seemed to stray further and further away from the ideals of the colony's founding fathers.[35] Continued emphasis on the providential aspects of Massachusetts history reminded wayward colonists of the power and glory of God.

In this discourse, Indian epidemics demonstrated the scope of God's wrath. They were used, in conjunction with stories of how God struck down the English, to frighten straying Puritans back into the fold. Puritan historians told story after story of colonists suffering God's judgment. In 1666, "the Lord threatened the Country with that infectious and contagious Disease of the *Small Pox*, which began at *Boston*, whereof some few died: but through his great mercy it is stayed, and none of late have died thereof." In his history of King Philip's War, Increase Mather described how God struck down the Indians with war and disease. But at times, particularly in the early part of the war, God also turned against the English: "*the Sword of the Lord* hath been drawn against this Land, in respect of Epidemical Diseases, which sin hath brought upon us; Sore and (doubtless) *Malignant Colds* prevailing every where." John Winthrop Jr., governor of Connecticut, died. Coffins passed each other on the streets of Boston. The message from God was clear: "if the Sword will not reform us, he hath other Judgments in store." By the end of the century, the English had suffered from many "Afflictive Providences": Indian wars, droughts, blights, fevers, smallpox, and the great fire. Joshua Scottow concluded that whereas once God "vomited out these Natives, to make room for us," the Lord "now hath vomited us out, to make room for them."[36] These narratives warned that God controlled disease among both Indians and English alike; health and safety could only be found through God.

Third, the signal of providence emerged more clearly to colonists over the course of the century as they increasingly recognized the disparate population trajectories of the two populations. As described in the previous chapter, John Smith, Robert Cushman, John White, and William Bradford had estimated that the epidemics of 1616 and 1633 claimed the lives of 95 percent of the Indians. During the second half of the century, historians made similar estimates. John Josselyn guessed that because of plague, and then smallpox, the three "*Sagamorships* of the *Mattachuset* . . . were brought from 30000 to 300." Gookin described how the Pawtucket, the Pequot, the Narragansett, and the Massachusett declined by 80 to 90 percent. Hubbard thought that the epidemics decimated the Indians, "not one in ten of the Indians in those parts surviving." Cotton Mather asserted that the "prodigious pestilence . . . carried away not a *tenth*, but *nine parts* of *ten*, (yea, 'tis said, *nineteen* of *twenty*) among them."[37] These estimates are clearly problematic, limited by inadequate informants and inability to differentiate between losses from epidemics, warfare, and migration.[38] But the accuracy of the estimates is less important here than the perception of decline.

Such estimates, which fit well into original narratives of Indians passing away to make room for the English, simultaneously evoked triumph and dismay from the colonists. The decline in Indian populations was made particularly striking by the opposite trajectory of the colonists' population, which experienced remarkable growth from 1640 into the eighteenth century. Edward Johnson described this well. While "such fearfull Desolations, and wonderfull Alterations" reduced the Massachusett from 30,000 to 300, the Puritans, "this poore Church of Christ," grew from seven to 7,750 souls. Mr. Moor, an English missionary in New York in 1705, also contrasted the decline of Indians with the growth of colonial populations: "the English here are a very thriving growing people, and ye Indians quite otherwise, they wast away & have done ever since our first arrival amongst them (as they themselves say) like Snow agt. ye Sun."[39] The contrasting fates of the populations allowed the ultimate message of the epidemics to coalesce around providential depopulation of American Indians.

Placing the population trajectories side by side, these authors perceived a natural, inevitable process. This doubly misrepresented what had happened. New England Indians died from epidemics and warfare initiated by English settlement. English populations grew from both "natural" reproduction and from continuing immigration. Both trajectories, unlike the melting of "Snow agt. ye sun," reflected social processes, not natural processes. It is easy to imagine the value of this naturalization to the colonists. Historian Joyce Chaplin has argued that English support of "an environmental view of disease," of natural processes of decline, "seems—sometimes—to have been both a denial of the demographic disaster taking place in the native populations and a strategic avoidance of the hypothesis of infectious transmission."[40] The rhetorical naturalization of depopulation absolved colonists of responsibility for what had happened.

One source of tension had begun to disrupt this reassuring world of providential decline. Over the century, colonists slowly but increasingly began feeling responsibility for American Indian demise. They feared that their arrival had changed the lives of the Massachusett, Wampanoag, and other groups in ways that increased their mortality. The Jesuits had quickly recognized that smallpox followed closely on their heels in Quebec. Realization came more slowly, or at least less openly, among the English. As discussed in the previous chapter, William Wood traced Indian epidemics to their changed diets, Roger Williams singled out alcohol, and Thomas Mayhew blamed the Capawacks' departure from "their old heathenish ways."[41] Daniel Gookin, superintendent of the Indians for the colony of Massachusetts, made the most substantial efforts to document and describe Indian decline. At times he made providential claims about Indian mortality, celebrated the destruction of the "insolent" Pequots, and suspected that "awful providences of God" had led to consumption and other diseases that killed Indian students at Harvard College. However, he and others did wonder whether those deaths could actually be attributed to their adoption of English food, clothing, and housing. But after suggesting that the English might have responsibility for the mortality, Gookin stepped back: "The truth is, this disease is frequent among the Indians; and sundry died of it, that live not with the English."[42] The English, he concluded, could not be held responsible.

Fear that the Indians might suffer as a consequence of English attempts to civilize them created a dilemma for the colonists. Indians could be segregated from the English and allowed to live separately, or they could be integrated into the new English society, but only after they had adopted the beliefs and practices of English culture. The English clearly believed that the best prospects for the Indians lay in adopting the presumed superior beliefs and practices of English life. The process of civilization, however, brought certain risks. Indian bodies would have to adapt to new foods and behaviors. During the instability of transition, disease could strike. English influences, instead of civilizing the Indians, could actually corrupt and sicken them. How could the colonists conduct a process that they knew threatened the people whom they hoped to save? This anxiety would remain an integral aspect of Indian policy for centuries.

Although this anxiety threatened to upset the New England colonies, it resolved as the Indians disappeared. New England Indians managed to maintain a significant presence in colonial life as late as the 1670s. Although both groups "retained their distinct cultural identities," historian James Drake has shown how they were bound together by "their shared social space and economy, as well as by their overlapping legal and political systems." The brutality of King Philip's War, which raged from 1675 to 1677, did irreparable harm to this society. The conflict was not simply one of English against Indians: Indians fought on both sides of the conflict. Colonists, however, quickly lost sight of this and began to see all Indians as enemies. Even Roger Williams, long a sympathizer with his Narragansett neighbors, enlisted in the army during the war and sold captured Indians into slavery.[43] As annihilation replaced assimilation as the goal of colonial policy, colonists escaped from the civilizing dilemma by abandoning what few hopes they had once held for integrating American Indians.

By the end of the war, the relations between English and Indians had been radically transformed. War and displacement reduced Indian populations by nearly 70 percent. Meanwhile, between 1670 and 1680, the colonists' population grew from 52,000 to 68,000. Whereas Indians had formed 25 percent of the colony's population in 1670, by 1680 they contributed only 10 percent. Drake believes that wartime racial hostility, in conjunction with these population trajectories, opened a gulf between the two groups. Such "racial ostracization" sowed the seeds of "a new frontier mentality." Jill Lepore has made a similar argument. English victory created stark boundaries between English and Indian land, people, and culture. Whereas Plymouth colonists once feasted with

Massasoit, they mounted the severed head of his son—Metacom (King Philip)—on a stake at the gates of Plymouth.[44]

Meanwhile, other concerns commanded colonists' attention. Colonial political leaders struggled against the machinations of James II, who dissolved charter of the Massachusetts Bay Company in 1684 and placed the colony under the control of New York governor Edmund Andros in 1686.[45] Religious leaders battled the declining religious spirit of second and third generations of settlers. As colonists grappled with their own internal problems, Indian policy, whether regarding land disputes or conversion efforts, became a less pressing concern.

The era in which colonists and Indians shared their struggle for existence had passed. As colonists thrived, Indians died. War, marginalization, and population decline estranged the Indians from the English. Whereas colonists had once responded to Indian epidemics with empathy, religious and political opportunism, or even nascent feelings of responsibility, indifference to Indian decline became increasingly common in the late seventeenth century. The contrasting fortunes of the two groups suggested that the colonists' ambitions for civilizing the Indians had been naïve. Ambivalence about Indians' role in the colonists' new state gave way to realization that there might be no need to include the Indians in the state.

Just as the initial instability of colonization had fueled a proliferation of disease narratives, the growing stability of English colonial populations allowed a consolidation of narratives. As the initial diversity of explanations was distilled into a memory of providence, the basic fatalism of Puritan minds readily accepted the inevitable demise of Indian populations. Increasingly lost in a wilderness of providential narratives, New England Indians seemed doomed to exist only in Puritans' histories.

Even this powerful vision, however, would trigger opposing narratives. As Indian epidemics continued into the eighteenth century, missionaries, traders, and soldiers recognized specific behaviors and social conditions that left Indians susceptible to smallpox and other diseases. A dawning sense of the contingency of disease fueled a new discourse about Indian epidemics, one that assigned humans both increasing responsibility for causing disease, and increasing capacity for managing disease. Colonists and settlers would find new ways to deploy disease to serve the interests of their expanding state.

3

Frontiers of Smallpox

DURING THE EARLY encounters of colonization, colonists and American Indians had been impressed by how much more the Indians suffered from epidemics. Indians frequently concluded that the colonists must have had control over disease. Ensenore, Squanto, Canonicus, and many angry Huron accused English and French colonists of sending smallpox and other epidemics into their midst. They believed that the Europeans had a "secret understanding" with disease that let them store it in barrels, load it into guns, and shoot it throughout their villages. Colonists, such as Roger Williams, always pleaded their innocence, arguing that "the plague and other sicknesses were alone in the hand of the one God."[1] Perhaps out of honesty, or perhaps out of faith that such affairs truly were in the hands of God, they denied that they had any such power over disease.

The colonists' relationship with disease, and its control, soon changed. As smallpox followed traders, soldiers, and settlers across the Appalachian frontier into the interior valleys of North America, Europeans and Americans continued to witness devastating epidemics among American Indian populations. But during these encounters, colonists took more responsibility over disease. When the Delaware and Shawnee besieged the British garrison at Fort Pitt in 1763, a local trader, William Trent, gave their chiefs blankets exposed to smallpox, hoping to spread the disease among the Indians. When the Blackfeet and Assiniboine surrounded American Fur Company traders at Fort Union in 1837, Charles Larpenteur and other company officials tried to prevent the spread of smallpox with quarantine and inoculation. No longer leaving smallpox to the hand of God, people attempted to assert control over the dread disease.

How can these new responses be understood? The colonists' ideas about disease had begun to change. Although providence still played a role in explaining disease, humans seemed increasingly responsible for its patterns of distribution. Explorers, traders, missionaries, and soldiers attributed Indian epidemics to specific behaviors, or to ways in which Indians interacted with their environments. These ideas inspired attempts to control the spread of smallpox. Missionaries preached that health could be found through conversion and adoption of civilized (European) culture. Traders offered or withheld trade. Everyone marveled at the potential offered by the emerging technologies of inoculation and vaccination. The ways in which these people responded to smallpox, and eventually deployed it, also reveal their startling ambivalence towards American Indians. Just as Indians could be enemies, converts, or customers, smallpox could be used to encourage cultural change, infect enemies, or protect economic assets. As differential mortality seemed to foretell the outcome of encounter, smallpox became a dangerous and unpredictable tool of the imperialist state, serving the needs of religion, commerce, or war whenever Indians threatened the prosperity and security of expanding American society.

Frontiers

The episodes at Fort Pitt in 1763 and Fort Union in 1837 provide two defining moments in the history of smallpox on the western frontier. William Trent and Charles Larpenteur witnessed the spread of smallpox into the Ohio and Missouri river valleys. Though separated by over seventy years, they faced similar situations. As smallpox raged inside their forts, they stood on the walls and looked out onto groups of angry and frustrated American Indians. They had to decide what to do about these Indians, and about smallpox. But aside from these parallels of circumstance, did they truly have much in common? Had their worlds changed so much between 1763 and 1837 that meaningful connections cannot be made? These questions, discussed in this chapter, must be answered before the episodes at Forts Pitt and Union, discussed in the next chapter, can be understood. The answers depend on an understanding of the frontier.

The nature, even the existence, of the American frontier has been one of the most contested questions of American historiography. Frederick Jackson Turner first defined the frontier in 1893 as the place (actually, a place constantly moving westward, more of a process than a geographical location) in which European civilization encountered North American savagery and produced a uniquely new American culture. Subsequent historians have argued that the frontier was irrelevant compared to the economic and industrial development of the east, or that Turner's hypothesis was ethnocentric and simplistic. Recent historians have focused on more nuanced, local models of cultural interactions, typified by Richard White's "middle ground."[2] It is possible to accept these critiques and still see the concept of the frontier as relevant in certain cases. Although the broad political and economic contexts in which Trent and Larpenteur operated were radically different, the stakes and exigencies of their local worlds were surprising similar.

In 1763 British colonists inhabited a narrow strip of land, pinned between the Appalachian mountains to the west and the Atlantic Ocean to the east. They had won rights to the vast interior from the French at the conclusion of the Seven Years War. But according to the Treaty of Easton of 1758 and the Royal Proclamation of 1763, English colonists were bound to stay east of the crest of the mountains, leaving the interior to the American Indians. By 1837 this line of demarcation had been long since abandoned. Even before the Revolutionary War, British colonists had poured across the mountains into the Ohio Valley. Half a century later, after the Louisiana Purchase and explorations of Meriwether Lewis and William Clark, American settlers had spread across the interior, with towns springing up along the Mississippi River and tentative explorations reaching west across the high plains toward the Rocky Mountains.[3]

The nature of American medical institutions had undergone similar transformations. In 1763 medical facilities in the colonies remained limited, with neither hospitals nor medical schools. The first hospital, in Philadelphia, opened in 1765. By 1837 medical institutions had proliferated, even into the new states of the Mississippi Valley. The government had also slowly begun to take a more active role in public health. Where once government institutions had only acted during times of epidemics, the federal government had now begun sponsoring efforts to prevent disease by subsidizing vaccination, even funding campaigns to vaccinate the eastern Indians.[4]

The transformations are demonstrated in the travels of German aristocrat Alexander Philip Maximilian, Prince of Wied-Neuwied. Maximilian arrived in Boston on 4 July 1832. Like John Smith two centuries before, he described the harbor islands "covered with corn, or beautifully green as in England." Numerous villages adorned the bays and inlets. But now there was a lighthouse and telegraph, and where Smith had found abundant Indians, Maximilian found none: "The stranger in Boston looks in vain for the original American race of Indians." By September Maximilian had reached Pittsburgh. The site of the once isolated and primitive Fort Pitt was thriving, "an old, large, but by no means handsome town." Its 12,000 inhabitants had developed coal mines, manufacturing, and trade. When he reached St. Louis the following spring, he was entertained by General William Clark (of Lewis and Clark fame), superintendent of Indian affairs. When he finally encountered American Indians, on the Missouri River in April 1833, they were Delawares and Shawnees, long since displaced from the east, whose parents or grandparents might have fought at Fort Pitt in 1763.[5]

Despite the many differences between William Trent's Fort Pitt and Charles Larpenteur's Fort Union, the two traders would have found much in common in each other's lives. Both lived in outposts "remote in the western wilderness." Fort Pitt sat 200 miles of mountains and wilderness west of Carlisle and the frontier of English settlements. A 1760 census found only 149 people, but by 1763 the garrison had expanded. Under the command of Swiss mercenary Simeon Ecuyer, it held 330 soldiers, traders, and backwoodsmen. This "farthest outpost of Anglo-Saxon civilization in the Ohio Valley" had a sawmill, a tanning yard, a coal mine; fields of corn, turnips, hay, and other vegetables; and herds of cattle and livestock. Life could be hard. On 7 and 8 March 1763, a flood destroyed many of the fortifications. Ecuyer ordered the residents to repair the walls and gardens, without much success: "Our people complain a great deal since this last order. They do not understand why they should work without pay, and what they do they do with an ill grace." He had no love for the residents, "everyone here (except the garrison) is the scum of nature." Despite such hardships, the garrison did have something of a social life. As Ecuyer noted in a letter to his commander, Henry Bouquet, "P:S: I forgot, Sir, to tell you that we have a club every Monday and a ball every Saturday evening, made up of the prettiest ladies of the garrison. We regale them with punch, and if it is not strong enough, the whiskey is at their disposal. You may be sure that we shall not be completely cheated."[6]

Fort Union and the other posts of the American Fur Company (by 1837 renamed Pratte, Chouteau, and Company) existed in similar isolation. St. Louis, founded by the French in 1763, was first reached by steamboat in 1817. Steamboats entered the Missouri River two years later. By the early 1830s, the company had a string of forts on the Missouri River. Fort Clark sat nearly 1,800 miles up the Missouri River from St. Louis. Forts Union and McKenzie were further yet (Figure 1). Fort Clark was quite simple, with square wooden walls, blockhouses at two corners, and low, one-story buildings. Life could be miserable, particularly in the long winters (Figure 3). Francis Chardon, who directed the fort from 1834 to 1843, captured this in his journal in January 1836: "One Single word *lonesome*—would suffice to express our feelings any day through the Year—We might add—discontented—but this would include the fate of all Mankind . . . [life] is like a dreary expansive waste—without one green verdant spot on which Memory loves to linger." Rats were a constant problem. Life, however, could occasionally be festive. At the Christmas feast of 1834, Mandan warriors, company traders, their Indian wives, and their mixed-blood children shared meat pies, pheasants, and coffee, a sight which "would of astonished any, but those who are accustomed to such sights." Fort Union, the center of activity of the company, "the principal and handsomest trading-post on the Missouri River," was more hospitable. Its gated walls housed roughly 100 employees, their Indian wives and children, and Indian trappers. Its residents enjoyed white bread, fresh milk, butter, cheese, fruit, corn, game, beef, fowl, vintage wines, and fine brandies. They entertained themselves with hunts, horse races, lacrosse games, cockfights, formal parties, and "Indian and halfbreed girls on call."[7]

These outposts of the British Army and the American Fur Company existed in a world of Indians. Like the American Indians encountered by Bradford and Winthrop, their lives had already been trans-

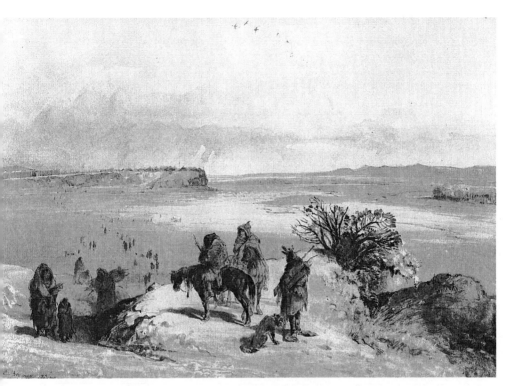

3. *Mih-Tutta-Hang-Kusch, Mandan Village* by Karl Bodmer, 1833–1834. This watercolor shows Mandan villagers hunting and collecting firewood in winter. Fort Clark and the Mandan village are visible on the distant bluff overlooking the frozen river. The group was nearly eradicated by smallpox only four years later. (By permission of the Joslyn Art Museum, Omaha, Nebraska. JAM.1986.49.382.)

formed by decades of interaction with Europeans. The Delaware and Shawnee who fought at Fort Pitt were immigrants to the forks of the Ohio River. Native to the Delaware valley of eastern Pennsylvania, the Delaware had been pushed westward by European immigrants. Beginning in 1702 they had moved into the Susquehanna and Ohio Valleys. The Shawnee faced similar pressure, migrating west from the Delaware valley and north from the Cumberland valley in the 1720s. By the 1740s, Delaware and Shawnee were establishing themselves in the upper Ohio valley. They had to negotiate with both the Six Nations, similarly being pushed westward across New York, and with the Miami and other native tribes of the Ohio valley. All of these groups had to contend with the determined efforts of Moravian missionaries who worked to convert and civilize them. Richard White has described the turbulence and violence of this fragile "middle ground," where the French, the British, and the American Indians all struggled to survive through "a process of creative, and often expedient, misunderstandings."[8]

The tribes of the Missouri Valley had suffered similar disruptions. The Mandans ("or See-pohs-kah-nu-mah-kah-kee, 'people of the pheasants,' as they call themselves") were well known by 1837. They had hosted Meriwether Lewis and William Clark in the winter of 1804 and 1805, painter George Catlin in 1832, and Maximilian with his Swiss artist, Charles Bodmer, in 1833 and 1834. Decades of war with the Dakota and other Sioux, displaced from Minnesota by eastern tribes, had forced the Mandan to migrate and consolidate. Disease had further reduced their population, from as high as 15,000 in the eighteenth century, to 3,600 in 1780 and 1,600 before 1837. An agricultural tribe, they lived in two "beautifully situated" villages. The many travelers who visited the Mandan left starkly contrasting visions of the romance or misery of their lives.[9]

The Blackfeet had a history of less peaceful relations with Europeans. They gained access to guns and horses early in the eighteenth century and quickly became the dominant military force on the northwest plains. They first met French traders around 1750. The British Hudson Bay Company established a trading post in 1780; smallpox followed in 1781. In 1806 Blackfeet hunters attacked Lewis as he returned from the Pacific Ocean. In 1811 they destroyed a post built by the Missouri Fur Company. During the 1820s they blocked the efforts of other fur traders to initiate trade. Only in 1830 did Kenneth McKenzie successfully establish relations with the Blackfeet; David Mitchell founded Fort McKenzie two years later. When Maximilian visited them in 1833, they remained a powerful tribe, recently pacified, but still a substantial threat. The other tribes who traded with the company— Arikara, Minatarees, Sioux, and many others—fell between the extremes of the peaceful Mandan and threatening Blackfeet.[10]

The presence of these tribes, from the Delaware to the Blackfeet, forced the British, French, and Americans into a series of ambivalent relationships. All of these American Indian groups remained powerful. In contrast, the soldiers and traders on the frontiers of the Ohio and Missouri rivers were stationed in small outposts. They lived beyond the periphery of European settlement, with little access to the vast resources of their towns and cities. Regardless of their feelings about the

Shawnee or Mandan, the soldiers and traders depended on them for safety, for trade, even for companionship. They saw the Indians as allies who deserved protection, but the whites were often unwilling to enforce the protection they granted. They might interact kindly while at peace, but it took little to trigger ferocity in war. With the Removal Act of 1830, the government began a campaign to move the Indians beyond the Mississippi in order to save them, even if that meant destroying their lives.[11]

The Ohio and Missouri river frontiers had one more thing in common: smallpox was everywhere. Decade after decade, it devastated American Indians as the sites of their encounters with the Europeans moved westward. After the great epidemic of 1633 and 1634, it struck again and again, first in New England and then in the southern and western colonies, in 1638–1640, 1662–1663, 1669–1670, 1688–1691, 1696, 1702, 1716–1717, 1721, 1730, 1738, 1746–1747, 1755–1760, and 1764–1765. It had reached the far northwestern plains by the 1780s, striking the Arikaras and Blackfeet. An epidemic began in the central United States and spread by 1802 along the Missouri Valley into the Pacific Northwest. The Omaha were devastated, as were the Ponca, Oto, Iowa, Arikara, Gros Ventres, Mandan, Crow, and Sioux. Some tribes lost as much as 80 percent of their populations. Smallpox struck the Great Lakes and northern plains in 1810 and 1811. In 1815 and 1816 it spread along the Red River and Rio Grande. In 1819 and 1820 it followed the White River into South Dakota.[12]

Just as Winthrop and Bradford described the horrors of smallpox in New England in 1634, many European observers witnessed the devastation in the eighteenth and nineteenth centuries. In the summer and fall of 1831, smallpox ravaged the Pawnee tribes. John Dougherty, the United States Indian agent at Cantonment Leavenworth, wrote that "their misery defies all description." No one younger than "thirty-three years of age escaped the monstrous disease." Half died. The horror of the epidemic challenges the imagination of a modern reader: "They were dying so fast, and taken down at once in such large numbers, that they had ceased to bury their dead, whose bodies were to be seen, in every direction, laying about in the river, lodged on the sand bars, in the hog weeds around their villages, and in their corn caches; others again were dragged off by the hungry dogs into the prairie, where they were torn to pieces by the more hungry wolves and buzzards. Their misery was so great and so general, that they seemed to be unconscious of it, and to look upon the dead and dying as they would on so many dead horses." Catlin described how this epidemic also decimated the Omahas, Otos, Missouri, Sioux, Osage, Konzas, and Puncahs. Maximilian met scarred survivors, Omaha, Oto, and Iowas, "much marked with the small pox."[13]

Only five years later, smallpox struck again. From 1836 to 1840, reaching its height in 1837 and 1838, the epidemic again spread through the Missouri Valley. Some historians consider this "perhaps the most severe episode of any disease among North American Indians, although it may very well only be the best documented." Over 15,000 Indians died along the Missouri River: 6,000 to 8,000 Blackfeet, Piegans, and Bloods; 2,000 Pawnee; several thousand Mandan; over 2,000 Arikara and Minetaree; 1,000 Crow; and 4,000 Assiniboine. Chardon, who witnessed this epidemic among the Mandan, later told Audubon that "the small-pox had never been known in the civilized world, as it had been among the poor Mandans and other Indians. Only *twenty-seven* Mandans were left to tell the tale." By 1850 the cumulative impact was clear. Henry Schoolcraft, who compiled an encyclopedia about the American Indians, believed that "No disease which has been introduced among the tribes, has exercised so fatal an influence upon them as the small-pox."[14] The remarkable susceptibility of American Indians to smallpox continued to shock observers well into the nineteenth century.

Exhortation

Seeing similar depopulation, seventeenth- and eighteenth-century Puritan historians, such as Edward Johnson, William Hubbard, and Cotton Mather, reassured themselves that the devastation was directed by the hand of God. Mr. Moor, an English missionary in New York in 1705, responded similarly. He described how the Indians had wasted away since English arrival, "like Snow agt. ye Sun." He had little doubt about the cause: "God's providence in this matter seems very wonderful." The decline of American Indian populations was particularly striking in contrast to the tremendous growth of the colonists' population. In 1764 Thomas Hutchinson went so far as to abandon his usual skepticism about Puritan mythology: "Our ancestors supposed an immediate interposition of providence in the great mortality among the Indians to make room for the settlement of the English. I am not inclined to credulity, but should not we go into the contrary extreme if we were to take no notice of the extinction of this people in all parts of the continent . . . They waste, they moulder away, and as Charlevoix says of the Indians of Canada, they disappear."[15]

Change, however, was in the air. After commenting about the likely role of providence, Moor wondered about the possible contribution of "their drinking Rum, with some new Distempers we have brought amongst them." A slow shift toward emphasizing behavioral and natural explanations of differential mortality reflected a general change in understandings of the natural world. Over the long span in which smallpox dominated American Indian mortality, the natural world and its diseases became gradually demystified for colonists and settlers. Consider two contrasting accounts of Indian rain dances. In 1623 Edward Winslow and the other Plymouth colonists prayed for rain and, when it came, bragged that the "soft, sweet, and moderate showers" brought by their prayers were better than the "storms and tempests" brought by Wampanoag conjuration. By 1832 Catlin observed Mandan rain dances and saw their "*hocus pocus* and *conjuration*" as a scam that would eventually succeed, ensuring the fame and fortune of whichever lucky medicine men happened to begin the ceremony at the right time: "when the Mandans undertake to make it rain, *they never fail to succeed*, for their ceremonies never stop until the rain begins to fall."[16]

Narratives of disease underwent similar transformation. Cholera, which spread into the Missouri Valley in 1833 and 1851, demonstrated this well. When Maximilian reached Fort Clark in 1833, he feared that cholera, "having prevailed on the lower Missouri," might reach the fort. Fortunately, these fears "proved to be groundless." Catlin believed that the spread of cholera had been halted by the Indians' low salt and "simple meat diet." While steaming down the Missouri the following spring, Maximilian's boat encountered another steamboat with passengers suffering from cholera. When his boat was forced to take on several of the passengers, he again feared contagion: "It was by no means pleasant to us to be obliged to receive passengers from this boat." When cholera broke out "with great virulence" on the steamer *Yellowstone*, local Missouri residents demanded that the boat leave the state. In 1851 cholera struck another steamer, only to recede when the boat reached "the purer air of the prairie country of the upper river." The recovery did not last: "the crew and voyageurs drank freely of a miserable article of whiskey, which resulted in a return of the epidemic." One person died. In response, "the boat was thoroughly fumigated and no further cases occurred."[17] These outbreaks demonstrate several styles of explanation, including contagion, diet, environment, and behavior. Specific acts put people at risk, while other acts could alleviate the disease.

As with the early colonists, environment and weather received considerable attention. James Kenny, a Quaker trader at Fort Pitt, traced ague to "getting my feet wet in ye Dew," "Epidemick Cold & fever" to the "Air got midling Cool," and a "fever" to a fishing trip. Chardon described how hot days in St. Louis could be "a real *fever* and *Ague* breeder." In 1834 Colonel Dodge led a military expedition to pacify the Comanche. His "army of men from the North," sent into "this Southern and warm climate, in the hottest months of the year," suffered greatly. Half of the group, including officers and horses, suffered "a slow and distressing bilious fever," which they attributed to a "fatal miasma which we conceived was hovering about the mouth of the False Washita." They also suffered from "poisonous and indigestible water." One third died within four months; Catlin believed another third would likely die. To these lists of colds, fevers, and rheumatisms, historian Bernard De Voto added "dreads and melancholies specific to the tenderfoot in the plains and mountains, a true neurosis, usually mild but sometimes severe."[18]

These same patterns of explanation appeared in the responses to smallpox and other diseases among American Indians. Many missionaries and traders, who lived and traveled with Indians, concluded that the harsh conditions of their lives put them at risk of disease. David Zeisberger, a Moravian missionary among the Iroquois in New York, believed that "Indians are not less, rather more, subject to disease than Europeans, their rough manner of life and the hardships of travel and the chase being contributing causes." They waded across rivers, regardless of snow or ice; they chased deer from morning until night, never stopping to eat. John Heckewelder, who continued Zeisberger's work, also emphasized the relationship of their diseases to the hardship of Delaware lives: "The disorders to which the Indians are most commonly subjected are pulmonary consumptions, fluxes, fevers and severe rheumatisms, all proceeding probably from the kind of life they lead, the hardships they undergo." He traced "intermitting and bilious fevers" to their towns, "situated near marshy grounds or ponds of stagnant water." Catlin, who had observed that smallpox was "far more fatal amongst the native than in civilized population," did not think the Indians suffered "some extraordinary constitutional susceptibility" to the disease. Instead, their suffering resulted from "the exposed lives they live, leading more directly to fatal consequences." Edwin James, a physician who accompanied the Yellowstone Expedition to Colorado in 1819 and 1820, believed that the storms and drastic temperature changes seen on the high plains and Rocky Mountains were a particular problem. Maximilian traced Mandan winter catarrh to "the frequent and sudden changes of temperature." This was exacerbated by their indifference to the freezing environment: "Rheumatism, coughs, and the like, are frequent, because they go half naked in the severest cold, and plunge into ice water."[19]

Diet could also be a major problem. Hutchinson suspected that the smallpox epidemic of 1633 might have been exacerbated by Massachusett diets, which furnished "greater quantities of morbifick matter." He had been told that a devastating smallpox epidemic on Nantucket in 1763, which killed 235 of the 320 Indians on the island, was caused by lack of corn and consumption of unripe pumpkins and squash. Zeisberger believed that the Iroquois' lack of "abundance and variety of nourishing food" made their bodies weak. They also suffered from diarrhea because "they know nothing of dieting and continue to eat whatever they wish." Heckewelder believed that Delaware disease was exacerbated by "the nature of the food that they take." For instance, their autumn fevers coincided with "the season of the wild plum, a fruit that the Indians are particularly fond of." Their diet caused worms in children, made them unable to endure manual labor, and gave them inordinate fondness for alcohol. Catlin wondered whether the "unexampled fatality" of smallpox could be traced to Indians "living entirely on animal food," but he left this "for sounder judgments than mine to decide."[20]

Such explanations simultaneously attributed disease to the conditions of Indian lives and to the choices Indians made about how to behave in those conditions. Other explanations focused solely on behavior, fueling a debate about etiology that placed blame for the diseases on their victims. Many observers discussed the harm of Indian healing practices. Chardon stated this most clearly: "A young Woman died at the Village last Night—or more properly speaking, was Killed by the *Doctors.*" Although surveyor John Lawson, Heckewelder, Texas settler David Burnet, Catlin, and trader Josiah Gregg all acknowledged that Indian healers had great skill with herbal remedies and simple external wounds, Zeisberger saw many patients who were overdosed: healers "make mistakes, namely, in not properly measuring doses and often needlessly torturing patients." Meanwhile, the magical and religious aspects of American Indian healing received universal condemnation. Lawson mocked the "Grimaces, antick postures, which are not to be matched in Bedlam." Burnet believed that the "hideous noises" produced in their rituals, "the object of which is to *scare away* the disease," was "better calculated to affright than to soothe." Catlin described how, in the rare cases when the patient "unaccountably recovers" after such "frightful rattles" and "songs of incantation," the healer would proclaim success. But should the patient die, the healer would argue that "it was the will of the Great Spirit that his patient should die."[21]

The therapeutic use of sweat baths and plunges in cold water received particularly extensive discussion. Zeisberger, Maximilian, and Catlin all believed that such baths "were, unquestionably, a great means of health." Catlin, for instance, described use of baths for fevers, "without the fatal consequences which we would naturally predict." According to one Indian informant, sweat baths opened the pores to let bad fluids out; a quick jump in cold water then closed the pores so that no nutritive juices escaped. However, many observers believed that sweat baths were remarkably dangerous in cases of smallpox. Lawson and James Adair blamed many smallpox deaths on this practice: jumping into water, "shutting up the Pores, hinders a kindly Evacuation of the pestilential Matter, and drives it back, by which Means Death most commonly ensues." Zeisberger, who generally praised sweat baths, cited Dr. McClure who believed that "the treatment was quite fatal" for smallpox. Catlin described how victims of smallpox "ignorantly and imprudently plunge into the coldest water, whilst in the highest state of fever, and often die before they have the power to get out." David Burnet, Josiah Gregg, Francis Chardon, and Father P. J. De Smet all agreed that sweat baths and cold plunges were "invariably fatal" for smallpox. Many historians, following these leads, have continued to argue that this behavior contributed to the severe mortality.[22]

Another genre of victim blaming appears in cases of smallpox transmitted when Indians scalped and plundered Europeans or other Indians. The most infamous case occurred after the French siege of Fort William Henry in upstate New York in 1757. The English, outnumbered and afflicted with smallpox, had surrendered. The French granted generous honors of war and allowed them to retreat. But the Indians, promised scalps and plunder by their French allies, attacked the retreating English. As described by the French general, the Indians soon paid the price: they caught the contagion and "died of the smallpox on their way home." This story, and its sense of retributive justice, has been repeated by many historians. A similar case occurred on the northwestern plains in 1781 when a Piegan band encountered a camp of their Shoshoni enemies. Piegan scouts found the camp silent. Though they feared a trap, they attacked. No one resisted: all were dead or dying, victims of smallpox. Piegans looted the Shoshoni camp. Two days later, they too succumbed to smallpox.[23]

These behavioral and environmental explanations of susceptibility to disease did not mean that disease had become secularized. Disease had not been removed from the domain of theology and placed into the natural world. Instead, these naturalized, behavioral accounts of disease continued to serve the moral purposes of missionaries and other observers. They simply worked in different ways: disease, no longer a sign of providence, became a tool of moral exhortation.

Zeisberger focused on sex and alcohol. He described how "Venereal diseases have during the last years spread more and more, due, doubtless, to their disorderly life." Increasing use of alcohol, "through which unquestionably many evils have crept in," only made matters worse. Heckewelder believed that "the introduction of ardent spirits among them" led to "vices which have brought on disorders which they say were unknown before": the "shameful complaint." Alcohol, and the "vicious and dissolute life" it brought, caused not only syphilis, but also low fertility and consumption. Such concerns were not limited to missionaries. Elbert Herring, commissioner of Indian affairs in 1833, believed that alcohol "tends inevitably to the degradation, misery, and extinction of the aboriginal race." Edwin James described how the Omahas suffered from a pain in the chest, a consequence of their excessive indulgence in tobacco. Maximilian found that "Gonorrhoea is very common" among the Mandan.[24]

These theories had a clear consequence: if vice brought disease, morality would bring health. Heckewelder believed that health could be obtained by working hard and avoiding "the vices of the white people."[25] By describing the sinful roots of disease, these writers encouraged the Indians with whom they worked, as well as their white audiences, to reform their behavior to maintain their health.

Two aspects of such moralizing must be noted. First, American Indians did not always accept these claims. Cherokee medicine men did blame a 1739 outbreak of smallpox on the sins of their people, notably adultery, and an old Shawnee man blamed the 1762 "Epidemical disorder" on an excess of pride: "he sd its Sent from God upon them for they are very Proud." But they rejected other similar explanations. In 1717 Governor Hunter of New York tried to explain that the Iroquois, like Christians, should see epidemics as "punishments for our misdeeds and sin, such as breaking of covenants & promises, murders and robbery, and the like." Dekanissore, the Iroquois leader, did not agree. The Iroquois were "apprehensive that ye great mortality which we had among our people last fall, of the Small Pox, has been sent us from Canistoge, Virginy, or Maryland." They planned "to send some of our people thither to discover if possible who has been the occasion of sending that contagion among us & to see to disswade them from such pernicious practices for the future." In the early 1840s, Catlin witnessed a debate in London between an English minister and a visiting Ioway delegation. The minister demanded that the Ioway acknowledge smallpox as divine punishment. The warchief had a quick reply: "If the Great Spirit sent the small pox into our country to destroy us, we believe it was to punish us for listening to the false promises of white men. It is white man's disease, and no doubt it was sent amongst white people to punish *them* for their sins."[26]

Second, even as these writers blamed epidemics on American Indian behaviors, they acknowledged that Europeans were the ultimate cause of the suffering. Indians always seemed healthy before contact with Europeans. Heckewelder noted that as recently as the middle of the eighteenth century, "the Indians were yet a hardy and healthy people, and many very aged men and women were seen among them, some of whom thought they had lived about one hundred years." Edwin James found that the diseases of the Indians near the Rocky Mountains were "far less extensive and appalling" than those of whites, with whom they had had little contact. Burnet and Maximilian described the remarkable constitutions of the Comanche and Blackfeet. Catlin believed that the Indians, in their original state, "undoubtedly are a longer lived and healthier race, and capable of enduring far more bodily privation and pain, than civilized people can." He suspected that this fortitude was the product of their native life style, not an inherent difference in their constitutions.[27]

The contrast between pre-contact health and post-contact disease led many observers to a seemingly inescapable conclusion. Zeisberger believed that the Delaware "caught the contagion" of smallpox from Europeans. They had also learned "much evil" from whites, especially from traders who taught them "the habit of drinking to excess." Heckewelder agreed that "Our vices have destroyed more than our swords." He described "a melancholy feeling, arising from the comparison which forces itself upon my mind of what the Indians were before the Europeans came into this country, and what they have become since, by a participation in our vices." The traveler Timothy Flint wrote in 1820 that "it must be admitted, that this depopulation has been accelerated, if not entirely produced, by Europeans." Catlin believed that 12 million Indians had died over 250 years, the consequence of European arrival: "White men—whiskey—tomahawks—scalping knives—guns, powder and ball—small-pox—debauchery—extermination." He feared that this record of destruction, "an unrequited account of sin and injustice that sooner or later will call for *national retribution*," would haunt all Americans on Judgment Day.[28]

The examples demonstrate how beliefs about smallpox and differential mortality served a wide range of moralizing agendas. By emphasizing behavioral etiologies, writers placed responsibility on the American Indians as the proximate cause of their own illnesses. If Indians abandoned sinful behaviors, they would be healthier. Many of these same writers noted that American Indians had been healthy in their original state; they had lost this health to the corrupting influences of the worst aspects of white society. By emphasizing this narrative of corruption, writers placed responsibility on whites as the ultimate cause of Indian illnesses. White populations, therefore, had an obligation to live more sober and temperate lives. Finally, by placing white society at the root of Indian disease, the writers also attempted to create an obligation for the colonial and federal government to intervene.

Belief that disease could be predictable and preventable, and suspicion that whites were often the source of American Indian epidemics, made smallpox a central issue in the diplomatic dialogue between Indians, settlers, and government officials. Initial interventions were quite limited. When Dekanissore, the Iroquois speaker, argued that smallpox and been sent to the Iroquois in 1707 from "Canistoge, Virginy, or Maryland," Governor Hunter of New York offered only sympathy: "I am very sorry for the loss that has happened by the Small Pox to the brethren, or any of your friends and allies." In September 1733, with smallpox among the Iroquois and English in New York, both sides exchanged condolences and gifts. Governor William Cosby empathized with the Iroquois: "Brethren, I understand with concern that you have had a great mortality among you by the small pox, and lost many of your people and hear that you are greatly grieved, therefore I wipe off the Tears from your eyes open your understandings, wash off your blood and condole the death of all people who have lost, that we may behold one another with joy. *Gave three strings of Wampum and a Belt.*" Three days later the Iroquois returned the favor: "We do in like manner condole the deaths of all your people who died since our last conference, you have also had a decrease among you . . . *Gave a string of Wampum.*"[29]

Such exchanges were not limited to the English. When Gaichoton, orator and chief of the Seneca, complained about the impact of smallpox, Pierre Rigaud de Vaudreuil, governor and lieutenant general in New France, expressed his sympathies. When Indian warriors caught smallpox after sacking the English captives at Fort William, French General Montcalm complained that "This is a real loss to us, and will cost the King considerable in consequence of the expenses it will occasion at the posts to treat them, cover the dead and console the widows."[30]

These smallpox condolences often reflected multiple interests. In July 1733 Governor Jonathan Belcher of Massachusetts wrote to the Penobscot that "I have great pleasure at the news of your health & welfare." While Belcher might have been genuinely empathetic, he was certainly thankful because these Penobscot served as an essential buffer, protecting English settlements against other tribes who, fleeing smallpox in Canada, raided the English frontier. In 1747 the French governor of Canada sent a messenger to the Onondaga "in order to condole the death of all those who dyed last fall & winter of the Small Pox &c." The English doubted this motive. William Johnson told New York's Governor Clinton that the French ambassador hoped to find out why the Onondaga had transferred allegiance to the English. Despite the French gift of an enormous belt of wampum, the Five Nations remained loyal to the English. French diplomats went so far as to circulate rumors among the Cherokee that English conjurers had sent smallpox among them.[31]

Concern with smallpox also shaped the timing and outcome of conferences between Europeans and Indians. Endemic smallpox in the Carolinas made the Cherokee and Creek reluctant to attend meetings in Charles Town. The Provincial Council of Pennsylvania frequently modified conference plans to minimize Delaware exposure to smallpox. In 1756 smallpox in Bethlehem forced the relocation of the council fire to Springitsberry, where the Indians "might Escape the Infection & be well Entertained." A conference in Philadelphia in April 1757 ended prematurely when Indian representatives caught smallpox and had to return home; when the governor learned of smallpox among the delegation from the Six Nations, he agreed to bring the negotiations to a rapid close. Smallpox also shaped military relations between the two groups. As historian D. Peter MacLeod has shown, recurrent smallpox epidemics during the 1750s hindered French efforts to recruit Indian warriors. Hutchinson, watching from the other side of the conflict, happily reported that the epidemic-induced weakness of the Indians led them to seek peace with the English.[32]

Interest in protecting Indians from white sins and contagions continued into the early nineteenth century. Indian sympathizers came to believe that the best way to protect American Indians from further degradation would be to set aside lands as a preserve for them. Commissioner Herring described how the Indians "seemed to be fast sinking in the overwhelming wave of white population." Fearing this, and motivated by both "national sympathy" and a sense of "incalculable debt," the federal government instituted Indian relocation, a policy "for their protection and perpetuation." The government hoped that by moving Indians west, relocation would protect them from whites and the "multitudinous evils, under the operation of which they were rapidly dwindling in numbers and deteriorating in morals."[33]

Although Indian relocation, which will be discussed in later chapters, had many economic and political motivations, it did also reflect this desire to quarantine the Indians from white society. The federal government hoped to move the Indians to lands where they would be insulated from the fatal influences of civilization. The new explanations of smallpox that had evolved on the frontiers of the late eighteenth and early nineteenth century had found yet another way to serve the evolving needs of federal Indian policy.

Technologies

Changing smallpox remedies, however, had already begun to take federal responses to Indian epidemics in a different direction. In December 1801 an enthusiastic President Thomas Jefferson told Chief Little Turtle and other members of a Miami delegation that "the Great Spirit has made a gift to the white men in showing them how to preserve themselves from the smallpox": vaccination. After vaccinating members of the delegation, he gave them vaccine matter with instructions to use it among their people. This, he explained, "would finally extirpate that disease from the earth."[34] Vaccination (with cowpox), and the earlier techniques of inoculation (with smallpox), created an opportunity to mitigate smallpox, a dominant contributor to the disparity in health status between Indians and whites. Initially, however, these technologies did neither. Instead, they served as precedents for the uses of smallpox on the battlefields and at trading houses on the Ohio and Missouri Rivers.

The story of inoculation has been told by many historians. The technique appeared in India, sometime in the early Christian era; it then spread through Asia and Africa. The procedure, in its most basic form, was simple. Pus or a scab taken from a person suffering from smallpox was rubbed on the skin of a healthy person. Sometimes the recipient's skin was cut or abraded to allow for a deeper exposure to the contagion. The recipient would then develop a case of smallpox, hopefully one more localized, less severe, and less scarring than a natural case. Once the induced case had resolved, the patient would be forever immune to natural smallpox. There was, however, a significant problem: inoculation left its recipients contagious for several weeks, capable of spreading smallpox to people they encountered. Inoculation was thus a delicate gamble of risk and benefit.[35]

Reports of inoculation had appeared in Europe by 1670. It had been discussed at the Royal Society of London by 1700. In 1714 an enthusiastic description of the technique appeared in the *Philosophical Transactions* of the Royal Society. Cotton Mather, who read this report, had also heard about the technique from Onesimus, his African slave. Inoculation was first used in England in April 1721. After testing it on six prison inmates in August, two royal princesses were inoculated in April 1722.[36] Meanwhile, Mather had initiated the first use of inoculation in the American colonies, in Boston in July 1721. Mather, the great expounder of Puritan providence, believed that God wanted humans to take such control over disease.

As the ensuing chaos in Boston showed, inoculation became extremely controversial in the colonies. When smallpox appeared in Boston, Mather encouraged local physicians to inoculate. None responded. When he convinced surgeon Zabdiel Boylston to inoculate, the town exploded in controversy. Some townsfolk feared that the practice would disseminate smallpox. Others challenged the morality of intervening against smallpox, God's chosen judgment. Selectmen banned the procedure. Physicians and mobs denounced Mather and Boylston. One enraged citizen lobbed a grenade into Mather's living room. The attached note read: "COTTON MATHER, You Dog, Dam you: I'l inoculate you with this, with a Pox to you." By the spring of 1722, half of all Bostonians (5,889 out of roughly 11,000 or 12,000) had suffered from smallpox; 844 had died. Meanwhile, Mather and Boylston had inoculated 242 patients, with only 6 deaths.[37]

Such data, however, did not settle a debate born of deep fears of a terrible disease. In 1722 the Massachusetts House of Representatives passed a bill banning inoculation. Virginia made inoculation a criminal offense. In other areas, particularly in Philadelphia, it became increasingly popular in the second half of the century. The procedure was welcomed more enthusiastically in England: in 1755 the College of Physicians in London endorsed the practice; the British army used it widely. Performed carefully, inoculation had a death rate as low as 1/1,000.[38]

The new technology of inoculation raised a host of complicated problems. It gave colonists the ability to collect, store, and cause smallpox. Some devout colonists remained concerned about meddling with God's province. Most saw the debate in more practical terms. Did inoculation really grant lifelong protection against smallpox? Did the potential benefit justify the known risks of the procedure? It was not simply a matter for individuals to decide. Every act of inoculation put others at risk of contagion, creating a complicated calculus of risk and benefit. Recognizing the potential threat to public health, professional societies and governments struggled to regulate the practice. This was well demonstrated in George Washington's decision to inoculate the Continental Army. Military leaders had witnessed the havoc wrought by smallpox in Boston in 1775 and Quebec in 1776, and suspected that British troops deliberately spread smallpox among American troops. Needing to protect his soldiers, Washington decided to inoculate them in February 1777. The procedure was conducted with few deaths among the soldiers. The citizens of Morristown, New Jersey, however, paid a price: sixty-eight members of a Presbyterian church used as an inoculation hospital died.[39]

The controversy swirling around inoculation limited its application among American Indians. Many colonists felt responsible for the severe mortality Indians suffered from smallpox. Inoculation gave them the capacity to take prophylactic action. Yet this combination of capacity and responsibility did not lead to intervention. Little evidence suggests that the English ever tried to inoculate Indians in North America during the eighteenth century. Historians have not criticized them for this, since inoculation remained such a controversial procedure among the colonists. Spanish colonists, however, made a different calculus of inoculation. A Carmelite missionary along the Amazon river in western Brazil inoculated his parishioners during an epidemic in 1728. Inoculation was practiced widely among the Indian and European populations of Spanish America from the 1760s into the 1800s.[40] This discrepancy suggests that more nuanced assessments of English colonists' decisions are needed. Decisions did not simply reflect beliefs about the safety and efficacy of inoculation. They also reflected ambivalence about the role of American Indians in English and American society.

The calculus changed with the appearance of vaccination. The striking protection milkmaids had against smallpox had long been part of the folklore of the English countryside. Edward Jenner, recognizing this potential, transformed folk knowledge into medical practice. He guessed that deliberate infection with cowpox would grant protection against smallpox. Since cowpox caused only a minor illness in humans, this technique, which he called vaccination, provided the same benefit as inoculation with less risk to its recipients. Furthermore, since vaccination used cowpox and not smallpox, it did not share inoculation's risk of spreading smallpox. By 1796, through a series of experimental infections with cowpox followed by challenge with smallpox, he had demonstrated the value of vaccination. The technique spread to continental Europe in 1799. By 1800 Jenner had performed over 6,000 vaccinations.[41]

News of vaccination reached the United States no later than 1799, when Boston physician Benjamin Waterhouse read a copy of Jenner's paper. He vaccinated his son and several servants as soon as he obtained samples of cowpox in July 1800. Thomas Jefferson was similarly enthusiastic: he personally vaccinated his family, relatives, and friends. He also sponsored Waterhouse's efforts and disseminated vaccine material to anyone interested. After vaccination was demonstrated in Philadelphia in April 1802, it was endorsed by a group of fifty physicians, including Benjamin Rush, who had observed the 15 percent mortality from smallpox among the Continental Army. Although these observers recognized vaccination as a tremendous improvement over inoculation, it remained controversial. It could also be difficult to implement: Waterhouse and other advocates of vaccination long struggled to ensure a steady supply of active vaccine.[42]

Despite such obstacles, vaccination gradually won acceptance. In May 1812 the United States Army began vaccinating recruits; by 1818 all soldiers not already vaccinated were vaccinated immediately. In February 1813 Congress passed a law to encourage vaccination: the president was given the authority "to appoint an agent to preserve the genuine vaccine matter." Mail privileges were also bestowed: "all letters or packages, not exceeding half an ounce in weight, containing vaccine matter, or relating to the subject of vaccination, and that alone, shall be carried by the United States' mail free of any postage." Further evidence of the enthusiasm over vaccination can be seen in one popular textbook, Robert Thomas's 1822 *Treatise on Domestic Medicine*. Thomas described how smallpox, "a painful, loathsome, and fatal disease" killed one out of every six people. Inoculation could protect individuals, but it put communities at risk. Vaccination, however, could protect 999 of 1,000 people, without any danger.[43]

Vaccination, accepted more enthusiastically than inoculation, was brought to American Indians. President Jefferson led the way, vaccinating Chief Little Turtle's delegation in December 1801. In 1803, as he planned the expedition of Lewis and Clark, he saw another opportunity for vaccination. Jefferson gave the explorers detailed written instructions, including the request that they carry "some matter of the kinepox, inform those of them with whom you may be of its efficacy as a preservative from the small-pox; and instruct & incourage them in the use of it." He also provided Lewis with a supply of vaccine.[44]

Others were not far behind. In 1803 King Charles IV of Spain sent the Expedicion de la Vacuna (also known as the Balmis-Salvany Expedition) to bring vaccination to every port in Spanish America. By 1806 the expedition reported that it had vaccinated 100,000 Europeans and Indians from South America to New Mexico. In 1803 British officials in Canada sought vaccination for the Abneki. In 1807 Edward Jenner sent a copy of his book on vaccination to the Five Nations. At their council in November 1807, representatives of the Five Nations sent their thanks, and a string of wampum, to Jenner: "We shall not fail to teach our children to speak the name of Jenner and to thank the Great Spirit for the bestowing upon him so much wisdom and so much benevolence . . . we beseech the Great Spirit to take care of you in this world, and in the land of spirits."[45]

Even the best intentioned plans could be tricky to execute, especially amid the difficult conditions of frontier life. Lewis, for instance, quickly realized that his supply of vaccine was inactive. In October 1803 he wrote to Jefferson from Cincinnati: "I would thank you to forward me some of the Vaxcine matter, as I have reason to believe from several experiments made with what I have, that it has lost it's virtue." Lewis never received a new supply. He made no subsequent mention of vaccination in his journals.[46]

The traders of the American Fur Company fared little better in 1837. When officials at Fort Union decided to inoculate the Assiniboine and Blackfeet at Fort Union, they turned to "Mr. Thomas' medical book." They found bewildering and complicated recommendations for the management of smallpox. Fever required a special diet: "panado, gruel, arrow-root moistened with milk, plain bread pudding, salep, tapioca, calf's feet jellies, roasted apples, chicken, or light veal broth; and where the fever is on decline, and is accompanied by considerable debility, beef tea." Specific beverages were needed, including

"water, lemonade, thin gruel, barley-water gently acidulated with orange or lemon juice, common tea, or that made from balm or mint."
Other symptoms (nausea, headache, sore throat, cough, irritability, de-
lirium, livid spots, pustules) required medicinal resources ranging from
lemonade and roses, to Peruvian bark, opium, laxatives, purgatives,
leeches, and effervescing saline. Special measures had to be taken to
prevent the spread of the contagion, including fumigation with nitric
acid, muriatic acid, and sulfuric acid. Meanwhile, medicine cabinets
were quite limited, at least at Fort Clark. When Maximilian visited in
1833 and 1834, he "examined all the medical stock of the fort" and
found only "a handful of elder flowers, and rather more of American
camomile," and "some common remedies."[47]

Vaccination was no less complicated. Fluid was supposed to be collected from a pustule of a person with cowpox on that person's ninth
day of illness, and only when the fluid was transparent. The material needed to be used before it dried out. As recipients recovered from
vaccination, they had to be treated with purgatives such as mercury,
jalap, and rhubarb. Since company officials lacked vaccine material,
they turned to inoculation. Thomas had promising things to say about
the technique: it "is a fact, fully and long established," that inoculation
was safer than natural smallpox and "highly beneficial to *individuals*."
Imagine their dismay when, turning the next page, they found that
Thomas disavowed inoculation: "Disapproving, as I do, of keeping up
the smallpox by inoculation, I shall refrain from laying down any rules
for its performance, and do strongly recommend vaccine inoculation in
its stead."[48]

Decades of changing ideas about smallpox had left the fur traders in
a difficult position. Puritans' notions of providence acting through natural mechanisms had given way to theories of disease that emphasized
misbehavior (alcohol, venery, wading across icy streams, sweat baths)
as the proximate causes of smallpox and disparities in health and mortality. American Indians, introduced to such misbehavior by their
contact with European settlers, suffered excruciating epidemics. Understood in this way, the disparity in health status demanded intervention. Motivated by humanitarian concern, and feeling more than a little
responsible for what had happened, missionaries, explorers, traders,
and government officials all sought ways to alleviate Indian suffering.
Missionaries placed smallpox in a moral framework in which health

could be obtained through temperance and moderation. Government officials shaped their diplomatic discourse around smallpox, providing presents and condolences to preserve the loyalty of their afflicted allies.

Into this world came the new technologies of inoculation and vaccination, specific measures that could be deployed to prevent smallpox. These techniques, with the power to transform the relationships between humans and smallpox, brought new responsibility. Inoculation required a difficult calculus of benefit and risk. Vaccination required a safe supply of the vaccine and a sophisticated regimen of supportive medical care. Both proved to be imperfect technologies in the many situations where ideal conditions did not exist. These imperfections had powerful consequences for American Indians. Although inoculation and vaccination had the potential to reduce the susceptibility of American Indians to their greatest scourge, the precarious mix of economic and political interests of colonial and federal Indian policy generated different outcomes. Just as differentials existed in the prevalence of smallpox, differentials quickly appeared in the utilization of smallpox technologies. This elusive promise of control would appear clearly in the uses of smallpox at Fort Pitt and Fort Union.

4

Using Smallpox

BY THE SECOND HALF of the eighteenth century, the relationship of humans to smallpox had changed fundamentally. Diseases
were increasingly seen as the result of specific behaviors, from exposure
to dangerous environments to indulgence in sinful pursuits. Many colonists assumed that the high mortality of American Indians reflected
their many forms of misbehavior. These damaging ways of living,
however, were recognized as the consequence of contact between the
white and Indian populations. Just as colonists had new understandings
of why smallpox occurred, they had new abilities to contain its afflictions. If colonists in Boston had watched helplessly as smallpox struck
during the seventeenth century and fought bitterly over the appearance
of inoculation in the 1720s, they had reached an uneasy détente by the
1760s. Thomas Hutchinson praised inoculation, "to which many thousands owe the preservation of their lives."[1] Those many thousands,
however, were only the white inhabitants of the English colonies. The
potential benefits of inoculation had not yet been brought to the Indians who lived within and beyond English settlements.

These tensions appeared dramatically on the western frontiers. In
1763 the traders and officers at Fort Pitt struggled to turn smallpox to
their advantage by disseminating it among Delaware and Shawnee
forces. In 1837, officials of the American Fur Company inoculated
Blackfeet and Assiniboine traders to minimize the spread of the epi-

93

demic. It is tempting to single out these episodes as crucial steps towards biological warfare or the eradication of smallpox. But even the seemingly most emblematic stories contain a complex mix of interests and motivations. The local needs of frontier life turned smallpox, and its control, into a calamity or ally in war, an obstacle or asset in trade.

If new understandings and technologies of smallpox created a space in which the disease became an instrument of war and trade, it remained a potential space. Smallpox never yielded easily to human designs, especially when those designs were compromised by ambivalence about whether Indians were friend, foe, or opportunity. These ambiguities played out at Fort Pitt and Fort Union, and in the efforts to vaccinate American Indians in the early nineteenth century. Even as the government tried and failed to incorporate American Indians into the social and political domain of the United States, its vaccination campaigns faced challenges of motivation and implementation. In the eighteenth and nineteenth centuries smallpox swept unchecked, arguably accelerated, into the interior river valleys of North America.

War

When William Trent and Sir Jeffrey Amherst each decided to spread smallpox among American Indians, they ensured their infamy as pioneers of biological warfare. Their efforts, however, have frequently been misunderstood. The episode must not be seen as an isolated act of unusual brutality. Instead, the commerce in smallpox at Fort Pitt was simply another way that the disease was put into the service of trade and empire.

The basic narratives of deliberate infection at Fort Pitt are quite clear. In the bitter conflicts of the Seven Years War, France and Britain battled for control of global empires in Europe, India, the Caribbean, and North America (where the conflict has been known as the French and Indian War). By the time that Britain emerged victorious, Amherst, commander in chief of British forces in North America, had added the vast lands of Canada to the empire. Only the Indian tribes, formerly allied to the French, continued the fight. In the spring of 1763 they attacked British garrisons along the Great Lakes and the Ohio River valley (Figure 1). Fort Pitt faced a siege by Delaware and Shawnee warriors. On 23 June 1763 Colonel Henry Bouquet,

Amherst's field commander on the New York and Pennsylvania frontier, told Amherst about a setback at Fort Pitt: "unluckily the Small Pox has broke out in the garrison." Captain Simeon Ecuyer, in charge of the garrison, "has built an Hospital under the Draw Bridge to prevent the Spreading of that distemper."[2]

Over the next week Amherst and Bouquet developed plans to deal with "the infernal treachery of the vilest Brutes." Bouquet awaited reinforcements that would allow him to "extirpate that Vermine from a Country they have forfeited, and with it all claim to the rights of humanity." Amherst ordered Bouquet to show no mercy: "I Wish to Hear of *no Prisoners*, should any of the Villains be met with in Arms." On 3 July Bouquet reported that the Indians had captured the British posts at Presque Isle, Le Bouef, and Venango. This loss gave Amherst "great Concern." In a letter to Bouquet on 7 July he added his infamous postscript: "Could it not be contrived to Send the *Small Pox* among those Disaffected Tribes of Indians? We must, on this occasion, Use Every Strategem in our power to Reduce them." On 13 July Bouquet responded enthusiastically: "I will try to inoculate the ____ with Some Blankets that may fall into their Hands, and take Care not to get the disease myself." On 16 July Amherst confirmed their intent: "You will Do well to try to Innoculate the *Indians*, by means of Blankets, as well as to Try Every other Method, that can Serve to Extirpate this Execrable Race."[3]

These letters show a shared desire to infect the Delaware with smallpox-infected blankets. But there is no evidence that either Bouquet or Amherst ever attempted to do so. Nor is there evidence that Bouquet passed this order to his subordinates. Neither Bouquet nor Amherst ever mentioned the idea again. As historian Bernhard Knollenberg concluded regarding Bouquet and Amherst, "execution of the intent is not supported even by circumstantial evidence."[4]

Had Bouquet sent Amherst's suggestion to Fort Pitt, it would have come too late: the attempt at deliberate infection had already been made. Ecuyer noted that smallpox broke out on 16 June: "We are so crowded in the fort that I fear disease, for in spite of all my care I cannot keep the place as clean as I should like; moreover, the smallpox is among us." On 22 June the Delaware and Shawnee made a fierce attack; Ecuyer dispersed them with his howitzer and cannon. On the morning of 24 June two Delaware chiefs, Turtle's Heart and

Dr The Crown To Sim. Trent &Comss. for Sundries had by
Order of Capt. Simon Ecuyer Commandt

1763 June				£
To Sundries for the Militia Vizt				
84 Tomhawks		10/	42.0.0	
6 large Tin Kettles		10/	3.0.0	
1 Canteen			0..3.0	45.3.0
To Sundries delivd the following Expresses Vizt				
Vossee & his Comerad 2 ps Legins	a6/	20.12.0		
1 Britchclout		0.8.0		
Cash		1.0.0	22.0.0	
Yazly 2 dressd Deerskins	a15/	1.10.0		
1 Blanket 20/ & Cash 3/6		1.3.6		
			2..13.6	
Thompson & Johnston 1 dressd Deerskin			0..15.0	
Isaac & John Cox 2 ps Legins	a6/	0.12.0		
2 Britchclouts 8/		0.16.0		
2 ps garters 1/6		0.3.0		
3 Linnen Hankhs		0.10.6		
1 dressd Deerskin		0.15.0		
2 Ruffles &c		15.0.0	17.16.6	
Abrm Bidler 1 ps Mochesons			0..7.6	23.12.6
To 1 Box Candles for the Guard &c wt 121 lb Wt a2/3				13.12.3
To Sundries got to Replace in kind those which were taken				
from people in the Hospital to Convey the Small pox				
to the Indians Vizt				
2 Blankets	a20/	2.0.0		
1 Silk Handkercheif 10/ & 1 Linnen do 3/6		0.13.6		2.13.6
				£ 85.1.3
				13.12.3
				71.9.0

Fort Pitt Augt 13th 1763

I do hereby Certify that the above Articles amounting to Eighty five
Pounds One Shilling & three pence Pennsylva Curry were had for the
uses above mentioned

S. Ecuyer Capt Commandt

Philadelphia May 22. 1764

Deduct pr 27/ of the Kings Horses employd eight days
carrying your Skins from Fort Pitt to Fort Bedford a 2/6 8 days ... 27:0:0

£ 58..1.3

Maumaultee, demanded the surrender of the British garrison. Both sides claimed that they had reinforcements en route, that resistance was futile, and that they would never back down. Both sides also offered promises of friendship. Ready to depart, the Delaware demanded "a little Provisions and Liquor, to carry us Home." Ecuyer complied: "The above Provisions was granted to them & they set off Home about 2 oClock that Night." Trent, who ran the local trading post, described a different gift for the departing chiefs: "Out of our regard to them we gave them two Blankets and an Handkerchief out of the Small Pox Hospital. I hope it will have the desired effect."[5]

It is unclear who joined Trent in this act. Neither Alexander McKee, the Indian agent at Fort Pitt, nor Ecuyer mentioned Trent's gift. The act, however, was later endorsed by Ecuyer and the British high command. Trent billed the British government for expenses during the siege in June (Figure 4). The total, £85 1s 3p, included £2 13s 6p for "Sundries got to Replace in kind those which were taken from people in the Hospital to Convey the Smallpox to the Indians," specifically two blankets, one silk handkerchief, and one linen handkerchief. Ecuyer certified the bill on 13 August 1763: "the above Articles amounting to Eighty five Pounds One Shilling & three pence Pennsylva: Currcy: were had for the uses above mentioned." On 24 May 1764 L. S. Ourry, quartermaster general, refused to pay for candles, and deducted £27 for transport costs, but approved the other charges. General Thomas Gage, who replaced Amherst as commander in chief, approved the modified bill on 13 August 1764.[6]

The Bouquet-Amherst exchange has been a fixture of the historical record since its discovery by Francis Parkman in 1870. The role of Trent and Ecuyer did not did not emerge until later. The episode has received tremendous attention as "history's first documentable case of biological warfare."[7] Identifying Amherst's intent and Trent's act as bi-

---

4. The Crown to Levy, Trent & Company for sundries had by order of Capt. Simeon Ecuyer, Commandant, June–August 1763. Trent billed the British Army £2 13s 6p for "Sundries got to Replace in kind those which were taken from people in the Hospital to Convey the Smallpox to the Indians." Ecuyer accepted the charges: "I do hereby Certify that the above Articles . . . were had for the uses above mentioned." This bill confirms both the intent of Trent's gift and the approval of the British command. (Bouquet Papers, ADD.21654 f168. By permission of the British Library.)

ological warfare, a term with very specific meanings in the twentieth century, confuses what the episode reveals about the relationship between the English, Indians, and smallpox in the eighteenth century. Was smallpox a special form of weapon, reserved for special circumstances of military desperation or ethnic hatred? Did the use of smallpox arise from belief that Indians were peculiarly vulnerable to its ravages? These questions can only be understood within the specific contexts of the attempt.

When Trent deployed smallpox to defend Fort Pitt, he sought to protect a fort that, although it had existed for only ten years, had become a cornerstone of empire. As late as 1740, the Mississippi Valley remained a land of American Indians, with fewer than 1,000 French soldiers and fur traders maintaining French claims to half a continent. English traders entered the Ohio valley in the 1740s. To defend French claims, the Marquis Duquesne, the governor-general of New France, built forts from Lake Erie to the Mississippi River in 1752. The Virginia government sent Major George Washington to demand that the French withdraw. Rebuffed, he selected the forks of the Ohio River as a promising site for a British fort. Trent, then a captain in the Virginia militia, began construction in 1754. Three months later, in the first overt act of the Seven Years War, the French seized the fort, fortified it, and renamed it Fort Duquesne. British forces tried, and failed, to retake the fort in 1754 and 1755. As hostilities spread throughout the Americas and beyond, France declared war in 1756. British forces turned the tide in America in 1758, when they captured Fort Frontenac and cut French supply lines between Montreal and Fort Duquesne. Promising to respect Delaware, Shawnee, and Iroquois land claims in the Treaty of Easton, the British convinced them to abandon the French. The French had to destroy the fort and retreat. General John Forbes and Lieutenant Colonel Henry Bouquet took possession of Fort Duquesne in November 1758 and renamed it Pittsburgh. By 1760 General Jeffrey Amherst had forced the surrender of all French forces in Canada.[8]

Peace on the frontier did not last. The French had maintained Indian loyalty with a generous policy of assistance and gifts. The Indians, recovering from years of damaging warfare, assumed that the English would continue this policy. The Ottawa, for instance, demanded that the English at Detroit provide "a smith to mend our Guns and

Hatchets, and a Doctor to attend our People when Sick." Since Amherst no longer needed Indian support against the French, he rejected such requests. When warriors demanded gifts at Fort Pitt in April and December 1762, Bouquet could not comply. Discontent grew as the British strengthened garrisons and allowed settlers to flood into the Ohio valley. The garrison at Fort Pitt began hearing rumors that the Delaware and other tribes planned to attack. Inflamed by Pontiac, a Delaware prophet who called for a renunciation of European presence and products, tribes from Michigan to New York rose up against the English. The Ottawa attacked Detroit on 9 May 1763. The Delaware and Mingo attacked Fort Pitt on 28 May. By late June, the British forts and garrisons at Michilimackinac, Venango, LeBouef, Presque Isle, Sandusky, and La Baie had been destroyed. English settlements had been burned. Detroit remained besieged by the Ottawa, Fort Niagara by the Seneca, and Fort Pitt by the Delaware and Shawnee.[9]

This attack caught the British off guard. Postwar troop reductions had left Amherst with only one battalion, Bouquet's Royal Americans, overextended in thirteen forts between New York and Michigan. Amherst initially thought that he could "Chastize" any tribe. But as fort after fort fell, he became enraged and dreamed of an English world free of those "Inhuman villains": "I Wish there was not an Indian Settlement with a Thousand Miles of our Country; for they are only fit to Live with the Inhabitants of the Woods, being more nearly Allied to the *Brute* than the *Human* Creation." Although Henry Bouquet had developed sympathy towards the Indians during the uneasy peace at Fort Pitt from 1758 to 1763, and had encouraged Amherst to adopt a more lenient gift policy before the war, he came to share Amherst's vision. Angered by the events of June, he too hoped "to extirpate that Vermine from a Country they have forfeited, and with it all claim to the rights of humanity."[10]

In such a context, it is not difficult to understand the motivation of Amherst and Bouquet. The Indian attacks had undermined their conquest of Canada. Even though Bouquet knew that the British presence violated the Treaty of Easton, he and Amherst felt that they had been attacked without justification. Defeated at six forts, they had to use all possible means to defend their remaining positions. But is it surprising that they turned to smallpox? Not at all.

Historians have written vividly about the brutality of colonial war-fare. Wars "were waged with a macabre intensity not seen in Europe for generations." The English "did not curtail cruelty or carnage but rather sought to maximize them." Brutality was especially marked to-wards Indians. Warfare "took on a tone of barbarism perhaps not wit-nessed in the Western world since antiquity." Indians, who had tradi-tionally practiced limited warfare, learned from the European example and responded in kind. Villages and corn fields were burned; women were raped; victims were scalped; terror was the goal.[11]

Such brutality was perpetrated at Fort Pitt. When the Delaware at-tacked on 29 May, they scalped two of their victims. Ecuyer, creative in the fort's defense, set beaver traps to trap Indians. When he described the traps to Bouquet, he added "I would be happy to send you one, with a savage's leg in it, but they haven't given me that satisfaction." On 11 July a member of the Pennsylvania Assembly suggested that Bouquet hunt the Indians with trained war dogs. He recommended this plan to Amherst: "As it is pity to expose good men against them I wish we would make use of the Spanish Method to hunt them with English Dogs."[12] Such dogs, however, were not available. With these prece-dents, use of smallpox seems less shocking. It could cause a horrible death, but so did being scalped or devoured by dogs. It would strike civilian populations, but that was a goal of warfare. The one unique aspect of smallpox (and it is unclear whether Trent or Amherst under-stood this) was that this weapon, once introduced, could propagate itself.

Soldiers were certainly very familiar with smallpox, which had long been as much a part of war as marching and muskets, determining the success or failure of many campaigns. Some historians have suspected that there was "a backwoods tradition of this sort of germ warfare." Ac-cusations certainly existed, from Ensenore, Squanto, and Canonicus, to Dekanissore in 1717, and to French accusations that the English in-fected the Cherokee in 1738 and the Micmac in 1744. Historian Eliza-beth Fenn has documented many accusations of deliberate infection during the Seven Years War: the Potawatomi accused the British, while the Ottawa and the British accused the French.[13] The garrison at Fort Pitt knew smallpox well. Most must have known of the precedent of in-oculation, with its demonstration that smallpox could be collected and transmitted. Some might have heard rumors of attempts at deliberate infection. Desperate for a way to raise the siege, two sets of British defenders independently found smallpox to be an obvious choice. When Trent billed the army for the costs of the attack, three levels of the British command signed off without complaint. And although they did not mention Trent's gift, Bouquet and Amherst praised Ecuyer for taking "all the Precautions which art and Judgment could Suggest for the Preservation of this Post."[14]

Although deliberate infection might have been a natural outgrowth of the events at Fort Pitt, there are two surprising aspects of this episode. First, the attack could not have arisen from belief in some unique American Indian vulnerability. In the seventeenth century, accusations of deliberate infection had arisen from Indian observations that they suffered while Europeans remained unscathed. But this was not the case at Fort Pitt. The attempt was possibly inspired, and certainly made possible, by the outbreak of smallpox among the British garrison. Bouquet feared that handling smallpox would put himself at risk, telling Amherst that he would "take Care not to get the disease myself." This sense of mutual vulnerability occurred repeatedly on the western frontier. Amherst and Trent did not see smallpox as a magic bullet that would only kill Indians. Instead, faced with smallpox among their own forces, they tried to share it with their enemies.[15]

Second, the attempt at deliberate infection did not depend on racial hatred between Indians and Europeans. Cultural and religious gulfs certainly exacerbated the savagery of frontier warfare. Higginbotham has suggested a gradient of savagery, with British forces being cruelest to Indians, less cruel to the French and Spaniards, and least cruel to the Americans during the Revolutionary War. Some have even argued that attacks with smallpox could have happened only in the context of Indian-European conflict. Elizabeth Fenn has shown that this is not true. During the Seven Years War, the British believed that the French had tried to send smallpox to Halifax. During the Revolutionary War, American officers believed that the British attacked them with smallpox at Boston, Quebec, Virginia, New Hampshire, and Yorktown. One British officer even published a military manual that advocated shooting American rebels with smallpox-dipped arrows.[16] It is certainly possible that while these ideas circulated in the contexts of British-

American warfare, the act was only executed in cases of British-Indian warfare. But it is equally possible that many attempts were made in a variety of contexts without surviving in the historical record.

While the attitudes of Amherst and Bouquet seem clear, William Trent presents a more complicated problem. Trent had the longest experience on the Pennsylvania frontier, having entered the Indian trade in 1750, served as an agent of Virginia in 1752, begun construction on Fort Pitt in 1754, assisted in the negotiations at Easton in 1758, participated in the capture of Fort Duquesne, re-entered the Indian trade, and remained active in Indian diplomacy. Since Trent left little record of his attitude towards the Indians, it remains unclear whether he saw them as friends or as people to be seduced with alcohol and trapped into debt. The siege, however, elicited a clear response. Eighteen traders and eighty-eight servants were killed or taken captive in June; traders' losses totaled more than £45,000. Trent did not watch passively. He organized the civilians into a militia company, helped Ecuyer set beaver traps, and attempted to infect Turtle's Heart and Maumaultee with smallpox. Was he angered by the betrayal of his former customers? Was this simply more hostility towards people he had long sought to exploit? Did he hope that smallpox, by hastening the end of hostilities, would allow him to re-open trade more quickly? Whatever his motivation, he acted like a practical merchant and billed the military for his expenses.[17]

One last ambiguity is the impact of Trent's gift. Bouquet arrived with reinforcements on 10 August and broke the siege. Did smallpox contribute? Three witnesses in 1764 and 1765 reported smallpox among the Delaware and Shawnee. Most historians interpret these reports as evidence of the success of Trent's attempt. However, the existence of smallpox could also indicate that the disease had already become endemic, or that it reached the Delaware and Shawnee through multiple routes. The most direct evidence suggests that Trent's blankets had no impact. One month after the gift, Turtle's Heart and Maumaultee returned to negotiate at Fort Pitt. They made no mention of smallpox among their people. Two days later the Delaware and Shawnee began a fierce attack that lasted for five days and five nights. Trent's gift neither weakened the tribes nor triggered accusations of deliberate infection.[18]

Gone were the days when Thomas Hariot could deny English control over smallpox, arguing that "our God would not subiect him selfe to anie such praiers and requestes of men."[19] By 1763 the English had taken some responsibility for smallpox and its distribution. The disease could be stored, packaged, transported, and inflicted. It could be sent to an enemy with an expectation of successful infection. The gift of blankets, existing within the frameworks of trade and diplomacy that tied British and Indians together, subverted these relationships in an effort to keep them apart. Yet as shocking as the attempt might seem, it elicited no alarm from its witnesses. Smallpox remained routine enough on the frontier to be unsurprising when used as an act of war. It did, however, remain elusive enough to defy attempts at control.

Trade

Officials of the American Fur Company put smallpox to very different uses in 1837. The epidemic began innocuously. The *St. Peter's*, the steamboat of the American Fur Company, left St. Louis on its annual trip up the Missouri River on 17 April. A passenger suffering from a fever boarded just south of Fort Leavenworth. By the time the steamer reached Council Bluffs, the fever had evolved into smallpox and spread to several other passengers. Three Arikara women boarded the *St. Peter's* at Council Bluffs. These women were infected by the time the steamer reached the Sioux agency at Fort Pierre on June 5. Officials and trade goods, dispersed at Fort Pierre, spread the disease to the Yankton and Santee Sioux. Jacob Halsey, en route to his new position as director at Fort Union, boarded the *St. Peter's* around 6 June. By June 17, as the steamer approached Fort Clark, the outbreak of smallpox appeared to have wound down. Nothing seemed amiss when the steamer reached Fort Clark on 19 June. The merchandise was unloaded, "all hands a Frolicking." The three Arikara women disembarked to join their tribe camped nearby. The *St. Peter's* left the next day.[20]

When the *St. Peter's* reached Fort Union on 25 June, "the mirth usual on such occasions was not of long duration": Halsey had caught smallpox. Although he had been vaccinated previously and now suffered only a minor case, the damage had been done. Trade had brought smallpox far up the Missouri Valley, and the results were devastating. The "detestable pest" broke out at Fort Union within days of Halsey and the arrival of the *St. Peter's*. Several workers died and twenty-seven others were soon sick. Smallpox soon spread to the Indians surrounding the fort. Halsey suspected that "the air was infected with it for a half mile without the pickets." Others argued that an Indian had stolen an infected blanket. The epidemic eventually receded from Fort Union, but among the Blackfeet and Assiniboine it was "raging with the greatest destruction imaginable at least 10 out of 12 die with it."[21]

Smallpox did not appear near Fort Clark until mid-July. On 14 July, in the midst of a heat wave, a "young Mandan died to day of the Small Pox—several others had caught it." On 17 July a thunderstorm broke the heat wave, but smallpox continued: "An other case of the small pox broke out to day at the Village." It spread throughout Mandan villages, and then to the nearby Arikara (Rees). Four Bears, the Mandan chief, caught smallpox, allegedly condemned the treachery of the traders, and died on 30 July. The tribes began fatalistic dances: "they expect to all die of the small pox—and as long as they are alive, they will take it out in dancing." By late August more than 50 Mandan men had died, and uncounted women and children. Smallpox appeared within Fort Clark on 13 August, devastating traders' Indian wives and children. Chardon caught the disease, but cured himself with whiskey and nutmeg. His own son died on 22 September. By the end of September, "it has distroyed the seven eights of the Mandans and one half of the Rees Nations." It continued to spread throughout the winter.[22]

A similar story played out at Fort McKenzie. Andrew Culbertson had sent a keelboat to collect trade goods from the *St. Peter's* at Fort Union. Smallpox appeared on the return trip and reached Fort McKenzie in late July. Two traders soon died. The Blackfeet, "undeterred by the spectacle, still insisted upon the opening of trade as usual." They dispersed after five days of trade. Smallpox soon erupted within the fort: "Scarcely one of its eighty-five or ninety occupants escaped an attack of greater or less severity." Indian women at the fort were especially hard hit. The disease soon emerged among the nearby Blackfeet.[23]

The epidemic left scenes of gruesome desolation at each fort. Victims died remarkably fast: "The patient, when first seized, complains of dreadful pains in the head and back, and in a few hours he is dead: the body immediately turns black, and swells to thrice its natural size." The few who remained healthy were unable to bury the dead. As corpses were dumped over bluffs or thrown into the river, rotting bodies created "a stench beyond description." Many Indians "gave themselves up in despair" and took their own lives. Some identified the traders as the source of their suffering and became hostile. The Mandan and Gros Ventres threatened to kill Chardon. Arikara warriors attacked a company boat sailing from Fort Union to St. Louis in the spring of 1838. Although the Blackfeet were angry, Forts Union and McKenzie faced fewer threats.[24]

By the time the epidemic died down in 1838, it had laid waste the upper Missouri Valley. As an anonymous witness described, the "destroying angel has visited the unfortunate sons of the wilderness with terror never before known, and has converted the extensive hunting grounds, as well as the peaceful settlements of those tribes, into desolate and boundless cemeteries." Abandoned villages covered the plains, "no sounds but the croaking of the raven and the howling of the wolf interrupt the fearful silence." Estimates of overall mortality ranged between 10,000 and 250,000. Between 7,000 and 8,000 Blackfeet died. The Mandan fell from 1,600 to 30.[25]

Many whites believed that the Plains Indians had met their doom: "It seems to be irrevocably written in the book of fate, that the race of red men shall be wholly extirpated in the land in which they ruled the undisputed masters, till the rapacity of the Whites brought to their shores the murderous fire-arms, the enervating ardent spirits, and the all-destructive pestilence of the small-pox." The epidemic transformed the political situation of the region. Before 1837 Americans had feared war with the Blackfeet, "the bravest and most crafty of all the Indians, dangerous and implacable to their enemies." Smallpox destroyed this threat: "Every thought of war was dispelled, and the few that are left are as humble as famished dogs." The government's "vast preparations for the protection of the western frontier are superfluous: another arm has undertaken the defence of the white inhabitants of the frontier; and the funeral torch, that lights the red man to his dreary grave, has become the auspicious star of the advancing settler, and of the roving trade of the white race."[26] Smallpox, once again, had facilitated white settlement.

Was this devastation inevitable? Most historians have assumed that it was. However, it is possible that the remarkable mortality reflected contingent circumstances. The Mandan, prevented from hunting by hostile tribes, experienced a near-famine that left them vulnerable. Historian Clyde Dollar has argued that a combination of cold, rainy weather and smoke from prairie fires, along with poor sanitation and overcrowding, created a "high contagion probability." Contingent factors also protected other tribes. The Gros Ventres, likely inoculated by previous exposure to smallpox, lost only 200 people. The Crows "did not take it at all, carefully keeping themselves during its progress beyond reach of infection."[27]

The federal government had different explanations. An 1838 inquiry, reflecting the belief that humans could be responsible for the distribution of their diseases, focused on human factors. The commissioner of Indian affairs concluded that the Indians "general want of medical advice and neglect of precautionary measures, added to their irregular and exposed modes of living, made them certain victims of the scourge."[28] Could more appropriate responses have prevented the epidemic? Was such control over smallpox possible? The acts of the traders provide a host of suggestive answers.

Once they recognized the presence of smallpox on the *St. Peter's*, the traders attempted to prevent an epidemic. First, the traders tried to quarantine each of the forts. Chardon begged the Gros Ventres to stay away from Fort Clark and sent them ten pounds of tobacco as compensation. When smallpox appeared inside Fort Union, officials locked the gates to prevent anyone from fleeing and spreading the contagion. Halsey sent a messenger to the Assiniboine to warn them not to approach the fort; when they arrived, traders attempted to scare them off by showing them a sick child "whose face was still one solid scab." When smallpox appeared on the keelboat en route to Fort McKenzie, its captain stopped the boat and sent a warning upriver. Culbertson "immediately decided to leave the boat there till the disease abated and cold weather set it." However, "five hundred lodges" of Blackfeet, awaiting the trade goods at the fort, ignored warnings that they risked an epidemic and demanded that the keelboat be brought to the fort. Although the disease broke out almost immediately, the Blackfeet, "undeterred by the spectacle, still insisted upon the opening of trade as usual."[29]

Second, even as they tried to contain the epidemic, the traders worked to treat its victims. Although Chardon spent most of his days simply observing the devastation of the Mandan, he did try to cure some with Epsom salts, or with a decoction of "Magnisia, peppermint, sugar lead, all Mixed together in a phial, filled with Indian grog." At Fort Union, officials organized a hospital, but to little avail: soon "the whole stock of medicines was exhausted." Vaccination could have been a decisive response. Officials at Fort Union did consider vaccinating people within the fort, especially the Indian wives of the traders, but they had no vaccine matter. In its absence, they "decided to inoculate with the smallpox itself." Guided by Thomas's *Domestic Medicine*, they inoculated "30 Indian squaws and a few white men." According to Larpenteur, these efforts were fruitless: inoculation "proved fatal to most of our patients." Culbertson, at Fort McKenzie, also resorted to inoculation. Although "the precaution came too late to have its usual efficacy," it "greatly lessened the mortality in the fort."[30]

If these accounts are reliable, they document considerable effort to contain smallpox. Such efforts were not limited to the traders. Many Arikara sought relief through dreams and sacrifices. One inadvertently cured himself by rolling in hot ashes. The Gros Ventres tried to protect themselves by quarantine, refusing Mandan and Arikara visitors. One Mandan father even saved his son with improvised inoculation: "An Indian Vaccinated his child, by cutting two small pieces of flesh out of his arms, and two on the belly—and then takeing a Scab from one, that was getting well of the disease, and rubbing it on the wounded part, three days after, it took effect, and the child is perfectly well."[31]

The actions of the traders have long been scrutinized by historians. Most assessments have ranged from "careless" to "criminally negligent." One argued that the traders "deliberately sacrificed" the Indians. Another concluded that the 1837 epidemic "appears particularly horrible because such high mortality was preventable." Many historians have sympathized with the traders: "the hapless actors in this tragedy acted out their parts as dictated by chance and their own human frailties of limited understanding of invisible forces." Lacking vaccine, the traders "were left with few alternatives." That they made any efforts at all suggests that they accepted "responsibility for the welfare of the Indians even in the midst of disaster."[32]

This focus on the traders' responses to the epidemic overlooks the responsibility of the traders, and possibly the Indians, for the epidemic itself, especially their willingness to risk lives to preserve trade. Like their French, English, and Dutch predecessors in New France, New

England, and New York, fur traders were drawn into the upper
Missouri Valley by "a mercenary motive—the commercial value of the
harmless and inoffensive beaver." Established by French traders in the
eighteenth century, the Missouri trade evolved through wars and epidemics. By the time steamboats reached the Missouri River in 1819,
the trade had become fiercely competitive, with bankruptcies, mergers,
and acquisitions. In 1837 Pratte, Chouteau, and Company, a descen-
dant of John Jacob Astor's American Fur Company, controlled the river
from Fort Pierre to Fort McKenzie. The federal government granted
these traders considerable autonomy. Although it had enacted prohibitions against selling alcohol to American Indians, it placed a member of
the American Fur Company in charge of the Missouri subagency: the
"great farce had begun."[33]

The relationships between traders and American Indians relied on
economic opportunism and co-dependency. The Indians had access to
resources (beaver skins and buffalo fur), which traders could buy from
them and then sell at a profit on American and European markets. In
exchange the Indians received textiles, alcohol, tobacco, and firearms.
These interactions created many auxiliary economic relationships. The
traders depended on Indian hunters and farmers for meat and corn.
Traders, scientists, and explorers hired Indians as guides in the wilderness. Artists used them as subjects for portraits. However, this was no
multicultural utopia: both sides contested the terms of the trade. The
relationship also contained marked asymmetries, especially the differential mortality that had shocked settlers for centuries. Appearing in
this world, smallpox threatened everyone and created new meanings
and opportunities.

Given their dependence on the American Indians, it is remarkable
that the traders allowed smallpox to reach the trading posts. Catlin, in
New York City at the time of the epidemic, assumed that smallpox
must have been recognized too late: "for if they had known it to be
such, I cannot conceive of such imprudence, as regarded their own interest in the country, as well as the fate of these poor people, by allow-
ing their boat to advance into the country under such circumstances."
But smallpox had been recognized before the *St. Peter's* reached Fort
Pierre. Culbertson accused Captain Bernard Pratte of "a reckless disregard of consequences" for continuing upstream.[34] But many other traders followed Pratte's example.

The traders faced a difficult situation. Conditions on the upper Missouri allowed only a single steamboat roundtrip each summer. Had Pratte turned back, the posts would have been left without supplies for an entire year. The traders accepted the risk of an epidemic and took steps to prevent it with self-quarantine, treatment, and inoculation. However, they repeatedly acquiesced to (alleged) Indian demands that the trade continue. This was reciprocal risk: American Indians were put at risk because of the trade, while the company was at risk because of its dependence on trade. Inoculation served all interests, humanitarian and opportunistic.

Officials, tragically, did not bring their efforts to fruition. Thousands died. Were the traders constrained by Indian threats? Did they make only halfhearted efforts because of their ambivalence towards the Indians? Or were their interventions incapable of halting the airborne contagion of smallpox? Some surely acted impulsively, without reasoned plans, responding to the horror of the moment.

If it is difficult to assign meanings to actions taken during the heat of the epidemic, it becomes easier to see meaning in actions taken in its aftermath. First, the traders blamed the outbreak on the Indians, claiming that smallpox appeared when Indians stole blankets from dying traders. Second, as the dust settled, they turned the epidemic itself into an economic opportunity. Maximilian, for instance, who had wintered with the Mandan before the epidemic, realized that the mortality made his observations "especially valuable." As his English translator and his editor explained, the "almost total extinction of these tribes greatly enhances the value and importance" of his writings.[35] These men might have been advertising the ethnographic value of the observations, but commercial value could not have been far from their minds.

The starkest opportunism came from the traders. During the epidemic, company officials complained that, with Indians sick and dying, buffalo survived unhunted. Chardon noted that "The whole country north and south is one sollid mass of Buffaloes, and sorry to say, no Indians to kill them." Halsey described how fur production would suffer: "The loss to the company by the introduction of this malady will be immense in fact incalculable as our most profitable Indians have died." David Mitchell worried that profits "will be a mere drop in the ocean." The traders, however, were quick to find a silver lining. Mitchell suspected that financial problems in the eastern cities the previous year had hurt the company's fur sales, leaving it with residual inventory. If news of the epidemic and impending fur shortage reached the fur markets, prices would skyrocket: this "will no doubt have a tendency to enhance the value of Robes that are now at market."[36]

Events did not turn out as expected. Hunters provided abundant furs in 1837 and 1838. Larpenteur suspected that the Indians, expecting to die, sold their own robes to have money for "a frolic till the end came." Culbertson thought that the survivors might have sold "robes belonging to the victims of the small-pox that would under other circumstance have been retained for use." What happened next is most remarkable. Suspecting that many of the furs came from victims of smallpox, and familiar with the idea that contaminated blankets could transmit smallpox, the traders shipped thousands of these robes east. As Culbertson later confessed, "they were purchased and shipped down the river with an utter neglect of any precaution to prevent the retransmission of the disease back to its starting point." As had happened at Fort Pitt, this commerce in smallpox had no apparent impact: "It is surprising that the introduction into the eastern markets of so many thousand of small-pox infected robes was not followed by a general prevalence of the epidemic throughout the United States." Baffled by this observation, Culbertson, like so many before him, turned to providence: "Certainly the ways of Providence are mysterious and past finding out. A single infected blanket stolen by an Indian results in the annihilation of whole tribes, strewing the plains with tens of thousands of victims; while the wholesale introduction into the States of thousand[s] of robes taken from the decomposing bodies of these victims is not followed by any appreciable injurious consequences."[37]

The facility with which the traders responded to the epidemic, their ability to transform the epidemic into economic opportunity, suggests that the devastation surprised no one. As their attempts at self-quarantine showed, they had no doubt that they could, and did, introduce the disease. This conflict penetrated all aspects of the fur trade: traders came to the Indians for furs, knowing that their presence threatened both Indians and their supplies of furs. When smallpox appeared, it laid bare the dangers and asymmetries in the relationships of whites and Indians. Perhaps traders believed that their understanding of smallpox and their nascent ability to control it with vaccination could mitigate the risk. Their hubris claimed thousands their lives.

Vaccination

The absence of vaccination during the 1837 epidemic is both puzzling and revealing. Back east, the epidemic had been contained by "a general vaccination of persons of all ages." The tribes of the Missouri Valley had heard that such a remedy existed and accused the traders of withholding it. The traders, however, had no vaccine to withhold. It was not until November, five months into the epidemic, that Halsey wrote to company officials in St. Louis asking for vaccine: "Pray send some Vaccine matter had Mr. Mitchell brought some thousands of lives might have been saved."[38]

The company did eventually act. By June 1838 David Mitchell was vaccinating the Gros Ventres at Fort Union. The federal government responded as well. According to the commissioner of Indian affairs, "every exertion was used to vaccinate as generally as possible." A physician, sent on this "benevolent errand" vaccinated "about 3,000 persons." Canadian officials had better luck. Before the outbreak, the directors of the Hudson's Bay Company had stocked their trading posts with vaccine. When fleeing Assiniboine and Blackfeet brought smallpox into central Canada in September 1837, company agents quickly vaccinated nearby tribes, saving many from death.[39]

If these stories are reliable, then the crucial difference between the American and Canadian epidemics was the decision by Canadian officials to provide trading posts with vaccine. Why had Americans not taken this precaution? As discussed earlier, vaccination of the Indians had gotten off to a promising start. Thomas Jefferson vaccinated a visiting Miami delegation in 1801 and instructed Lewis and Clark in 1803 to carry vaccination across the continent to the Pacific Ocean. Lewis, however, had to abandon this quest even before he crossed the Mississippi River. His failure was the harbinger of many more to come. Although vaccination had won acceptance in official circles in the United States by 1815, sustained efforts to vaccinate American Indians did not come quickly.

Vaccination was certainly hampered by the limited role of the federal government. The early republic had few institutions devoted to American Indians. In 1789 President Washington established an ad hoc Indian Section in the War Department. In 1790 Congress began requiring licenses for the Indian trade; it appointed a superintendent of Indian affairs in 1806 to supervise this regulation. The first specific Indian appropriation came in 1819 when Congress allocated $10,000 for teaching Indians "the habits and arts of civilization." During the Monroe Administration, Secretary of War John Calhoun appointed Thomas McKenney head of a new Indian Bureau. The office, including McKenney, two clerks, and a messenger, opened in 1824. Ten years later, on 30 June 1834, Congress officially established the Office of Indian Affairs (also known as the Indian Bureau). It faced many obstacles: inconsistent treaties, ill-defined authority over field personnel, and lack of uniform accounting procedures. Congress transferred the Indian Bureau to the newly created Interior Department in 1849.[40]

These institutions initially showed little concern for Indian health. In 1802 the army instructed its physicians to curb smallpox and other diseases among American Indians near the army posts. Whether the doctors were acting to protect soldiers or aid Indians, the Indians at least received some care from physicians. Health and sanitation did receive attention during Indian removals, but not enough to prevent tremendous mortality. A new era began in 1832 when a treaty with the Winnebago included a promise to provide medical care. Similar treaties followed. The Interior Department demonstrated increasing concern for Indian health, but again emphasized protecting agents and their families.

During this period, the push for vaccination largely came from private sources. In 1818 W. A. Trimble, who had traveled among the Comanche, encouraged Calhoun to implement vaccination, "a course dictated by humanity." The Reverend J. Morse made a similar recommendation in 1821. In 1819 the government sponsored the Yellowstone Project, an effort to explore and fortify the Missouri River. Although Calhoun's instructions made no specific mention of vaccination, he did refer expedition leader Stephen Long to Jefferson's instructions to Lewis and Clark, which had recommended it. In 1820 the team received "a box containing a quantity of vaccine virus, transmitted to the exploring party, for the purpose of introducing vaccination among the Indians." The box, however, was not sent by the government. Instead, it came from Sylvanus Fansher, a Connecticut man who tried to make a living by promoting vaccination. The team physician, Edwin James, soon realized that the effort had proved fruitless: the keel-boat containing the vaccine had sunk en route and "the box and its contents, although saved from the wreck, was thoroughly drenched, and the virus completely ruined." When the team later encountered a party of Pawnees, they could only educate them about the procedure.[41]

British and Spanish authorities had more success. Canadian Indians were vaccinated during an outbreak in 1823. During an epidemic on the California coast in 1828, Governor Encheandia coerced James Pattie, an imprisoned American trader, to vaccinate the Spanish missions. Pattie traveled from San Diego to San Francisco, vaccinating, by his count, 23,500 Spaniards, Indians, and Russians. Although a more plausible estimate is between 3,000 and 6,000, this was an impressive accomplishment.[42]

The epidemic of 1831 and 1832 finally spurred the United States government into action. Smallpox appeared among Pawnee and other midwestern tribes in 1831. As described by John Dougherty, the United States Indian agent at Leavenworth, "their misery defies all description." Such reports shocked government officials. In March 1832 Congress asked Lewis Cass, the secretary of war, to provide information about "the spread and ravages of the small pox among any of the Indian tribes." Cass sent vivid descriptions and forwarded letters from agents and missionaries calling for vaccination to "prevent the desolating ravages of this dreadful disorder." On 5 May 1832 Congress passed an act that called for vaccination of the Indians: the secretary of war would provide vaccine matter, physicians would be sent "to the remote Indians," and agents would convene their tribes and "use all proper means to persuade the Indian population to submit to vaccination." The whole plan would cost only $12,000. Within a week, Cass sent vaccine and instructions to the agents, encouraging them to persevere. He also assigned a value to this lifesaving procedure, $0.06 for each Indian: vaccination of 100 Indians was "considered equal to a day's service, and for which the surgeon will be entitled to a compensation of six dollars."[43]

By November the plan was underway. Despite delays and occasionally inactive vaccine, Dougherty had hired two physicians who vaccinated over 2,000 Omaha, Otoe, Iowa, and Sioux at Council Bluffs. Elbert Herring, commissioner of Indian affairs, reported that most Indians accepted the procedure: "It is gratifying to know that the Indians have every where, with one exception, received the persons selected to perform this duty, with gratitude of the Government." The main problem had been inactive vaccines. During the first year, $8,192.50 was spent, and 10,206 Sioux, Potawatamies, Miamies, Illinois, Winnebagoes, Menomonees, Sacs, Foxes, Choctaws, Osages, Shawnees, Kickapoos, Cherokees, Chippewas, Ottawas, Creeks, Ohio, and Seminoles were vaccinated (at an actual cost of about $0.80 each). Herring expected that all remaining Indians would be vaccinated in the next season, without needing to spend the full $12,000. By 1834 $9,439.40 had been spent; subsequent reports made no further mention of the act. In 1836 a treaty with the Ottawa and Chippewa included an annual budget of $300 for vaccination.[44]

The next year smallpox struck many tribes, including those of the upper Missouri Valley. Five years of vaccination efforts had not had the impact that Cass and Herring had thought: thousands of American Indians died. As described earlier, the epidemic did re-inspire vaccination, which began in the spring of 1838. In the fall Crawford sought an appropriation of $5,000. Sylvanus Fansher (who did not specifically mention the epidemic) petitioned Congress to establish a permanent vaccine institution for the army, navy, and Indian Department. According to missionary Isaac McCoy, these efforts had little impact: "as it had happened in cases of vaccination which immediately followed the passage of the law for that object in 1832, the effect was too feeble and unsystematic."[45]

Many historians have condemned the failure of the 1832 campaign. At a rate of $0.06 per person, the government program could have protected nearly 200,000 American Indians. But this effort had not reached the upper Missouri Valley. Many observers blamed Indian hostility to vaccination. Maximilian met Puncahs who "had manifested distrust" and refused vaccination. Catlin believed that the government succeeded only with tribes that had already experienced the disease: "amongst those tribes in their wild state, and where they have not suffered with the disease, very little success has been met with in the attempt to protect them, on account of their superstitions, which have generally resisted all attempts to introduce vaccination." Historians have often accepted these explanations.[46]

Such resistance, however, was not insurmountable. Dougherty and Herring both described Indians accepting the procedure. Maximilian noted that Major Bean had vaccinated 2,600 Indians despite resistance.

Other factors must have limited the impact of the program. As noted above, cases of vaccine failure were common, with Halsey, Culbertson, and many others catching smallpox despite previous vaccinations. The United States Army long struggled with this problem. Although the army had begun vaccinating all new recruits in 1812, smallpox remained a serious problem during the Civil War, especially among black soldiers whose case rates were more than six times those of white soldiers.[47] Even when the government had good intentions, strong motivations, and adequate resources, vaccination could fail to control smallpox.

It is far from clear that the government had such good intentions and strong motivations toward American Indians. Throughout the early nineteenth century, the federal government struggled to define the role of Indians in the United States. Many officials and missionaries believed that the Indians could only be saved if their savagery were converted to civilization. They knew this was no easy task: "Every day's observation shews that the near association of the white and red man is destructive to the latter." The government also had little patience for these efforts. The 1819 appropriation for civilizing the Indians was given only a decade to work before the government adopted a new solution: relocation. By moving Indians away from the influence of white society, relocation, it was hoped, would allow the civilizing process to proceed more gradually. Led by President Andrew Jackson, the government removed the Choctaw, Cherokee, and other southern tribes across the Mississippi River. Many historians have rejected this rhetoric of civilization as a justification of land theft and westward expansion.[48] Regardless of motivation, Indian relocation was one of the greatest disruptions ever perpetrated by the federal government on American Indians. It also provided the context for the vaccination campaigns of the 1830s. Perhaps vaccination helped assuage the guilt of an expansionist and destructive United States.

In this setting, vaccination could never have been a simple act of medical philanthropy. Ambivalence took a particularly high toll on the upper Missouri. Federal policy in the 1830s focused on Indians east of the Mississippi. The 1836 annual report of the commissioner of Indian affairs classified these tribes as planning to relocate, already relocated, or not relocating. These were the tribes that had received vaccination in 1832. The western tribes, including those of the upper Missouri, were classified as "Indigenous Tribes within Striking Distance of the Western Frontier." Between 1815 and 1831, these tribes had killed or injured 230 Americans and destroyed nearly $150,000 of property. Historian David Ferch has suggested that these "losses may have left the Secretary fearful of sending men too far up the Missouri or indifferent to the fate of these northern plains hostiles."[49]

The government thus differentiated two sorts of Indians: those within the reach of the federal government, who were to be moved beyond the Mississippi, and those who threatened the government. Only the former received vaccination. When Cass planned the 1832 campaign, he noted that "no effort would be made . . . under any circumstances . . . to send a Surgeon higher up the Missouri than the Mandans, and I think not higher than the Aricaras."[50] The fate of the Mandan suggests that vaccination, and the moral community of the federal government, had not even reached them.

This pattern of neglect is consistent with government policy that left the upper Missouri tribes in the hands of the American Fur Company. The distance, geographic and conceptual, between the government and those tribes was so great that news of the 1837 epidemic, which was in full swing by July, had not reached the commissioner of Indian affairs by the following December. The tribes were even beyond the reach of company officials in St. Louis: Halsey asked for vaccine in November 1837, but received none until June. Similar failures to contain outbreaks among remote tribes occurred repeatedly in the nineteenth century.[51] Too much prairie, too many miles of river, and too many cultural barriers stood between officials and their responsibility to intervene.

Much had changed from the time when Daniel Gookin had worried about the deaths of Indian students at Harvard College. Whereas Gookin debated the role of diet, housing, and providence, Cass and Herring emphasized environment and behavior. Whereas Gookin worked on his own as superintendent of the Indians, Cass and Herring oversaw a small but growing Indian Office, with congressional funding and treaty obligations to safeguard the health of American Indians. But much remained the same. Soldiers, traders, and government agents continued to witness dramatic disparities in mortality. The meanings of smallpox remained as complex as the relationships that bound American Indians to the expanding nation. Everyone recognized, or at least suspected, that the epidemics arose from the encounter between settlers and Indians. As force of numbers and economic resources increasingly gave white Americans the upper hand, disparities in disease reflected disparities in wealth and power.

The most significant development between Gookin and his nineteenth century successors remained elusive: control over smallpox. Inoculation and vaccination offered the promise that smallpox could be controlled by human action. These technologies might have lessened the disparities in smallpox mortality. Instead, they found other uses. Smallpox, through blankets, was given to the Delaware and Shawnee to induce an epidemic. Smallpox, through inoculation, was given to the Blackfeet and Assiniboine to protect traders' interests in the upper Missouri Valley. Smallpox, through vaccination, was given to eastern tribes with the expectation that they would be removed beyond white society. The disease resisted this control: imperfect technology and imperfect motivation undermined the desired outcomes. Smallpox cast in stark relief the many inconsistencies in American attitudes toward American Indians. Western tribes were enough a part of the growing nation to be exposed to its diseases, yet not enough a part of it to be within reach—physical and moral—of its medicine.

5

Race to Extinction

SMALLPOX HAD BEEN the scourge of American Indians ever since the arrival of Europeans in the Americas. William Bradford and Edward Winslow watched helplessly as the Massachusett succumbed in 1633. Jacob Halsey and Alexander Culbertson tried unsuccessfully to contain smallpox in 1837 by inoculating Assiniboine and Blackfeet. Five years after Congress had passed a bill calling for the vaccination of American Indians, somewhere between 10,000 and 150,000 died from smallpox. With limited motivation and limited resources, government officials and private activists had consistently failed to contain the devastation of smallpox. This would all change.

By the 1880s government officials had begun to respond quickly, possibly effectively, to outbreaks of smallpox among American Indians, containing epidemics with quarantine, fumigation, and vaccination. This new enthusiasm for Indian health, however, had its limits: it did not extend to tuberculosis, which had begun to replace smallpox as the dominant cause of American Indian morbidity and mortality. Tuberculosis emerged during the nineteenth century as the government, motivated by desire for Indian lands and by dreams of incorporating Indians into American society, moved American Indians onto reservations. This transition did not go smoothly, especially for the Sioux. As they endured the transition from nomadic hunters to settled farmers, they faced a devastating epidemic of tuberculosis. By the 1890s rates of tuberculosis among the rural Sioux exceeded those among the darkest slums of eastern cities.

Although tuberculosis had replaced smallpox, the old disparities in health status survived: American Indians continued to suffer more severely than whites despite the change in the dominant disease. Physicians, soldiers, and government officials sought explanations for both the new disease and the persistent disparities in morbidity and mortality. They re-evaluated long-familiar theories of behavior and environment in light of new ideas about heredity and bacteriology. Most significantly, they assessed the meaning of the outbreak of tuberculosis. They found that tuberculosis reflected past interactions between Americans and American Indians and foretold possible futures of each group. While some saw the epidemic of tuberculosis as the transient agony of a race undergoing the passage to civilization, others saw it as the last step on the American Indians' road to extinction. This debate determined the direction of Indian policy.

Changes

The apparent mastery of government officials over Indian smallpox did not come easily. Physicians and government officials in the United States had quickly recognized the promise of vaccination for American Indians. Within five years of Edward Jenner's description of vaccination, Thomas Jefferson had vaccinated Chief Little Turtle and sent vaccination across North America with Meriwether Lewis and William Clark. Philanthropists and missionaries advocated widespread Indian vaccination. In 1832 Congress appropriated $12,000 for such programs. This effort, however, did little to avert the disastrous epidemic of 1837 in the Missouri Valley. Imperfect technology, complicated logistics, Indian skepticism, and limited motivation all undermined these efforts.

Such epidemics of smallpox and other infections had appeared among the Plains Indians even when the tribes had lived beyond the American frontier. The Lakota Sioux, for instance, whose records contain only a sparse history of the tribe, described measles in 1782, 1801, 1818, and 1845, and smallpox in 1837 (possibly) and 1850. The reservation system that emerged after the Civil War only made matters worse.[1] Epidemics of acute infectious diseases, especially smallpox, measles, whooping cough, and diphtheria, were common. The Indian Service, which had been unable to contain the epidemic of 1837, gradually gained familiarity with such outbreaks and developed mechanisms for managing them.

Consider several examples. Smallpox, measles, chicken pox, and a mysterious fever struck the Chippewa on their reservation in northern Minnesota in the winter of 1883. James Walker, the agency physician, knew how to respond. Although he "had to threaten with a gun to get my orders carried out," he quarantined affected cabins and vaccinated all of the nearby Chippewa. As temperatures reached 52° below zero, exhaustion clouded his thoughts: "going thru the forest on my snowshoes from one tepee to another, I could see skeletons dodging among the pine trees." But his efforts brought success: the epidemic did not spread beyond this initial outbreak. Praised by the commissioner of Indian affairs for preventing a larger epidemic, he was eventually decorated for his heroism by President Theodore Roosevelt.[2]

Similar stories and claims of success appeared repeatedly. When measles struck the Sioux reservations in 1888, agency physicians believed that isolation and quarantine saved countless lives. Fred Treon was "proud to say that out of one hundred and thirty cases treated in the schools not one proved fatal." He claimed similar success against influenza and whooping cough in 1890, and against measles in 1893. Quarantine in 1896 protected the Sioux on the Rosebud Reservation from measles that had appeared among neighboring white towns. Indian Agent John Harding used "strict quarantine" and "excellent care" against measles and whooping cough at the Yankton Reservation in 1899. Prophylactic vaccination and quarantine minimized the spread of smallpox from white settlers to the reservations at Rosebud and Sisseton. Smallpox reappeared in 1901 after a white settler near the Cheyenne River Reservation supposedly "gave his infected clothing to an Indian boy." Quarantine, vaccination, and fumigation minimized its spread. Although smallpox killed six Oglala at the Pine Ridge Reservation, James Walker quarantined infected camps, limiting the outbreak to only three additional cases. When cases of smallpox appeared in November 1902, physician Z. T. Daniel reported that "the Department liberally responded to our request in all particulars, furnishing whatever was required, physician, disinfectants, medicine, etc." He used formaldehyde gas, vaporized sulfur, and carbolic acid to fumigate houses. The police provided a "prompt and effectual quarantine." In addition, "vaccination was freely done, which mitigated the ravages of the disease, and the Red Man no longer doubts its advantages."[3]

These responses were, of course, imperfect. Measles spread at the Crow Creek Reservation in 1899 "in spite of stringent efforts to prevent it." A batch of vaccine used at Yankton in 1900 was "almost entirely inert, and did very little good." But severe mortality from smallpox was rare in the late nineteenth century. Outbreaks of measles and smallpox generally claimed few lives. Smallpox never again seriously threatened American Indians.[4] Agency physicians frequently claimed credit for this success, and agents and Indians apparently accepted their claims.

It is difficult to assess the physicians' claims of efficacy. They might have overlooked outbreaks and deaths. Declining mortality might have reflected efficacious intervention, less virulent strains of smallpox, or increasing acquired immunity among American Indians. Whatever the cause of declining mortality, the rapid and consistent responses to epidemics marked a dramatic change from the situation in 1837. Indians on reservations lived under the surveillance of government physicians and officials. Railroads overcame the geographic distance that had hindered intervention in 1837. Outbreaks triggered routine and powerful mechanisms of quarantine and vaccination. Such responses protected the reservations even as nearby whites died. Daniel believed that the Sioux owed a tremendous debt to the federal government: "this community ought to feel profoundly grateful to the authorities for their aid and interest in preventing the spread of such a terrible scourge as smallpox."[5] A polished system of medical surveillance and intervention had been created. Or so it seemed.

The decline of smallpox and measles, for which agents and agency physicians took credit, occurred in parallel with the rise of tuberculosis. By 1891 Daniel realized that tubercular diseases, especially consumption and scrofula, had become "the great destroyers of the Sioux."[6] Even as the federal government claimed success against smallpox, a new challenge had appeared. The problem began with the transition to reservations.

In our popular imagination the Sioux represent Indians incarnate: mounted warriors, bedecked with feathered war bonnets, hunting buffalo on the prairies of the Great Plains. This image actually reflects changes triggered by European colonization. When they first encountered Europeans around 1640, the Sioux were a woodland tribe, living in small bands along the headwaters of the Mississippi River. As colonists forced eastern tribes west across the Great Lakes, these tribes displaced the Sioux onto the prairies. The Lakota, the largest division of the Sioux, left Minnesota around 1700, crossed the Missouri River in 1750, and reached the Black Hills by 1775. In the 1830s they traded with the American Fur Company for whiskey and other goods. Whether protected by nomadic dispersion or by partial vaccination in 1832, they suffered less than other plains tribes in the smallpox epidemic of 1837. The Lakota exploited the ensuing chaos to expand their territory and population. With access to guns and horses, the Sioux dominated the high plains from 1830 to 1877. They had adapted remarkably well to this early phase of European colonization.[7]

They soon faced new challenges. By the 1820s the federal government had abandoned hopes of acculturating the eastern tribes and incorporating them into white society. This failure, and desire to seize the valuable lands of the Cherokee and other tribes, fueled Andrew Jackson's policy of Indian Removal: all tribes east of the Mississippi River would be moved to reservations west of the river, forever beyond the reach of white society. Advocates argued that removal would allow the Indians to become civilized in peace, sheltered from the aggressive aspects of white culture. Most historians see such claims as superficial justifications for land theft. Whatever its motivation, the policy generated countless tragedies. During the 1838 Trail of Tears, between one eighth and one half of the Cherokee died. Government officials, oblivious to such tragedies, reported in 1848 that removal had been completed successfully. Relocation, once accomplished, was soon undermined. In 1834 Congress had passed legislation that set aside all land west of the Mississippi, excluding Arkansas and Missouri, as Indian territory. But this line, like the Proclamation Line of 1763, never held. Indians stood between the settled lands of the east and the promised lands of California and the west. Settlers and miners poured into Iowa, Texas, and Minnesota. They moved the line west to the 95th meridian, and then west beyond that. Settlers took Indian lands and carved caravan routes and railroads across Indian territories.[8]

With the spread of Euro-American settlement throughout the west, the Sioux and other tribes who had once lived beyond the frontier of federal concern became the focus of Indian policy. In 1849 responsibility for Indian affairs was transferred from the War Department to the newly created Department of the Interior and its Bureau of Indian Affairs (BIA). Initial diplomatic efforts were optimistic. David Mitchell, former fur trader, now superintendent of Indian affairs at St. Louis, negotiated the Treaty of Fort Laramie in 1851. The Indians agreed to cease hostilities among themselves. Their lands were reduced and defined; the Lakota, for instance, received lands north of the Platte River and west of the Missouri River. The United States received the right to establish roads and military posts throughout the west. Indian leaders promised not to attack travelers, freight, and mail stages. In exchange, the Indians received gifts, annuities, and promises of protection against white depredations.

Peace, however, did not last. Gold strikes drew settlers into the western mountains. By 1864 Colorado, Nevada, Arizona, Idaho, and Montana had been established as territories or states. The Civil War exacerbated tensions. Distracted by war in the east, Abraham Lincoln did not enforce federal policies in the west. Wars were fought with the Sioux in Minnesota and Dakota, with the Cheyenne, Arapahoe, Kiowa, and Comanche in Kansas and eastern Colorado, and with the Apache and Navajo in Arizona and New Mexico. The Santee Sioux, on a reservation in Minnesota, had struggled with whites about hunting, trade, and annuities throughout the 1850s. When the U.S. Army withdrew from western posts, the Santee attacked, killing hundreds of settlers in 1862. With settlers demanding "exterminate or banish," the army crushed this uprising and shipped the Santee to the Crow Creek Reservation in the Dakota territory. Barren soil, scarce game, and alkaline water claimed the lives of one-quarter of the Santee during their first winter there. Some fled into Nebraska, only to be defeated by the Army and placed onto reservations at Sisseton and Devil's Lake.[9]

The Plains Sioux fared little better. In 1864 they joined Cheyenne and Arapaho raids against miners who invaded Indian lands in Colorado. After the army massacred Indian civilians at Sand Creek, public outrage forced a truce in 1865. But when the government tried in 1866 to extend roads across Sioux lands toward the gold fields of Montana, the largest group, the Oglala attacked again. A series of Sioux victories led by Red Cloud forced the government's peace commission to negotiate a second Treaty of Fort Laramie in 1868. The government abandoned its plans for the road; in exchange, the Lakota accepted lands west of the Missouri River in the Dakotas as the Great Sioux Reservation. Exhausted by the wars of the 1860s, the government sought a new Indian policy. Motivated by eastern missionary groups, President Ulysses S. Grant adopted a new "peace policy" that gave missionary groups substantial authority on the reservations. Despite such optimistic visions, warfare with the Sioux lasted into the 1870s.

The transition to reservation life did not go smoothly. The Sioux had to abandon hunting and adopt farming and ranching. Assistance promised by the government failed to materialize or was consumed by fraud and corruption. Tensions exploded in 1874 when an army reconnaissance mission led by General George Custer confirmed rumors of gold in the Black Hills: 10,000 miners and railroad surveyors violated the Treaty of Fort Laramie and swarmed onto Sioux lands. Failed negotiations led to war and the destruction of Custer's 7th Cavalry at the Battle of Little Bighorn on 24 June 1876. This defeat shocked the United States on the eve of its centennial. By autumn, however, the Sioux were low on rations and had lost interest in war. They surrendered their guns, their horses, and the Black Hills.

By 1876 nearly all American Indians had been subdued and confined on reservations. They faced a new world, as islands in a sea of white settlements. The Lakota were dispersed across several reservations in what would become South Dakota: the Oglala at Pine Ridge, the Brule at Rosebud, and other groups at Lower Brulé, Crow Creek, Cheyenne River, and Standing Rock. Despite government assurances, peace and prosperity did not follow. The 1878 Sioux Commission found them struggling on forsaken land: "no equal extent of territory east of the Rocky Mountains could be laid off so deficient in natural resources." The Sioux worked hard to cultivate this land, using "their hands for shovels and hoes." Crops, however, succumbed to hordes of grasshoppers and potato bugs. Horses and cattle perished during heavy winter snows. Indian agents claimed that the Sioux, unable to gather enough wood to cook or keep themselves warm, "fully appreciated the goodness of the government in providing for them" (Figure 5).[10]

Government officials remained optimistic. Commissioner E. A. Hayt praised the Oglala for taking "a long stride in the right direction toward complete civilization and eventual self-support." In 1887 Commissioner J. D. C. Atkins praised progress with farming, ranching, education, and culture, something "gratifying to every American patriot and to the humanitarian of any clime or country." However, by 1890 Commissioner T. J. Morgan believed that the whole reservation system had become "vicious," a world of fear, pauperism, fraud, and extortion. Tensions inevitably re-emerged. Indian agents complained that the Sioux, with no incentive to provide for themselves, exploited government aid. The government, meanwhile, bowed to pressure from railroads and settlers and acted unilaterally in 1889 to divide and reduce the Great Sioux Reservation. Motivated by a Paiute prophet who promised the return of Indian lands, dissatisfied Sioux at Pine Ridge joined the ceremonies of the Ghost Dance in October 1890. The new agent, named "Young-Man-Afraid-of-Indians" by defiant Sioux, called in the army. Many Oglala fled Pine Ridge and joined Sitting Bull in the Badlands. The army killed Sitting Bull when he was arrested in December. His followers surrendered, but were stopped at Wounded Knee by the 7th Cavalry. In the ensuing confusion, the army opened fire. Roughly 150 of the 340 men, women, and children, and 26 soldiers, were killed. Congress struggled long and hard to restore order and appease the Sioux.[11]

Peace brought the familiar mix of optimism and failure. In 1891 Commissioner Morgan expected that the "Indian problem" would be solved by 1900. The government implemented civil service reform and tried to replace ration allotments with wage labor. But the reservations remained bleak. In 1893 Charles Penney, the agent at Pine Ridge, despaired: "There is little to note in the way of improvement among the Indians. They are still the same shiftless, improvident people, and, withal, careless and happy, patient under hardship, and with a faithful trust in the future that is exasperating." Droughts destroyed crops. Alcohol increasingly ruined lives. Attempts at land reform simply allowed individuals to sell their lands to white settlers, further reducing tribal lands.[12]

Between 1850 and 1900 the Sioux experienced breathtaking change. The proud masters of the plains had been reduced by the army and federal policy to impoverished farmers and ranchers. This shattered group depended on the Bureau of Indian Affairs (BIA), whose apparatus existed to accomplish cultural alchemy: transform red hunters into white farmers. Always optimistic, the BIA believed that the Sioux could be integrated as equal members of white society. However, it attempted this transformation without realizing the magnitude of its task, and without

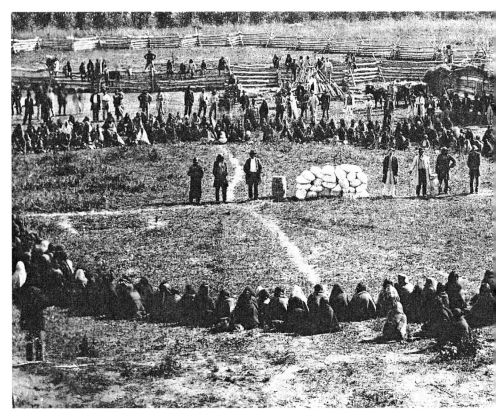

5. Government agent distributing food rations to the Sioux. The photograph shows a large group, in native dress, sitting in a circle around government agents with sacks of food. Note the primitive conditions on the reservation, with a mix of traditional tepees and new log and sod buildings. (By permission of the National Anthropological Archives, Smithsonian Institution, 56,630.)

the necessary resources or wisdom. As a result, the transition left the Sioux with the worst of both worlds. They lost their rich lives as buffalo hunters and found only poor lives as farmers. This change had an immediate impact on their patterns of disease. The transition state, the product of failed alchemy, left them vulnerable to the ravages of tuberculosis.

Tuberculosis had likely been present among American Indians for centuries. Paleopathologists have found evidence of tuberculosis in a Peruvian mummy from A.D. 700. Analysis of skeletal remains suggests the presence of pre-Columbian tuberculosis in New York, Tennessee,

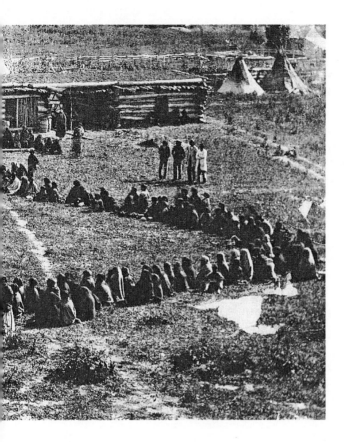

and the Missouri Valley. Some archeologists even interpret Kokopelli, the ubiquitous southwestern image of a hunchbacked flautist, as evidence of spinal tuberculosis. Early colonists, such as Paul Le Jeune and Roger Williams, described consumption among the natives of New France and New England. Caleb, for instance, a promising Capawack scholar, "died of consumption" after graduating from Harvard College in 1654. Despite its presence, tuberculosis was rare before the nineteenth century.[13] Tuberculosis began to increase mid-century. Thomas Williamson reported consumption among the Sioux and Chippewa at Lac qui Parle in Minnesota in 1846. Washington Matthews was "astonished" by its prevalence among the tribes of the Missouri and Yellowstone valleys. But such reports were inconsistent. Matthews found little tuberculosis among the Sioux in the Dakotas in 1865: "scrofula was not then observed among them, and consumption was but little known." Other observers compiled long lists of the predominant diseases among the plains tribes. These included smallpox, measles, dysentery, venereal disease, cholera, conjunctivitis, bronchitis, rheumatism, malaria, and drunkenness, but not consumption.[14] Within twenty years this had changed.

The link between tuberculosis and living conditions has long been recognized by epidemiologists and historians. René Dubos and Jean Dubos described tuberculosis as a "social disease." Paul Farmer has shown how tuberculosis and other diseases of poverty are "biological reflections of social fault lines."[15] It is not surprising that tuberculosis exploded on the Sioux reservations after 1876. Of the 152 annual reports from agents and physicians at the nine Sioux reservations that mention health conditions between 1877 and 1906, nearly 75 percent (113 of 152) cite tuberculosis (including consumption and scrofula) as the leading cause of mortality. Dr. Weirick reported in 1878 that "consumption and scrofula are the prevailing diseases" at Cheyenne River. By 1890, consumption and scrofula, unknown among the Sioux at Yankton "in their wild state," had "obtained a permanent hold on them and cause more deaths than all other diseases combined." It gave "a depressed, almost gloomy feeling to the people." Treon struggled to stop "this grim monster" at Crow Creek. Daniel believed that "it is practically the only disease that causes their large death rate and in its absence they would multiply and overrun the country." By 1903 he had developed a morbid fascination for the disease: "Its forms are multitudinous to almost infinity." Walker, alone in his optimism, wrote from Pine Ridge in 1906 that the "relative great death rate" caused by tuberculosis and "improper care of their infants" could both "be prevented by proper medical supervision."[16]

Many sources document the burden of tuberculosis among the Sioux. Agency physicians made monthly reports of cases treated and causes of death. Agents compiled this data and filed annual reports to the commissioner of Indian affairs. Tuberculosis dominated report after report: "this scourge of the Indians" caused 12 of 33 deaths at Devil's Lake in 1891, 26 of 47 at Crow Creek in 1893, 68 of 130 at Pine Ridge in 1901, and an average of 56 percent of the deaths at Yankton between 1901 and 1906. Standing Rock suffered the heaviest burden, with an average of 282 cases per year between 1879 and 1900, an incidence of roughly 70/1,000. Pine Ridge had a lighter burden, roughly 17/1,000 (Figure 6). Data on the overwhelming burden of Sioux tuberculosis also appeared in the *Annual Report of the Surgeon-General of the Army* and published reports by Treon, Joseph Graham, and Walker.[17]

This information allowed observers to compare tuberculosis rates between American Indians and other groups to highlight great disparities in health status. The surgeon general reported that the consumption hospitalization rate for American Indian soldiers was 35.62/1,000, compared to 4.34 overall, 3.27 for whites, and 4.42 for blacks. The "death rate from this cause alone among the Indians, 8.94, was greater than the death rate, 6.44, from all causes in the Army as a whole." Physician T. M. Bridges noted in 1895 that deaths from consumption among the Sioux "exceed in nearly every instance the death rate per 1,000 from all causes in more than 200 of our largest cities." O. M. Chapman found that the Sioux mortality rate at Yankton in 1903 and 1904 was "fully four or five times what it would be among an equal number of whites." In 1911 Joseph Murphy, the new medical director of the Indian Medical Service, reported that tuberculosis mortality was three times higher among Indians than among whites.[18]

None of the data were perfect. The single physician at Pine Ridge could not possibly collect comprehensive health data on the 6,000 Oglala there. Indians did not seek care for every illness. Even the seemingly simple task of collecting data on births and deaths was impossible: the allotment of rations motivated the Sioux to exaggerate births and conceal deaths. Agents complained that the Oglala raced from village to village on census days, swapping babies, "for the express purpose of defeating the census." A simultaneous count of all Sioux at Pine Ridge at 7:00 A.M. on 30 June 1886, conducted with police assistance, reduced their official population from 7,649 to 4,873, saving $50,000 "of beef alone" each year. Disease data were even less reliable. Some physicians underreported illness rates, either out of indifference to Indian suffering or out of a desire to make their ministrations appear more successful.[19] Others might have overreported morbidity to obtain more resources from the BIA. Such inaccuracy makes it difficult to interpret the four-fold disparity in tuberculosis rates at Standing Rock and Pine Ridge.

Diagnostic ambiguity further complicates the data. Physicians,

A.

Incidence of tuberculosis, 1879–1894

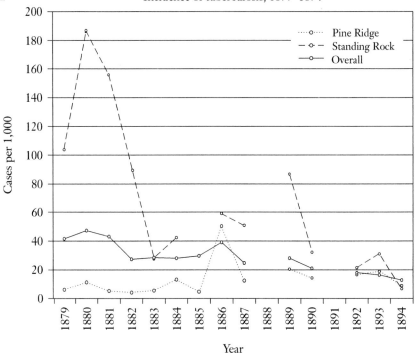

B.

Mortality rate, 1879–1906

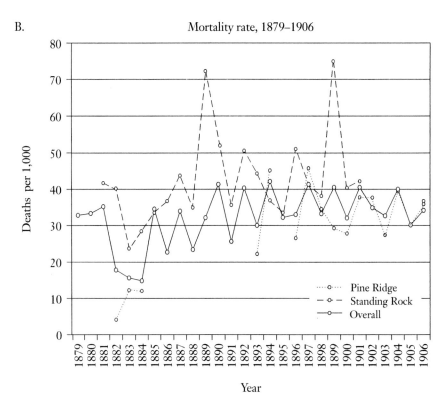

for instance, did not reliably distinguish between pneumonia and consumption. Furthermore, diagnoses underwent major changes between 1877 and 1906. With the discoveries of Jean-Antonie Villemin, who demonstrated the transmission of tuberculosis between rabbits in 1865, and Robert Koch, who isolated the tubercle bacillus in 1882, consumption and scrofula were reconfigured from constitutional diseases (along with cancer, anemia, and rheumatism) into infectious diseases: pulmonary and lymphatic tuberculosis. This change occurred slowly on the Sioux reservations. The diagnosis of "consumption" remained common through 1894, and continued to appear as late as 1906. The term "tuberculosis" appeared occasionally in the 1890s, but did not dominate reporting until 1897. Use of these diagnoses was, to some extent, constrained by the official nomenclature of the BIA. New reporting forms, issued in 1892, codified the change from constitutional to infectious disease.[20] With such changing theories, it is impossible to know how well a diagnosis of consumption in 1880 corresponds to a diagnosis of pulmonary tuberculosis in 1900.

Despite such limitations, the data do have tremendous value. Although they may not accurately reflect the burden of disease that modern doctors would recognize as tuberculosis, they do show that agents and agency physicians recognized severe morbidity and mortality on the Sioux reservations. They believed that tuberculosis, in its varied incarnations, dominated. They knew that the burden of tuberculosis had appeared quickly over twenty years. This knowledge fueled an extraordinarily varied discourse on the nature and causes of Sioux tuberculosis.

---

6. Incidence of tuberculosis and total Mortality on the Sioux reservations, compiled from the *Annual Report of the Commissioner of Indian Affairs*. Each graph shows data from two representative reservations (Pine Ridge, Standing Rock), as well as overall data from all nine Sioux reservations (Cheyenne River, Crow Creek, Devil's Lake, Lower Brulé, Pine Ridge, Rosebud, Sisseton, Standing Rock, and Yankton). The top graph shows that the reported incidence of tuberculosis varied widely between reservations, and that the overall incidence declined slowly over this fifteen-year span. The bottom graph shows that total mortality remained more or less constant, with tuberculosis responsible for roughly half of all deaths. Agents inconsistently reported population size, total deaths, and cases of diseases, leaving many gaps in the data.

Explanations

Prior to the creation of the reservation system, few Europeans and even fewer physicians had ever had extended contact with American Indians and their diseases. As discussed in the previous chapters, many accounts of Indian epidemics exist, but usually as incidental accounts in journals, natural histories, travel narratives, and missionary reports. These records are dwarfed by the vast outpouring of medical writing that followed the assignment of physicians to the Indian Agencies in the 1870s. In letters, monthly reports, annual reports, and publications, physicians, agents, and commissioners offered their explanations of why the Sioux had such a high burden of tuberculosis. At first pass their explanations seem remarkably similar to those of their seventeenth- and eighteenth-century predecessors. New emphasis, however, came to be placed on heredity. As tuberculosis threatened to push the Sioux to extinction, these etiological debates would have crucial implications for Indian policy.

Physicians had long wondered about the ways in which contagion and constitutional susceptibility interacted to produce disease. Villemin had shown that tuberculosis was a transmissible disease, and Koch had identified the causative agent. But neither discovery explained why tuberculosis affected only certain sorts of people, why many were exposed, but only a few fell sick. As Treon complained in 1889, "True, Koch has proven pretty conclusively that phthisis is a germ disease and is due to certain bacilli, but beyond that his microscope has failed to enlighten us with any degree of satisfaction."[21] The Sioux had many theories of their own. Sioux medicine men believed that disease occurred when a variety of creatures entered a person's body. Scrofula, with its characteristic swellings under the skin, was attributed to mice, moles, or gophers. Consumption was traced to worms that entered people's lungs and consumed their fat. Why did some get sick while others stayed healthy? Sickness followed a spiritual transgression or an act by an angry and arbitrary spirit.[22]

Physicians had different explanations of differential susceptibility. As late as 1920, the emphasis remained on old theories of predisposition. As George Bushnell, who had studied tuberculosis among the Sioux, explained "Of all those exposed to the infectious agent only those will fall sick whose resistance is low." What contributed to predisposition?

The interaction of a person's body and its environment created the diathesis, a susceptibility to disease that could be inherited or acquired by careless living.[23]

Observers recognized many conditions of Sioux life that decreased their resistance to tuberculosis. When buffalo were abundant, the Sioux had been "generally fine and healthy." But as buffalo became scarce, their health deteriorated: "This suffering from lack of sufficient food is another cause of phthisis." A. B. Holder blamed the government: "Rations furnished by the Government to Indian tribes are in most cases entirely insufficient to maintain health." Some physicians traced endemic consumption and scrofula to their "damp, unhealthy tepees" which typically housed "four or five persons and a similar number of canines." Most, however, believed that their adoption of western style housing was a turn for the worse. In tepees, at least, "they necessarily breathed plenty of fresh air." Log cabins, in contrast, were "poorly ventilated." With "noxious impurities thus constantly taken into the lungs," the Sioux fell victim to consumption. Furthermore, as Charles Penney complained about Pine Ridge, many reservations had been settled "absolutely without any attention to the laws of health. The whole ground is honeycombed with privy vaults and cesspools, abandoned and in use, and the earth is reeking with filth, covered and out of sight, but none the less certain to do its deadly work as soon as the wells shall be contaminated. A pestilence is sure to follow." The severe climate of the Dakotas did not help. In the winter of 1903 and 1904, snow stayed on the ground from September until May: "it is doubtless from this cause that the deaths exceed the births." The following winter was also severe. Many "contracted severe colds, and with their tubercular trouble caused their death."[24]

As had happened in Massachusetts, Pennsylvania, and the Missouri Valley, agents and agency physicians did not simply identify American Indians as victims of unfavorable environments, housing, and food. Instead, they emphasized the synergy of bad environment and bad behavior. Treon invited his readers to "push aside the curtain and peer into the 'tepi.'" They would find "filth," "a disagreeable odor," and "little or no ventilation." Throughout "the room hangs plenty of green beef, upon which the flies may light and deposit their quota of living germs to be taken into the stomach of these people." These houses were "the habitation of every imaginable vermin." Treon also described Sioux "'lousing' one another and eating the vermin." C. H. Kermott similarly believed that food, poorly prepared, became "a vehicle whereby many a parasitical and disease germ is carried into the system." Air in crowded houses was "polluted by the expectoration of tuberculous patients." Consumptive sputa and scrofulous pus turned Sioux homes into "veritable culture soils and hot-beds." Physicians encouraged ventilation, but complained that "It is almost impossible to secure these Indians' efficient cooperation in measures to prevent the spread of this disease."[25]

In addition to describing this baseline of unhealthful behavior in daily life, observers of the Sioux highlighted specific behaviors that left them susceptible to disease. Many condemned tobacco. Treon saw shared pipes as a vector for tuberculosis: "If it is true that the disease is sometimes communicated by kissing, is it not reasonable to suppose that the Indian habit of smoking the pipe and passing it from man to man until a dozen or more have had the end of the same pipe-stem in their mouth furnishes a common carrier for the bacilli of the disease?" Those who exchanged pipes for the new vice of cigarettes were not better off. As Daniel explained in 1903, cigarettes are "well known to be the most deadly form in which tobacco can be used, and in a people whose lungs are distinctly tubercular it is superlatively contraindicated." Sweat baths, especially when followed by a plunge in snow or cold water, had long been seen as a contributing factor to smallpox mortality. Fordyce Grinnell and Holder both believed that they were similarly dangerous for tuberculosis: "Its influence on the production of pulmonary diseases is only equaled by its influence in bringing them rapidly to a fatal conclusion." Dances were singled out as "disease breeders and hotbeds of other vices and indiscretions that sooner or later demand the attention of the physician." Many cases of consumption were "the result of this most pernicious practice."[26]

A common theory tied many of the specific causes together. Exposure to cold, wet winters had long been recognized as a cause of tuberculosis, pneumonia, whooping cough, and lung fever: "unnecessary exposure of the body to the cold and dampness of winter and spring are all productive of many fatal terminations." But cold, on its own, was less dangerous than an abrupt transition from heat to cold, or from dry to wet. Treon and James G. Wright both believed that the transition from overheated winter lodges to subzero temperatures outside bred lung diseases in children and adults. Such exposure did not help "overcome the tendency to consumption and other hereditary diseases among this people." Fear of such transitions motivated physicians' concern with both sweat baths and dancing. J. A. Stephan remarked that even in winter they would be "nearly in a nude state when dancing." When they stop, "they cool off suddenly, which produces lung fever and consumption."[27]

Observers also blamed Sioux attitudes. Richard Dodge criticized them for slipping into hopelessness, especially when sick: "Indians have plenty of courage and extraordinary endurance, but little of that rather indefinable quality called 'pluck.'" Matthews believed that such a "depressed mental condition is a potent auxiliary to consumption." According to Daniel, the ration system "begets idleness both of mind and body, and inertia is a fruitful source of disease." Such idleness was seen by others as "stupid indifference to the laws of health." Agent James McLaughlin condemned Sioux "disregard," or "ignorance, of the necessity of proper precautions and care." Others traced mortality "not so much to race characteristics as to nonconformity to health laws." Anthropologist Ales Hrdlicka, who saw similar conditions and tuberculosis among many tribes, concluded that "ignorance among Indians, as elsewhere, must be regarded as the most potent pathogenic agency." Chapman summarized such sentiments most clearly: "In almost every feature of their existence where sanitary matters are involved they are aggressive violators and consequently losers at every point of contact. The excessive mortality is but the sum total of all these influences combined—is the measure of their transgressions."[28]

These attempts to place responsibility for tuberculosis on the Sioux resemble earlier behavioral explanations of smallpox. But they existed in parallel with a new style of explanation, one that blamed tuberculosis on Sioux bodies. As historians have shown, heredity became one of the dominant explanations of disease in mid- to late-nineteenth-century Europe and the United States, even as the rise of tuberculosis in urban slums made the social roots of disease plainly visible. Not even the rise of germ theory slowed the rise of hereditarian thought.[29] As noted above, germ theory did not explain why some fell sick while others did not. Heredity provided a convenient answer.

Hereditary transmission of tuberculosis could occur through several mechanisms. Koch believed that parents passed a "disposition" for tuberculosis to their children. Graham believed that the bacillus could possibly be transmitted through semen, or across the uterine wall. If not transmitted before birth, it was transmitted soon after birth by nursing. These mechanisms made certain that tuberculosis would appear in children of tuberculous parents, "under the law that 'like produces like.'" Such theories were part of an extended debate about scientific racism. As historians have shown, racial theories of tuberculosis susceptibility were used to explain the gradient of susceptibility, from most resistant (Jews and other Europeans) to least resistant (Africans and American Indians).[30]

Agents and agency physicians made many claims about the hereditary origin of Sioux tuberculosis. J. F. Kinney identified consumption as the "result usually of hereditary scrofula." William McKusick and Daniel blamed inbreeding: "We all know the ill effects of breeding in too much of cattle, hogs, sheep, horses, chickens, dogs, etc. As a physiologist I believe the same rule holds good with the human race and is fully demonstrated in the Indian tribes of North America." Walker, analyzing twenty years of data at Pine Ridge, concluded that the "greater physical weakness of the Indian is inherent in his being." Even Charles Eastman, a Sioux and a trained physician, acknowledged that "the Indian had not become in any sense immune to disease." Because of the higher susceptibility of full-blooded Brule at Rosebud, Charles McChesney believed "it is only reasonable that an extra effort be made in their behalf or confess our policy of extermination." Daniel believed that American Indians could only be saved by interbreeding with other groups: they "will continue to die everywhere they go, of tuberculosis, until the race is so thoroughly crossed by 'foreign blood' that it will stamp out the tubercle bacillus, and when that is done the Indian race in its original purity will be no more."[31]

Despite such adamant claims, there was no clear consensus about the role of heredity. F. O. Getchell attributed the high burden of pulmonary disease "not to a weaker organization than the whites have, but to the fact that during the last generation they have changed their mode of living to an extent hitherto unknown to any class of people." Walker, who in 1900 made his own claims about inherent weakness, reversed his position by 1906: "There is no inherent peculiarity of the Indian which renders him more liable to infection with tuberculosis than is a white man under like circumstances." For Bushnell, who observed some of the first outbreaks of tuberculosis among the Sioux in

1881, susceptibility did not depend on racial background: "it is not a question of racial susceptibility or immunity," but a question of the history and level of "tuberculization" of individual groups. Walker and agent W. H. Clapp traced the better health of mixed-blood Indians not to their ancestry, but to their greater enthusiasm at "adopting the ways of civilization."[32]

It is possible, in a limited way, to quantify the contested role of heredity in accounting for the disparities in tuberculosis mortality. On the 152 annual reports that mentioned health concerns, 113 cited tuberculosis as the leading cause of mortality. Of these, 15 discussed the question of heredity (6 of these by Z. T. Daniel alone): 8 described tuberculosis as a hereditary disease, 5 blamed intermarriage, 1 advocated an infusion of fresh blood, and 1 denied the relevance of heredity. Meanwhile, these reports included 125 statements about the role of environment and behavior.[33] If asked why the Sioux suffered from so much tuberculosis, agents and agency physicians were far more likely to cite living conditions than racial susceptibility. These explanations, of course, were not mutually exclusive. Many agents and doctors expressed concern that all of these factors, working synergistically to create an epidemic of tuberculosis, drove the Sioux, and all American Indians, towards extinction. As noted by one agency physician in 1879, tuberculosis "is slowly but surely solving the Indian problem."[34]

Extinction

The specter of extinction was of vital importance. The proximate causes of Sioux tuberculosis were clear to anyone who looked: poor housing, poor food, harsh climate, poor hygiene, and suboptimal health behaviors. Such causes paralleled earlier discussions of disease outbreaks among American Indians. The debates in the late nineteenth century were distinguished by their concern with ultimate causes and ultimate outcomes. Was tuberculosis the inevitable product of hereditary inferiority, simply the final step on the Indian's road to extinction? Or was it a contingent product of the difficult transition from nomadic to settled life? Choice between these two narratives determined the course of Indian policy.

Concern with Indian extinction did not begin with tuberculosis. From Thomas Morton to Thomas Hutchinson, seventeenth- and eighteenth-century writers expressed amazement at Indian population decline. This continued into the nineteenth century. In their 1854 *Types of Mankind*, Josiah Nott and George Gliddon articulated an influential theory of racial difference. They believed that American Indians, inherently inferior to the Europeans, had been living in America on borrowed time. The arrival of the Europeans pushed them towards their destiny: "It is as clear as the sun at noon-day, that in a few generations more the last of these Red men will be numbered with the dead." Indian extinction seemed even closer at hand after the conflicts of the Civil War. A congressional investigation of Indian depopulation, chaired by Senator James Doolittle, issued its report in 1867. It identified many causes of decline: disease, intemperance, war, loss of land, and "the irrepressible conflict between a superior and an inferior race." In his testimony to the Doolittle Commission, General James Carleton invoked old, providential themes: "The causes which the Almighty originates, when in their appointed time He wills that one race of men—as in races of lower animals—shall disappear off the face of the earth and given place to another race . . . has reasons too deep to be fathomed by us. The races of the mammoths and the mastodons, and the great sloths, came and passed away: the red man of America is passing away!"[35]

Many observers shared this expectation of inevitable Indian decline. Fur trader Henry Boller believed that the spread of Atlantic and Pacific settlements towards the interior would inevitably crush the Indians: "As the affiliation of the two races is impossible, the extinction of the Indian is a question of time." V. T. McGillycuddy, the agent at Pine Ridge in 1885, believed that although the Reservation system had temporarily halted the decline of Sioux populations, "the rapid development of latent scrofulous and tubercular diseases, &c., will eventual 'evolute' 'Poor Lo' to a higher sphere in the happy hunting grounds, and, in obedience to the law of the survival of the fittest, the Sioux Nation as a people will be forced to the wall." Daniel believed that the "Indian is fading, he is disappearing; one by one they are passing over the divide by the tubercular route." Treon expected that the Sioux would be extinct within a century: "the great Indian problem will have been solved."[36]

These expectations of American Indian extinction buttressed parallel discussions about the fate of African Americans after emancipation. Nott, Gliddon, and many others had long believed that blacks were inferior to whites. They expected that emancipation would initiate a period of racial competition that would lead inevitably to the decline of African Americans. As the Reverend J. M. Sturtevant wrote in 1863, "Like his brother the Indian of the forest, he must melt away and disappear forever from the midst of us." Census data from 1870, 1880, and 1890 supported these suspicions, showing that African-American populations were growing more slowly than whites. By 1900 Walter F. Wilcox, chief statistician of the Census Bureau, concluded that blacks "will follow the fate of the Indians, that the great majority will disappear." As historians have shown, these theories "constituted a convenient rationale for new and more overtly oppressive racial policies." If black disappearance was inevitable, then whites had little need to civilize and improve them: "The new prognosis pointed rather to the need to segregate or quarantine a race liable to be a source of contamination and social danger to the white community, as it sank ever deeper into the slough of disease, vice, and criminality."[37]

Belief in the inferiority and eventual extinction of both blacks and Indians had potentially devastating implications for federal policy. If the government had fully accepted a future without Indians, then it would have felt little obligation to support those Indians who remained. The reservation system would have been transformed from a program of civilization to a place for palliative care.[38] Historians have long debated the impact of scientific racism on nineteenth-century Indian policy. Some argue that most Americans accepted the inevitable subordination and extinction of the Indians. Others believe that evangelical sentiments maintained faith that the Indians could be saved by bringing them to civilization. Among physicians of the Indian Service, there was a wide range of fiercely contested opinion. After all, the survival of a race seemed at stake.

Opposition to the narrative of extinction appeared quickly. In 1877 S. N. Clark submitted a report to the commissioner of Indian affairs about the state of Indian populations. His extensive review of government records suggested that Indian populations had been stable, at around 300,000, throughout the nineteenth century. His conclusion was clear: "the usual theory that the Indian population is destined to decline and finally disappear, as a result of contact with white civilization, must be greatly modified, probably abandoned altogether." He hoped that with his report "the necessity of their civilization will be at once recognized, and all efforts in that direction will be treated as their importance demands." Many others agreed. J. H. Hammond, superintendent of the Dakotas in 1877, rejected the inevitability of the "final extinction of the whole Indian race." Matthews believed that "the old notion of the red race being a dying race is incorrect. Ethnologically, it is a disappearing race; biologically, it is a living and increasing race." Grinnell, convinced that populations had stabilized, encouraged the government to focus on "amicable relations," and not extinction. W. A. Jones, commissioner of Indian affairs in 1900, was optimistic: "It is evident that with the humane treatment of this Government, and contrary to the predictions of many, the Indian is not dying out, is not becoming extinct." In Jones's vision, the Indian race would eventually disappear, not by dying but by "its absorption into the body politic of this country."[39]

The proponents of inevitable extinction had a simpler case. Everyone agreed that catastrophic population decline had occurred since European arrival in the Americas. Everyone agreed that the Sioux suffered rates of tuberculosis far in excess of those of the general population. Extinction seemed the logical outcome. Opponents of the extinction theory had to accept these two premises and turn them to a different conclusion: tuberculosis was not proof of inevitable decline, but a symptom of contingent transitions. Just as transitions from hot to cold and dry to wet could cause tuberculosis, the cultural transition from savage to civilized had pathogenic power.

These narratives had a clear beginning. The Sioux were healthy in their native state because "they were well fed, well clothed, and well housed in a climate almost unsurpassed, and always had that freedom of mind and thought unhampered by the bonds of civilization, roving wild and free in their happy hunting grounds, the undisputed possessors of the land." Reservations ended this health. Indians were "reduced to the condition of paupers, without food, shelter, clothing, or any of those necessaries of life which came from the buffalo; and without friends, except the harpies, who, under the guise of friendship, feed upon them."[40] These conditions created tuberculosis.

Since different Sioux groups made the transition at different times, the contrast between native health and transition disease could be clearly seen. In 1881 Bushnell cared for Sioux prisoners of war brought to live among Sioux already settled on a reservation. He observed "scrofulous youths from the Agency, their fleshless limbs fully clad, looking on wistfully at the dances of the warriors in the summer twilight . . . revealing in many instances a magnificent physique and a boundless vitality, which contrasted cruelly with the listless aspect of some of their spectators." Matthews contrasted the high rates of consumption among the Santee Sioux, long settled in Nebraska, and the Oglala Sioux, only recently settled at Pine Ridge. While 621 died at the Santee Agency in 1875, only 96 died at Pine Ridge. The conclusion seemed clear: "consumption increases among Indians under the influence of civilization—*i.e.*, under a compulsory endeavor to accustom themselves to the food and the habits of an alien and more advanced race." McLaughlin, Treon, McKusick, Getchell, and Eastman all described the pathogenic role of cultural transition. As L. M. Hardin described, tuberculosis "seems to make its greatest ravages on the present generation, whose civilization seems too rapid. The transition from a stage of savagery to that of prospective citizenship within one generation furnishes a good field of operation for the tubercle bacillus."[41]

Specific aspects of cultural transition were singled out as dangerous. One theme was contamination. General Sprague told the Doolittle Commission that as "soon as Indians adopt the habits of white men they begin to decrease, aggravated by imbibing all the vices and none of their virtues." Grinnell believed that insidious venereal diseases *"have destroyed more lives than the sword."* Even Commissioner Jones confessed in 1904 that "Civilization is not an unmixed blessing. It carries with it grave responsibilities and some undesirable tendencies. The Indian, while being fitted for citizenship, is absorbing vices as well as virtues, and weakness as well as strength."[42] To benefit from the blessings of civilization, the Sioux would have to learn to manage its curses.

Another theme was maladaptation. Old habits of living, suited for their former nomadic lives, caused new problems when the Sioux adopted a settled existence. Nat McKitterick noted that when the Sioux lived in tepees, "the laws of sanitation were easily lived up to; when the surroundings became uncomfortably dirty, the tepee was moved to some clean spot." Such informal mechanisms of sanitation were ill-suited to settled agricultural life. McKitterick continued: "since the advent of the log-house among them, things have changed; it is not practicable to move the house, and not being the most thrifty and industrious people in the world, the filth remains about the house." Bushnell believed that this accumulation of filth around the newly sedentary Sioux led to "a wide dissemination of tuberculosis."[43] Many practices, tolerable in their old lives, became dangerous in their new lives.

A third theme was mismanagement. Some proponents believed that civilization was, and could only be, inherently good. Trouble only occurred when civilization was improperly executed. Holder believed that had the Sioux been provided with good houses, good food, good clothing, and good education in hygiene, *his condition would at once and permanently be greatly improved as to health and longevity.* This had not happened. The government had mismanaged the civilizing process. The resulting "evils of imperfect civilization and misapplied efforts at civilization" did their damage.[44] Reservation conditions, a mockery of civilized life, created disease.

Indian schools, one of the core tools of the civilizing process, provided an emblematic dilemma. Many Sioux children were taken away from the reservations and sent to boarding schools, particularly to Captain R. H. Pratt's school at Carlisle, Pennsylvania. Agents and other government officials believed that the "instrumentalities of the school" were essential to a rapid civilizing process. But it quickly became clear that students at these schools suffered a tremendous burden of tuberculosis. Out of a student population of around 700 students, tuberculosis caused all 8 deaths in 1885, 9 of 11 in 1886, all 7 in 1887, 14 of 18 in 1889, and 5 of 6 in 1906. Many students returned to the reservations "suffering from consumption in its most advanced stage." Some officials believed that basic sanitary precautions, such as barring infected employees from the schools, could make the schools safe. Bridges was skeptical: "I infinitely prefer a good, strong, healthy, uneducated live Indian rather than the most highly educated dead Indian imaginable." Walker struggled to assess the value of schools, frequently changing his mind about their hazards. Pratt, perhaps defensive about the prevalence of tuberculosis at Carlisle, made the most interesting argument. Any claim that "consumption increases among the Indians under the influence of civilization" necessarily failed, because health data only existed on Indians already undergoing the civilizing process. In his version of an uncertainty principle, Indians could only be measured once they had been partially civilized, changing what was being measured.[45]

Even as they watched civilization undermine Sioux health, many agents and physicians maintained faith that the outcome would justify the costs. Graham saw civilization as the only salvation for the Sioux: it should "for their own good be forced upon them." Others were reassured that the Sioux always seemed on the verge of recovery. S. R. Riggs, a missionary among the Sioux in the 1870s, believed that "some families, we think, are beginning to recuperate." Grinnell reported that the preconditions for recovery (such as protection from vices, provision of medical care, incentives for industry) "are now realized in numerous tribes." J. M. Woodburn believed in 1889 that the "Sioux seemingly are on a fair road to become a healthy race, as compared with their condition eight or ten years ago. The young are extremely healthy, and civilized living and treatment do much for their general hygienic condition." Births equaled deaths for the first time at Crow Creek in 1893 and at Standing Rock in 1894, "a hopeful sign that the most trying part of their transition period has passed and that they are beginning to observe some of the more important laws of health." Sanitary conditions continued to improve at Standing Rock in 1901, "partly through the efficient work of the Government and partly through the willingness of Indians to profit by instruction." By 1915, Sioux populations were rebounding: "the race has reached and passed the lowest point of its decline, and is beginning slowly but surely to recuperate." They had survived the cultural transition.[46]

The transition narrative, as counterpoint to the extinction narrative, had clear meanings for federal policy. Riggs stated it clearly to Commissioner John Eaton in 1877: "We have no right to assume that they are a race given over to God to destruction, and we have less right to doom them ourselves." Instead, the government had deep obligations to American Indians. Contact between the United States and the Sioux had triggered the process of cultural transition. The adverse aspects of the early stages of transition had fueled epidemics of tuberculosis, creating dramatic disparities in health status. As a result, the government had the responsibility to guide American Indians through transition until their final integration into the general population. This was not a responsibility to be taken lightly. Getchell realized that of 1,132 recipients of land allotments at Devil's Lake in 1892, one third were dead by 1903: "This condition of things is not as it should be, and I shudder to think that perhaps the great Indian civilizing scheme, of which I am a part, is more responsible for the condition than appears on the surface to the casual observer."[47]

Until conditions of life supported healthy populations, the government was obligated to provide medical care. Smallpox and other acute infections had been contained despite terrible conditions on the reservations. Tuberculosis proved a more difficult challenge. Agents and physicians had no trouble accounting for its emergence in the early reservation period: disparities in tuberculosis mortality between whites and Indians reflected existing economic, hygienic, behavioral, and racial fault lines. Assessing the contribution of each factor, however, proved to be a complicated challenge, and assignment of etiological significance had powerful implications for the future of Indian policy and Indian populations. Officials agreed that the transition to reservation life had ultimately triggered the emergence of tuberculosis, but they disagreed about whether this transition could be survived. As the fate of American Indians hung in the balance, the government had to care for those who suffered the consequences of its policies. This daunting task fell to the agency physicians.

6

Impossible Responsibilities

IN 1837 no government physicians worked in the Indian lands west of the Mississippi River. By 1888 there were eighty-one agency physicians and two Indian hospitals. This change reflected fundamental transformations in American Indian health and health policy. With the confinement of the Plains Indians on reservations in the 1870s and 1880s, tuberculosis replaced smallpox as the scourge of American Indians. Echoing old disparities in smallpox mortality, tuberculosis caused far more morbidity and mortality among the Sioux than among even the urban poor of eastern cities. These changes created a difficult problem for the federal government: it remained committed to the civilizing process, even as it realized that this process had created the problem of tuberculosis, killing those it hoped to save.

Responses to tuberculosis appeared quickly. Physicians and Indian agents had little difficulty explaining its emergence. While old themes of behavior and environment persisted, a new issue, hereditary susceptibility, attracted considerable attention. Faced with an overabundance of explanations, observers had to choose which ones to emphasize. The ensuing debates about the ultimate causes of Sioux tuberculosis had far-reaching implications. Did tuberculosis signal the imminent extinction of American Indians, or did it simply reflect the transient struggles of the Sioux's passage from savagery to civilization? In either case, the dramatic emergence of tuberculosis was the product of a cultural transition that the government had initiated. The government accepted responsibility, bound itself through treaty obligations to provide medical care, and set out to alleviate the suffering caused by tuberculosis.

Government officials believed that long-term relief would come through economic development and the adoption of American cultural practices. This was, after all, a time of unashamed paternalism, of "ethnocentrism of frightening intensity."[1] But officials needed to manage tuberculosis and other diseases until social change brought health. This task of healing, enlightenment, and even redemption fell to the agency physicians. As they struggled to overcome the depredations of tuberculosis, they encountered severe obstacles of geography, resources, and the entrenched poverty of the Dakota reservations. They also faced an ambivalent, even hostile, bureaucracy. Congress, meanwhile, aware of the disparities in health status experienced by the Sioux, had to determine what resources would be made available for restoring the Sioux to health. As the fate of a race hung in the balance, government officials repeatedly accepted the challenge of combating Sioux tuberculosis, always unaware of the lessons of past efforts and failures.

Obstacles

Agency physicians only gradually gained their role on the front lines of federal paternalism. Army physicians had provided intermittent care to American Indians near army posts as early as 1802. The Bureau of Indian Affairs (BIA), established in 1824, initially paid little attention to health, except during relocations of tribes to reservations. In 1832 Congress funded a vaccination program and signed the first treaty that promised care by a physician. The 1849 transfer of the BIA from the War Department to the new Department of the Interior initially had little impact. A medical service was provided, but its focus remained on the agents, the employees, and their families. Federal involvement in Indian health slowly increased. By 1871, when Congress stopped making treaties with tribes, over twenty treaties promised some medical care. When these health provisions expired after five to twenty years, Congress began extending the treaties as "gratuity appropriations," acting unilaterally to provide health services. From the point of view of medical services, Indians had become "objects of national charity."[2]

Half of all Indian agencies had doctors by 1875. By 1882 there was generally one physician at each agency. The first two hospitals opened in 1885. Two more appeared by 1889. By 1888, 81 doctors treated some 200,000 American Indians. By 1900 there were 83 physicians, 25 nurses, and 15 hospital employees. The commissioners of Indian affairs were pleased with these physicians. In 1882 Commissioner Hiram Price noted that 75,078 Indians had been treated, with only 1,225 deaths: "the inference is that they have faithfully performed the duty assigned to them." The commissioners knew that these doctors were terribly overextended. Could one doctor really care for 6,000 Oglala Sioux at Pine Ridge? Commissioner T. J. Morgan saw the challenge optimistically: "There is opportunity for a large exercise of the self-sacrificing spirit which is characteristic of the medical profession."[3]

The challenge went deeper than simply providing medical care for thousands of people. The agency physicians also had a crucial, complicated role in the civilizing process. Their official job description listed their responsibilities: physician to employees and Indians; apothecary; nursing instructor; sanitary inspector; recorder of vital statistics; controller of epidemics; lecturer on physiology, hygiene, and first aid; and suppressor of medicine men. All had to be done with the "highest code of professional conduct." Since "Harmony is essential to the proper conduct of an agency," physicians were expected to "treat the agent with proper respect, promptly and cheerfully obeying all orders issued by him." Physicians even had to hire their own replacements if they desired a vacation. As historian Francis Paul Prucha concluded, the "physicians faced a difficult task."[4]

Commissioner Morgan did express sympathy for the agency physicians. The "duties devolving upon the physician are very severe. He has the work of a surgeon and physician, with the sanitary oversight of people with whose language he is unfamiliar and who are ignorant, superstitious, and predisposed to a great variety of diseases. He must be his own apothecary; he usually has no hospital and no nurses, and his patients have few of the most ordinary comforts of home, and little, if any, intelligent care in the preparation of their food or the administering of prescribed medicine. He is alone and has to cope with accident and disease without consultation, with few books, and but few surgical instruments." To ensure that his physicians would be up to this task, Morgan sought doctors who had graduated from "some reputable medical college," who were actively practicing, aged 25 to 45, "temperate, active, industrious, in sound health, and must possess a good personal and professional character." Married men were preferred. To ensure their dedication, they were forbidden from pursuing private practice while employed by the Indian Service.[5]

Many of the agency physicians had great confidence that they could perform their jobs well. They claimed success against both acute epidemics and routine ailments, winning the praise of many agents. W. T. Hughes, the agent at Standing Rock in 1878, reported, "Some very remarkable cures have been performed by our agency physician (who is a very skillful young gentleman) during the past year." The agents at Rosebud praised the "intelligent treatment" provided by their physicians. Physicians credited specific interventions. Fred Treon praised alcohol (inconveniently banned on the reservations) as the *"sine qua non* or sheet anchor in treating consumption among the Indians." A. Judson Morris successfully used the "Amick treatment" against consumption. Julius Silberstein controlled tuberculosis with "diet, air, exercise, and cleanliness—medication was a secondary matter—and with them good results are achieved . . . many cases have been and can be cured."[6]

Many agents also described the progress made by agency physicians against medicine men. Hughes explained that the physician's "success in treating the sick Indians has given them great confidence in him, and caused a large proportion of them to abandon the treatment of the medicine men." V. T. McGillycuddy believed that the Oglala at Pine Ridge were "rapidly losing faith in their native medicine men." J. A. Stephan described how the Sioux at Standing Rock were "fast becoming cognizant of the folly and absurdity of their art of healing." Commissioner Price believed that medicine men would disappear as older Indians passed "to the 'happy hunting grounds.'"[7]

Despite such enthusiasm, the work of agency physicians was hardly a complete success. As discussed in the previous chapter, tuberculosis persisted on the reservations as the dominant cause of continuing disparities in morbidity and mortality. Some of the Sioux came to recognize the physicians' limitations: "The people seem to realize that with the treatment we can furnish them in these cases, little can be accomplished in the hope of a full recovery."[8] Agency physicians had little difficulty explaining their limited impact. They identified many obstacles in their daily lives that conspired to make their difficult jobs even more challenging.

To begin with, the new agencies did not always have full-time physicians. In 1878, as Red Cloud's Oglala settled at Pine Ridge, they "had only such medical assistance as the surgeon of the [army] post can render outside his regular duties." Some agents struggled to provide care on their own, while most pleaded that physicians be appointed. The Sioux agencies were fortunate. Rosebud received a physician in 1877; Cheyenne River, Standing Rock, and Yankton in 1878; Lower Brulé, Pine Ridge, and Sisseton in 1879; Devil's Lake in 1880; and Crow Creek in 1882. Turnover, however, was high, and months could pass before replacements arrived. The presence of a physician, moreover, did not guarantee adequate care. Agents often complained about the "utter inefficiency" of their physicians. Commissioner Morgan worried that qualified candidates would have little interest in the "meager salaries" of the BIA. While some qualified physicians entered the service, he had to discharge others "for immorality, neglect of duty, incompetency, or unprofessional conduct." Even when qualified physicians arrived at reservations, they spent several years adapting to the unique demands of reservation practice. To overcome these problems, Commissioner Price sought "permanent medical officers of pronounced moral and temperate habits, of great will power."[9]

When an agency had the good fortune to receive a competent, dedicated physician, this physician faced thousands of patients, dispersed across the meandering canyons, creek beds, and badlands of an enormous reservation, with undependable roads and severe weather that made travel dangerous. Charles Eastman rode day and night, through wind and blizzards, "for I never refused a call." A single house call could take several days. A horseback tour made in 1897 to conduct health inspections of all seventeen schools at Pine Ridge took James Walker three months. Since the physician had to keep an office at agency headquarters open at all times, house calls were often impossible. James Brewster believed that 186 Sioux died without treatment at Standing Rock in 1892 because of the impossibility of visiting them at their distant homes. Travel by horseback was so central to physicians' work that Agent McGillycuddy requested that an appointee be "both physically & professionally qualified." Z. T. Daniel believed that simply providing him with horses and a wagon would bring about "a marked diminution" in mortality. Making heroic efforts in these conditions, physicians accumulated impressive mileage. In his first year at Crow Creek, Treon traveled 97 miles by foot, 94 by horseback, and

1,170 by wagon to treat 197 patients in their homes. An unnamed physician at Cheyenne River in 1899 set the record, traveling 6,000 miles to treat 1,000 patients.[10]

When physicians managed to get access to patients, they often had to treat them without medications. The physician at Rosebud in 1879 quickly exhausted his annual supply of drugs, leaving him "sorely perplexed." The doctor at Standing Rock in 1885 could not treat consumption and scrofula because the agency's medical supplies did not include "an alcohol stimulant, such as brandy or whisky." Eastman found the drugs at Pine Ridge "obsolete in kind, and either stale or of the poorest quality." Ralph Ross complained that drugs, shipped in midwinter, often arrived frozen, "which either spoils their efficiency or breaks the bottles and thereby wastes the medicines." Walker, who exhausted his annual supply within six months in 1904, wrote that "there have doubtless been many deaths among such persons that might have been prevented had they been supplied with the proper remedies." Surgical intervention was just as difficult, something Commissioner Price attributed to the "great aversion of the Indians to the knife." Treon and Daniel had to go to great lengths to convince Sioux patients to accept surgery. Many Sioux also distrusted hospitals: they avoided places where people had died; they missed the social life and familiar rituals of their camps; and they spurned hospital food. As Daniel wrote, "it is another world to them, and they dislike everything about a hospital on general Indian principles."[11]

Sioux who refused hospitalization faced treatment at home. J. Ashley Thompson blamed the death of many children at Pine Ridge on "the harsh practices of their relatives, a majority of whom have not the remotest idea of the indispensable nursing and ordinary hygiene." Treon complained that the Sioux "know nothing about nursing their sick, and to treat them in a dirty hut, or tepee, lying on a cot filthy with dirt or vermin, and their food of the coarsest and worst prepared imaginable is indeed discouraging." When he told one mother to keep her infant warm until measles resolved, she plunged the baby into a cold bath, "That night the child died." Even Eastman, who generally had excellent relations with his fellow Sioux, grew frustrated: "Much of my labor was wasted, moreover, because of the impossibility of seeing that my directions were followed, and of securing proper nursing and attention."[12]

Physicians also complained that the Sioux would not follow directions about prescriptions. Hughes noted that they "frequently cast the physician's medicine aside, without even tasting it." James McLaughlin described the opposite problem. Believing that if a little of a medicine is good, then more of it must be better, Sioux patients often took too much, "thereby defeating the desired effect and producing different results from that intended." Commissioner J. D. C. Atkins concluded that Indians simply lacked the necessary patience and discipline: "If the medicine is distasteful it will not be taken. If one dose does not cure, the patient is discouraged." Commissioner W. A. Jones believed that Indian "ignorance and superstition" made treatment impossible. Some physicians, however, found that the Sioux followed prescriptions more closely than whites.[13]

It is easy to imagine that other obstacles might have limited Sioux compliance more than these cultural and behavioral explanations. Inadequately educated by physicians, forced to travel great distances to receive care, and struggling to maintain subsistence, Sioux patients had little energy for following prescriptions. The physicians, however, saw this problem only in the most practical terms. Treon found it "very annoying" that the Sioux "have no idea of our plan of reckoning time." This prevented his patients from taking medications at the recommended intervals. W. L. Brown had a simple solution: "it would materially lessen the death rate among these people if they were provided with timepieces and taught how to use them."[14] If only medical care had been so simple.

Through all of this, agency physicians continued to grapple with medicine men, whose influence they were expected to destroy. McGillycuddy, who described medicine men as "barbarism personified," believed that "no efforts or means should be neglected to destroy his influence." Treon, who considered them "the most remarkable frauds imaginable," struggled against them during the 1888 measles epidemic, kicking one down the school stairs. Physicians had many specific concerns. Some medicine men distracted Sioux patients away from prescribed medicines. Others feigned illnesses, received medications from the physicians, and then passed these medicines along to their own patients. J. M. Woodburn worried that "should their cunning prevail and prescription given be of service, of course all credit would be ascribed to their own 'tom-tom' and 'noisy doings.'" He had to use "utmost tact and rigid questioning" to expose this duplicity. Amid this conflict, medicine men occasionally won grudging respect from the physicians. Woodburn confessed, "Some of their remedies are extremely efficacious." Eastman found them harmless at worst, which was more than he would say for most physicians. Walker studied their methods most closely and came to respect at least their powers of suggestion.[15]

This catalogue of obstacles provides a telling glimpse into the lives of agency physicians. Many approached their positions with enthusiasm and optimism, but when they arrived at the reservations, they entered a world of bewildering challenges. Patients were inaccessible, medicines unavailable, and nursing care inadequate. Medicine men undermined their authority and ministrations. Their lives must have felt like a constant struggle against geography and Indian intransigence. Meanwhile, they were also expected to serve as sanitary officers, school inspectors, and educators. This alone would have sorely tested physicians' "self-sacrificing spirit." All of this, however, was just the beginning of the problem. These struggles were simply the ones that physicians were willing to publish in their annual reports. Their personal correspondence with the Indian Office reveals another problem: their constant struggle against the dysfunctional bureaucracy of the Bureau of Indian Affairs.

Fordyce Grinnell, for instance, was an experienced agency physician when he sought reappointment to the Indian Service in 1881. He presented a sterling recommendation from a good friend, who happened to be an old neighbor of Commissioner Price. It described him as "a Christian gentleman," "a good physician, and a good man": "My head for a football if you are the least disappointed in him." Most important, Grinnell and his wife were both "intense republicans." Grinnell won appointment to Pine Ridge and arrived in June 1881. Although he quickly won praise from agent McGillycuddy, this did not last. Conflict started innocuously in 1882 with a dispute about whether Grinnell could keep private cows at the agency corral. Tensions escalated when agency employees called for an investigation of McGillycuddy's administration. McGillycuddy responded by accusing Grinnell of defying his authority and colluding with Red Cloud (Grinnell admitted to hosting Red Cloud for dinner). Grinnell suspected that McGillycuddy disliked him because he had shown sympathy for the Sioux, and because he and his wife did not "dance, play cards, or billiards, and are teetotalers, hence arises some lack of congeniality." The BIA investigator sympathized with Grinnell: "His only fault as an agency physician seems to lie in the fact that in some things he ventured to think differently than did Agt McGillycuddy." But when the controversy continued, Grinnell was forced to accept transfer to Rosebud, where he was welcomed in 1883. Fed up by continuing politics, he left Rosebud in 1885 and moved to the Pacific coast.[16]

George Underhill, who replaced Grinnell at Rosebud, fared little better. Underhill arrived in August 1885 and was warmly received by the agent, James Wright, who described him as "an able physician" and "a courteous gentleman." The feeling was not mutual. By June Underhill became concerned that Wright had fraudulently provided the Sioux with worthless cattle. Afraid to report this officially, he voiced his concerns to an old friend, S. S. Bloom. Bloom was outraged that Underhill, a Democrat, feared Wright, a Republican. He fired off a letter to the secretary of the interior and to President Grover Cleveland (the first Democrat elected since before the Civil War): *"This ought not be so* . . . Republicans *ought* to give way sometime." Bloom added that Underhill, unlike Wright, "has the best interests of the Indians, and the country, as well as the democratic party at heart." Wright was soon replaced. Although he won the conflict, Underhill did not enjoy the fruits of victory. Within a few months he suffered "a severe illness" and had to resign.[17] Wright was eventually avenged: restored as the agent at Rosebud in 1890, he served until 1895.

Similar struggles recurred time and time again. Fred Treon applied to the Indian Service in 1886 and, with the support of his congressman, won appointment to Crow Creek (at the expense of another physician from his own district). Treon lost his position after a single term, presumably to another political appointee. He immediately sought reappointment, submitting testimonials of his value to the Indian Service. Dr. James Lamb, his father-in-law and former partner, noted that Treon was "deeply interested" in Indian welfare. Furthermore, "it was very largely through his influence over them that they signed the treaty ceding their lands to the U.S." Treon also described the "wide field for scientific research" provided by Sioux consumption; he sent Commissioner Morgan reprints of his publications on this subject. Treon won reappointment in 1891 but, in a typical snafu, was not sent to the Sioux, with whom he was already familiar, but to the San Carlos Apache in Arizona. Disappointed by the climate, isolation, and salary, he convinced Morgan to shuffle a series of physicians and transfer him to Crow Creek. Once there, his career actually progressed rapidly: Treon was promoted to agent of the Crow Creek and Lower Brulé Consolidated Agency, a position he held from 1893 to 1897.[18]

Charles Eastman provides the most dramatic case. Three quarters Santee Sioux by birth, Eastman fled with his grandmother to Canada during the Minnesota uprising in 1862. He had planned a career on the warpath until he rediscovered his father (previously thought dead, actually imprisoned in the United States), converted to Christianity, attended mission schools in Dakota, graduated from Dartmouth College, and studied medicine at Boston University. After graduating in 1890, he applied to the Indian Service, submitting glowing recommendations: "he is to-day the finest object lesson of what Christianity and education will do for the Indian that can be found in this country." He won appointment, not to the Sioux, whose languages he spoke, but to the Mandan, Arikara, and Gros Ventres. Eastman immediately protested this waste of his Sioux heritage: this "will practically snatch from me that advantage which I could have over a white physician." His logic slowly overcame the bureaucratic inertia of the BIA: after complicated maneuvering, he was transferred to Pine Ridge.[19]

Eastman found Pine Ridge "a bleak and desolate looking place in those days, more especially in a November dust storm." Nevertheless, he felt "alive with energy and enthusiasm." He arrived just in time for the crises of the Ghost Dance and Wounded Knee. Able to speak the Lakota dialects, he gained the trust of Sioux leaders and became a crucial advisor to Commissioner Morgan. Once peace was restored, however, he ran afoul of Captain George LeRoy Brown, the military agent given control of Pine Ridge. The problem, which again began with a dispute about keeping private cattle on agency land, quickly escalated. Eastman accused Brown of embezzling reparation payments. Brown accused Eastman of insubordination. An investigation (a "farce" and a "white-washing" according to Eastman) cleared Brown. They continued to exchange charges of "wicked treatment," libel, absenteeism, and not being "Christian." Eastman complained to a friend, who complained to his senator, who reported the conflict to President Benjamin Harrison, who summoned Eastman to Washington, D.C., in January 1893. A second investigation, by the same inspector, again cleared Brown.

Eastman, offered transfer, quit the Indian Service altogether, "being utterly disillusioned and disgusted with these revelations of Government mismanagement in the field, and realizing the helplessness of the best-equipped Indians to secure a fair deal for their people." After a brief stint in private practice in St. Paul, Eastman eventually re-entered government service, holding a variety of posts, including agency physician at Crow Creek from 1899 to 1902.[20]

In these cases, bureaucratic conflict forced agency physicians to abandon their work. New physicians and new agents could always be appointed, but even when conflict was less severe, bureaucratic inertia compromised medical care. This happened with James Walker, who served as physician at Pine Ridge from 1896 to 1914. Walker, as described in the previous chapter, had worked at the Chippewa agency from 1882 to 1893, earning renown for his efforts against smallpox. In 1893, however, while confiscating contraband whiskey, he accidentally shot and wounded a Chippewa. Although the infantry eventually restored peace, Walker was transferred to the Colville Agency in Washington, to the Indian School at Carlisle, and finally to Pine Ridge. During the next ten years, he made a special study of tuberculosis. Rejecting traditional explanations, he argued that the Sioux had no particular affinity for tuberculosis and that tuberculosis was not caused by filth, diet, or alcohol. Instead, he traced everything to exposure and contagion. Before the reservations, the Sioux lived in well-ventilated tepees, spit into open fires, and moved before filth accumulated. In their new lives, they lived in crowded, filthy, unventilated cabins. Conditions that once protected them had been reversed. This made sick people sicker and increased the exposure of everyone to their sputum: "all the requisites for the propagation and spread of the diseases were supplied."[21]

Convinced that exposure was crucial, Walker set out to prevent consumptive sputum and scrofulous discharges from coming into contact with uninfected people. Despite "much annoyance and discouragement," he studied the methods of medicine men, obtained their cooperation, showed them tubercle bacilli under a microscope, and convinced them of the value of his "rational treatment." With their assistance, he tried to move people to cleaner homes, to increase their exposure to fresh air and sunshine, to segregate healthy and sick, and to destroy "products of the disease." An assistant physician, appointed in 1897, freed Walker to supervise his tuberculosis control program. Success came quickly. Walker's data showed a continuous decline in tuberculosis from 1897 to 1903, with incidence decreasing 49 percent and mortality 44 percent (from 24.88/1,000 to 13.45/1,000). The BIA, however, brought this program to a crashing halt in 1903: it reassigned Walker's assistant, giving each doctor full responsibility for half the reservation. With no one to cover his office practice, he had to abandon the control program. This was "a misfortune which has almost amounted to a calamity to these Indians." The program became "intermittent and ineffectual." By 1905 annual mortality had increased 62 percent. Predicting "evil consequences" from "entirely unnecessary" BIA meddling, Walker demanded additional assistants, but without success.[22]

Although mismanagement had killed his control program, Walker believed that his emphasis on exposure had been validated. Resigned to his clinical responsibilities, he tried another approach. He envisioned a sanitary camp, "where all that are infected with the disease should be collected and maintained, under competent supervision, until each case terminates." This camp of tents, much cheaper than a hospital, was endorsed by the agent and the commissioner. However, undermined by disputes between the agent and school staff, it was never built. This second defeat broke Walker's interest in tuberculosis control. Disillusioned, he pursued his interest in Oglala medical beliefs and mythology. By 1914 he had completed training and had become an Oglala shaman: "I was saluted by the older Oglala as the Holy Man."[23] That year he took a leave of absence and was retired by the BIA. Unable to deploy his expertise against tuberculosis, Walker had undermined a fundamental role of the agency physician and become a medicine man.

These episodes each represent a peculiar tragedy of the agency physicians. The conditions of reservation life had created an enormous burden of tuberculosis. The federal government accepted this burden and, probably naively, sent fewer than 100 physicians to care for over 200,000 American Indians. Had the system worked perfectly, the physicians would have faced only the obstacles of geography, poverty, and inadequate resources. However, the bureaucracy that should have supported health care often obstructed it. Even the most motivated advocates of Indian health were drawn into the system only to be broken by it. If these physicians met with failure, what happened at agencies whose physicians had less zeal? The BIA did little to encourage initiative or discourage complacency. Commissioner Price tried to institute central oversight in 1882, but Congress did not approve a medical inspector for the BIA until 1909. This system allowed tremendous negligence. When Eastman arrived at Pine Ridge in 1890, he found that his predecessor had simply sat at a window "to deal out pills and potions to a crowd of patients standing in line."[24] Perhaps this predecessor had once been as "alive with energy and enthusiasm" as Eastman, only to have encountered insurmountable resistance. While the system created and allowed powerlessness, tuberculosis persisted.

Resources

The epidemic of Sioux tuberculosis in the 1880s and 1890s was a product of the growth of the American nation. To make way for white settlement, the Sioux had been confined on reservations that could not support their populations. Vibrant health gave way to tuberculosis. But the United States remained a work in progress: although the government took responsibility for Sioux tuberculosis, it only provided a minimal Indian service to confront the problems the expanding country had created. The nation had become pathogenic, without finding a way to be therapeutic. This paradox appears clearly in the continuing efforts of agency physicians. They struggled to attract more resources to the reservations, only to find that the slow increase in personnel and facilities did little to help.

Year after year, agents and physicians requested more medical personnel. As early as 1882, McGillycuddy sought an assistant for Grinnell at Pine Ridge. In 1884 and 1885 he asked for two: "To expect one physician to properly attend 8,000 people, scattered over 100 miles of creek bottoms, is simply nonsense." Charles McChesney wanted three physicians at Cheyenne River since "this agency embraces in its boundaries nearly as much land as the State of Massachusetts . . . it is simply a human impossibility for one agency physician to visit the sick in this vast area." Commissioner Morgan understood the consequences of such understaffing: "the results are a large degree of needless suffering and hundreds of deaths." Even when assistants appeared, more were always needed. Walker believed that the conditions at Pine Ridge, if they existed among whites, would have profitably employed five or six doctors. L. M. Hardin wanted seven at Rosebud. All would have agreed with Walker that inadequate medical services on the reservations were "an error of grave import to these Indians." In addition to these frequent calls for additional doctors, agents and agency physicians requested apothecaries, nurses, and hospital stewards. Such requests were rarely met: physician staffing for all Indian reservations only increased from 64 in 1882 to 83 in 1900. An innovative BIA program, which sent "field matrons" to teach Indian women cooking, hygiene, child care, and nursing, helped but was always inadequate.[25]

The situation with hospitals was just as critical. This was a time of dramatic hospital construction throughout the United States. The total number of hospitals nationwide increased from 178 in 1873 (roughly 50,000 beds) to 4,359 in 1909 (roughly 420,000 beds). Agency physicians worked to bring this development to the Sioux reservations. In 1877 Hughes wanted a hospital at Standing Rock "where not only the sick could receive such treatment as the nature of their diseases might require, but the old and infirm could be carefully attended to there, many of whom die, without our knowing, from neglect." Cicero Newell believed that provision of a hospital at Rosebud in 1879 would be "an act of humanity." McLaughlin believed that hospitals would "be another convincing proof of the good intention of the government." Commissioners agreed that the benefits far outweighed their costs. For Morgan, the obligation seemed clear: "Common humanity dictates that some provision should be made in the way of hospitals and asylums." Requests came frequently, but little happened. Agents and physicians grew frustrated. By 1887 P. C. Barbour complained that "I presume it really unnecessary to ask for hospital advantages, as there seems no disposition whatever to furnish a much-needed convenience." J. M. Woodburn described how a "great many cases" died from "neglectful murder," from "Neglect of proper medical treatment and nursing. Nothing else killed them." Noting that a twenty-bed hospital could be built for less than $2,000, he demanded one "in the name of charity and humanity."[26]

Each year Commissioner Morgan submitted requests for hospital funding, but Congress refused: "I have been powerless to remedy a great evil, which in my view amounts to a national disgrace." Some slowly appeared. A hospital opened at Standing Rock in 1889, at Pine Ridge in 1892, at Crow Creek in 1892 (funded by private donors), and at Cheyenne River by 1895. Other agencies had less luck. By 1901, after fourteen years of ignored requests, the staff at Rosebud had lost hope: "we are forced to the conclusion that proper allowance is never to be made and that their civilization is to be correspondingly retarded." When hospitals were built, they won praise from agents and physicians, but never seemed adequate. In its first year the twenty-bed hospital at Standing Rock had "been of great benefit," but had been "taxed to its utmost capacity." The agent requested a special ward for consumption at that hospital but was apparently ignored. An asylum for mental illness, "a most humane and noble act on the part of the Government," opened in 1903 but was quickly overwhelmed.[27]

Frustrated by failures to achieve substantial reform of medical services, physicians could only pursue superficial changes. Brown, as noted earlier, believed that clocks could decrease mortality by improving compliance. Treon relied on disinfection and whitewashing, believing that "in this manner many of the germs of disease have been destroyed." Tuberculosis control at Indian schools received special attention. Anthropologist Ales Hrdlicka emphasized the importance of outdoor exercise, clean clothing, wood floors, clean swimming pools, nourishing food, weekly weighing, isolation of sick students, sputum disposal, open-air schools, suppressing alcohol, "combating ignorance," and, if possible, exterminating flies. He also warned about the dangers of shared cups and the mouthpieces of shared musical instruments. Another expert had similar ideas, adding that students should not be allowed to spit on floors or sleep with their heads covered. He also recommended that the "habit of expanding the lungs often should be encouraged." A third expert warned that "water-closets in the dormitories are a most pernicious evil."[28]

The most divisive effort at sanitary reform came with the slaughterhouse campaign of the 1890s. Whites had long been repulsed by the Sioux custom of butchering and eating raw buffalo and cattle. Physicians feared that such practices spread tuberculosis and other diseases. In 1890 Commissioner Morgan banned these customs and issued detailed instructions for the hygienic slaughter and distribution of beef rations. The order won praise from agency physicians, including Treon, who believed that it "will prove a great boon to these poor sickley people. They may consider it a hardship to give up the entrails, but the sacrifice will be to them a benefit in more ways than one." The Sioux, however, resisted and continued their traditional practices. Treon claimed victory in 1894: with the construction of a "new, commodious slaughterhouse," "the old degrading, demoralizing, filthy manner of slaughtering beef cattle for issue has received a death blow." But success remained elusive. At Pine Ridge, where the Oglala missed the sport of the hunt and the ritual of butchering, someone burned down the slaughterhouse.[29]

Year after year, agents and physicians called for more resources, producing a slow trickle of assistant physicians and small hospitals. They orchestrated campaigns against tuberculosis, from slaughterhouse hygiene to whitewashing, instructions about safe use of trumpets, and Walker's campaign to reduce exposure. Although officials generally seemed happy with the results, they continued to be concerned about the persistence of tuberculosis. Rates of tuberculosis began to increase as soon as Walker's program was dismantled. After twelve years as physician and agent, Treon felt that he had achieved no success: "I kept at the authorities with hammer and tongs along these lines, but nothing of consequence has been done." Eastman, who remained active in Indian policy from 1890 to 1915, saw little improvement. American Indian mortality (30/1,000) remained twice that of whites; 30,000 suffered from tuberculosis, with a case fatality rate "almost three times that among the whites."[30]

It is difficult to assess the accuracy of these impressions. Agency physicians reported how many cases of each disease they treated each year. If these data are accepted as a proxy of disease prevalence, then tuberculosis declined by 70 percent over fifteen years, from 47/1,000 in 1879 to 13/1,000 in 1894. Mortality data, however, tell a different story. Overall mortality rates remained stable, from 33/1,000 in 1878 to 42/1,000 in 1894 and 34/1,000 in 1906 (Figure 6B). Intermittent reports about the cause of mortality show the dominant role of tuberculosis, with the disease generally causing half of all deaths. With overall mortality and the contribution of tuberculosis both holding constant, the impact of the disease could not have decreased appreciably. This persistence is easy to understand. Thomas McKeown and many historians have argued that physicians had little impact on tuberculosis before the midtwentieth century. Even the value of major public health programs remains contested.[31] The agency physicians, however, were convinced that they could control tuberculosis. Its persistence produced growing frustration that adequate resources had not been allocated.

During this time, the BIA budget grew substantially. Annual expenditures rose by 60 percent, from $4 million in 1877–1878 to $6.4 million in 1894–1895. Personnel expanded from 2,102 employees in 1881 to 3917 in 1897. Education dominated this growth, increasing from 0.8 percent to 30.8 percent of the total budget. School personnel increased from 238 in 1881 (11.3 percent of all total BIA employees) to 1936 (49.4 percent) in 1897. Despite this increase in spending, medical appropriations remained low. The portion of the staff devoted to medicine actually decreased, from 2.9 percent in 1881 to 2.2 percent in 1897. Consider the 1884 budget. Congress appropriated over $5 million to the BIA. While subsistence programs received over $2 million, and schools nearly $700,000, medical personnel received roughly $75,000, medical supplies only $15,729, and vaccination only $246. Unspent appropriations ($295,324) actually exceeded the amount spent on health care. To put this in perspective, Woodburn was not given the $2,000 he requested to build a hospital at Rosebud in 1889. When Treon tried to build a hospital at Crow Creek in 1891, the Episcopal Society offered a building rent-free, and the agent provided furniture and rations. The BIA, however, would not provide the $118 required to convert the church building into a hospital. Treon had to turn to private charity.[32]

This lack of funding received bitter commentary from physicians and agents. Children and elders died at Devil's Lake from malnutrition: "This condition of affairs is wrong, for the Government of the United States is surely wealthy enough to provide these people with the necessaries of life when they are so unfortunate to be unable to obtain it for themselves." Hardin protested a 50 percent reduction in medical supplies at Rosebud in 1902, "an economy which can not but result seriously to both physician and patient." Only something as dramatic as an outbreak of smallpox motivated the BIA to provide generous funding. Many were especially angry about the generous funding provided to other BIA programs. McChesney complained that there "is annually expended thousands of dollars in the improvement and advancement of these Indians in other directions, but we seem to be content with expending a paltry few hundred dollars in their medical care and treatment." While other officials had assistants, or wagons with horses, physicians did not. F. O. Getchell noted that vast amounts were frivolously wasted on sports and marching bands at the boarding school at Devil's Lake, while tuberculosis rampaged unchecked. Students returned home either "in the coffin" or as "walking dead men" to spare the school burial costs.[33]

The disparity in funding between BIA and army medical services was particularly frustrating. While 8,000 Sioux had only Grinnell at Rosebud in 1884, "a mere handful of soldiers" at nearby Fort Niobara had a hospital with a nurse, steward, and two physicians. During military operations at Wounded Knee, the army provided three hospitals, eight surgeons, four noncommissioned medical officers, three hospital stewards, thirty-two privates, and five ambulances for 1,300 soldiers. Meanwhile, the 5,000 Oglala at Pine Ridge had only one doctor, Eastman, and no hospital. When hostilities began, the 7th Cavalry requested more medical officers and supplies, "all of which were promptly furnished." Once peace was restored, wounded soldiers were transferred to larger forts "by tourist sleeper on the railroad." Not only did the Indian service receive fewer medical personnel, it also offered substantially less compensation. At the time of Wounded Knee, agency physicians earned between $200 and $1,300, with an average annual salary of $1,062. Meanwhile, the entrylevel salary for a military physician was $1,600, with an average of $2,823 in the army and $2,693 in the navy. Dividing these salaries by the patient population served, Commissioner Morgan found the following values: $21.91 per soldier, $48.10 per sailor, and $1.25 per Indian.[34]

Observers condemned such indifference to the plight of American Indians. Richard Dodge described how famines or natural disasters in Ireland, India, and China inspired "lavish" donations from "our people, whose charitable instincts are as wide [as] the earth itself. It is only at our own doors, and towards a race whose care should be our peculiar duty, that we suddenly become incomprehensibly deaf to the appeals of those slowly but surely dying of absolute starvation." In the absence of spontaneous charity, officials sought new ways to increase interest in, and funding for, Indian health. One approach, which became common as white populations increasingly crowded the once remote reservations, stressed the threat posed by untreated Indian disease. O. M. Chapman described how "many whites have lost their lives from contact with consumption among the Indians." Since Indians had access to public schools, railroads, the trucking industry, and meat packing houses, "enough infection will be soon broadcast to increase the disease at an alarming rate."[35]

As will be seen in the next chapter, these efforts only slowly increased interest in American Indian tuberculosis. The indifference, curiously, seemed to have been limited to tuberculosis. South Dakota doctor Frank Creamer described this well: "If our settlers were in the midst of an epidemic of plague or diphtheria or some other dangerous disease, they would insist upon the strictest rules in dealing with such epidemic. But, since tuberculosis is a slow, sneaking enemy we allow it to steal upon our unsuspecting settlers and Indians and infect them with its slowly developing process, which in due course of time reaps its harvest." Physicians believed that this could have been prevented. Resources that might have helped overcome disparities in tuberculosis mortality certainly existed. Motivation did not.[36]

Rediscovery

Even if the government had provided unlimited resources, it is unclear whether it could have controlled tuberculosis. The disease persisted on the Sioux reservations for many reasons. Decades of effort to establish a firm economic base, especially at Pine Ridge and Rosebud, had failed. Poor land, harsh climate, bureaucratic ineptness, and Sioux complacency with the ration system all contributed to limited success with farming and ranching. Underfunding of the BIA medical services, compared to educational programs and military medicine, only made matters worse. Agents begged for physicians; some were provided, but never enough to meet the need. Physicians begged for hospitals; some were built, but they immediately overflowed with patients.

As demand for medical care continued to exceed the slowly growing supply, some agents and physicians began to realize that they faced a more fundamental challenge. They now understood that tuberculosis was not the product of a specific problem, whether behavior, housing, or heredity. Instead, it was the product of all of the conditions of daily existence that stemmed from the underlying problem of poverty. In 1886 J. F. Kinney identified scrofula and consumption at Yankton as diseases "of dirt and poverty." Ralph Hall attributed the bewilderingly high death rate in 1895 to "no cause except want and destitution." Learning that the "terrible scourge" of tuberculosis still caused half of all deaths, Chapman concluded that efforts at health education among the Sioux were futile: "He is too poor." On reservations nationwide,

Smithsonian anthropologist Ales Hrdlicka found that "Want and consequent debilitation" contributed to American Indian tuberculosis.[37]

The link between poverty and tuberculosis gained support from the few places where economic conditions improved. In 1905 the Sioux at Devil's Lake "had more to eat as a result of the money they have received, and this has resisted their common enemy—tuberculosis." But such successes were rare. Economic conditions at Yankton had also improved, but health did not: "they are doing almost nothing to better their condition from a sanitary point of view." Most reservations, meanwhile, remained mired in poverty. By 1911 Joseph Murphy, the first medical supervisor of the BIA, had lost hope for raising standards of living. He could only hope that improving "health and education in the schools" might help the younger generation.[38]

From this perspective, BIA efforts against tuberculosis could only have been stopgap measures. No number of physicians or hospital beds could have ended the disparate impact of tuberculosis on the Sioux. This situation left the federal government with a dilemma. By the 1880s it had taken responsibility for improving American Indian health. By the 1900s, however, it had proved unable to convert this responsibility into meaningful action against American Indian disease. Though aware of the failure, Congress did not provide adequate appropriations. What explains this curious mix of responsibility and failure? The government may simply have found satisfaction in having made an effort. It provided eighty-eight physicians for the reservations, where none had worked before. Year after year commissioners celebrated the number of Indians treated by these physicians. This alone seemed proof of the desire of the government to make good on its treaty obligations and moral responsibilities to provide care for American Indians. The actual impact of these efforts on morbidity and mortality may have seemed less relevant. After all, concern with the efficacy of medical systems did not emerge until the midtwentieth century, something discussed in the next chapters.

A second process of rationalization was also at work. The persistent inability of the BIA to reduce the burden of tuberculosis could have engendered a sense of futility amongst its staff. Something else happened instead. Each time that new physicians or officials confronted the challenge of tuberculosis, they managed to be either oblivious to the existence of past health campaigns or dismissive of these past efforts. This fueled a cycle of rediscovering the problem of Indian tuberculosis in the 1890s, 1900s, and 1910s, and then promoting, as new and original, the same old ideas that had already failed.

The process began by denying that adequate data on Sioux morbidity and mortality had ever existed. As discussed earlier, monthly reports from agency physicians had produced a wealth of data from the Sioux reservations by the 1880s. Later observers casually dismissed these data as worthless. Walker, for instance, believed that no useful data existed at Pine Ridge before his arrival: "It was not, however, until 1897, that any adequate sanitary records were compiled." As late as 1911, Murphy complained that "General statistics in regard to the prevalence of disease among Indians are either incomplete and far from accurate, or have not be compiled."[39]

Believing that adequate data had never existed, health officials in the early 1900s repeatedly set out to collect it. In 1903 Commissioner Jones, under pressure from Indian advocacy groups, undertook the first comprehensive health survey of all reservations and Indian schools. In 1908 Hrdlicka led another major survey: he collected data from physicians' annual reports and visited the five most heavily affected reservations, including Pine Ridge. Advocates hoped that new data would produce new ideas about tuberculosis. The resulting reports reached a series of conclusions. Jones found that tuberculosis was "more widespread among the Indians than among an equal number of whites," suggesting that Indians were more susceptible than whites. The prevalence was attributed to failure to control sputum, poor sanitation, poorly prepared food, intermarriage (of related Indians, and of Indians to whites), crowded dormitories, alcohol, and poor medical care. Failure of medical care arose "from causes relating principally to the Indian himself." Jones saw this report as a call for action that could guide government efforts against "the great white plague." He emphasized hospital construction and school sanitation. Hrdlicka made similar sanitary recommendations about school hygiene, diet, flies, and musical instruments, asking that no effort be spared "to bring the Indian medical service to the highest degree of efficiency and dignity." With such steps, "speedy progress can be made in preventing and curing tuberculosis among the Indians."[40]

Hrdlicka presented his findings at the Sixth International Congress on Tuberculosis, held in Washington, D.C., in September and October

1908. He attracted the attention of Commissioner Francis E. Leupp, who gave an address at the Congress and identified tuberculosis as "the greatest single menace to the Indian race." In his annual report, he described the "urgent necessity of doing more than has ever been done" against Indian tuberculosis, "not only for their own sakes but because the infected Indian community becomes a peril to every white community near it." Leupp recommended a series of measures, from sanitary camps to preventing shared wind instruments (that "medium of evil"). He also took the long-awaited step of appointing a medical supervisor for the Indian medical service. His appointee, Joseph Murphy, shared his excitement: "The crusade against tuberculosis is one of the greatest works which the present generation has so far attempted." Blaming the Indian Service "for the continuance of the condition," he remained confident that tuberculosis, like smallpox, cholera, and yellow fever, "once scourges to the world, are preventable." Murphy had a simple plan: health education, special diets (extra milk and eggs), and sputum control. Many shared his enthusiasm. Frank Creamer believed that "Tuberculosis among the Indians can be wiped out in time if we go at it in the right way, and the Government is the proper channel through which to work."[41]

This excitement eventually triggered action by the president and Congress. In 1912 President William Howard Taft decried the "very unsatisfactory" health conditions on reservations: "In many parts of the Indian country infant mortality, tuberculosis, and disastrous diseases generally prevail to an extent exceeded only in some of the most insanitary of our white rural districts and in the worst slums of our large cities." The government, "guardians of the welfare of the Indians," had to act. He praised Leupp's efforts, "the most vigorous campaign ever waged against diseases among the Indians," and thanked Congress for an emergency appropriation of $12,000. He then requested a further appropriation of $253,350 to expand the Indian medical service and improve its efficiency: "it is believed that the tide can be turned, that the danger of infection among the Indians themselves and to the several millions of white persons now living as neighbors to them can be greatly reduced."[42]

All of this optimism shared the belief that meaningful efforts had never been tried in the past. Dismissing the quality of prior health data, officials convinced themselves that the problem of tuberculosis had not been recognized previously. Downplaying the existence of agency physicians for the past thirty years, they demanded that physicians be appointed. Time and time again, they emphasized the novelty of their health campaigns. In 1911 Murphy claimed that only "within recent years" had anyone realized "the importance of considering the necessity for action" to improve American Indian health. Taft believed that "little attention had been given to the hygiene and health of the Indians." In 1923 tuberculosis expert George Kober praised Murphy, who "inaugurated practically the first intensive health campaign among the Indians" and initiated "intelligent and progressive health work." When officials did acknowledge the past failures of government efforts, they dismissed them as irrelevant to the current campaign. Robert Valentine believed that prior efforts had been stymied by "the small force and inadequate funds at our disposal." Historians have generally accepted this mythology. Even Prucha, very familiar with the Annual Reports of the nineteenth century, wrote that the Commissioners "found no occasion to devote any space to health until 1904 . . . and then 1908."[43]

Despite this faith in novelty (of data, of recognition of tuberculosis, of enthusiasm for preventive efforts), little was actually new in 1906 compared to 1896, or even 1886. Disparities in tuberculosis status persisted. Hrdlicka had brought American Indian tuberculosis to the attention of an international meeting in 1908, but reports about Sioux tuberculosis had been appearing in the medical literature since the 1880s. Leupp did create the position of medical inspector, but commissioners had worked to improve the quality of the medical service since the 1880s. Taft did petition Congress for large sums of money for Indian health, but past presidents had been personally involved in the struggles faced by agency physicians in the 1880s and 1890s. Physicians did increasingly recognize the importance of Koch's discovery of the tubercle bacillus, but knowledge of the bacteria had little impact on theories of etiology or plans for eradication: Grinnell, Treon, Walker, and Murphy would all have agreed about the decisive roles of nutrition and sanitation.

If nothing was new, then why did the discourse of novelty emerge? It could be that the burden of tuberculosis among the Sioux became newly intolerable as tuberculosis receded from its position as the leading cause of morbidity and mortality among the general population. The spirit of progressivism also contributed. The progressive movement engendered a new confidence that humans could improve the conditions of their existence and defeat infectious diseases. This confidence made the deadly persistence of infectious diseases unacceptable. Unfortunately, physicians and public health officials had little to offer against Indian tuberculosis in 1910, except perhaps better funding, than they could have offered in 1880. Efforts to improve living conditions and health behaviors had all been tried, year after year, on agency after agency, by a series of motivated and well-intentioned agency physicians, without success. By forgetting, or never even knowing, that past efforts had failed, officials of the progressive era could maintain their enthusiasm for old programs of sanitation and health education. If such efforts against tuberculosis merely ran on a treadmill to nowhere, then this cycle of ignorance and rediscovery prevented government officials from getting bored of the scenery.[44]

Presented with the problem of Indian tuberculosis, agents, physicians, commissioners, and even presidents had to act. With few available interventions, they had two basic options. Some proceeded stalwartly with the effort to improve health conditions, indifferent to efficacy, reassured that the effort had been made. Others convinced themselves that the programs were new, that their efforts against Indian tuberculosis bore no resemblance to what had come before. Thus armed, they marched proudly into the twentieth century and embarked on their "crusade against tuberculosis." This crusade would chase tuberculosis from the high plains of the Dakotas to the high deserts of Arizona. Along the way, the crusaders would accept a crucial responsibility. Unlike their predecessors, they did not find satisfaction simply in making efforts against tuberculosis. Instead, they accepted the requirement that they demonstrate their efficacy. This would become the new measure, and motivation, of success.

$$7$$

Pursuit of Efficacy

THE RISE OF TUBERCULOSIS among the Sioux in the late nineteenth century had challenged physicians and government officials in the United States. First, they had to explain the appearance of tuberculosis in the sparsely settled prairies and mountains of the western states, environments so different from the eastern urban slums in which tuberculosis typically thrived. Although researchers generated an abundance of explanations, from the squalid conditions of reservation life to the contested vigor of Indian bodies, many observers ultimately recognized tuberculosis as a symptom of the transition from nomadic to settled life, a process initiated by the government. Second, after accepting this responsibility for tuberculosis, the government had to manage its consequences. Agency physicians, assigned this task, struggled against reservation conditions and the crippling ambivalence of the federal bureaucracy. Unable to attract needed resources, they could neither treat tuberculosis amid reservation poverty nor improve the underlying economic conditions.

As these struggles against American Indian tuberculosis persisted into the twentieth century, their focus shifted from the high prairies of the Dakotas to the high deserts of the southwest. Tuberculosis was initially rare among the Navajo. By 1950, however, this had changed: tuberculosis mortality on their reservation in Arizona dwarfed that of the general population. This was just the tip of an iceberg: the Navajo suffered remarkable rates of many diseases, from tuberculosis to ear infections, pneumonia, diarrhea, and trauma. As physicians worked to explain the broad scope of Navajo ill health, old theories of behavior, environment, and race all found support. New ideas also emerged. Instead of tracing Navajo disease to a transition from savagery to civilization, researchers would increasingly recognize Navajo ill health as a consequence of failed economic development. Although the Navajo were officially part of the modern United States, their economy, culture, and health status more closely resembled those of impoverished and underdeveloped areas throughout the globe.

The existence of such conditions within the United States offended a country fresh from the military, technological, and moral triumphs of World War II. Navajo veterans, exposed for a few years to a better life, refused to accept the conditions they found when they returned to the reservation. Postwar economic crises on the reservation exacerbated their discontent. The overwhelming burden of Navajo suffering finally triggered government intervention. But even as Congress committed itself to economic development, a new technology—antibiotics—appeared that promised a simpler solution to the problem of tuberculosis. This gave the government unprecedented confidence that it could solve the problem that it had created. The pursuit of efficacy and the promise of antibiotics converged on the Navajo.

Persistence

Walsh McDermott, one of the nation's leading tuberculosis experts, first learned about Navajo tuberculosis in January 1952. He was embarrassed by his prior ignorance. As he later told the Navajo Tribal Council, "I am ashamed to say that I did not know then how much tuberculosis there was out here among the Navajos."[1] This lack of knowledge was astonishing. Government agencies and independent physicians had long called attention to tuberculosis, especially the growing epidemic among the Navajo. Decades of effort, however, failed to raise the problem of American Indian tuberculosis onto the national agenda. The isolation of the Navajo—a condition that allowed tuberculosis to persist in the first place—allowed it to persist in anonymity.

Over the nineteenth century the initial indolence of tuberculosis among American Indians had given way to the devastating epidemics of the reservation period. First among the Chippewa, then among the Sioux and other tribes of the High Plains, tuberculosis began to dominate mortality. James Walker had provided some hope: a careful program of education and sanitary reform reduced rates of tuberculosis. His ideas came at an exciting time. Ales Hrdlicka's documentation of the burden of Indian tuberculosis generated tremendous interest at the 1908 International Congress on Tuberculosis. Joseph Murphy, the new medical supervisor of the Bureau of Indian Affairs (BIA), believed that the "crusade against tuberculosis" was one of the "greatest works" of his generation. President Taft committed the government to action. In 1912 Congress responded with an emergency appropriation of $12,000. The BIA organized campaigns against trachoma, infant mortality, flies, alcoholism, handicapped children, and tooth decay. A program for hospital construction began in 1914. By 1918 there were 87 hospitals on Indian reservations with a total capacity of 2,411 patients.[2]

Such progress produced great pride. Tuberculosis expert George Bushnell believed that these facts "disclose the working out of an enlightened policy in obscure and remote places and doubtless under many difficulties of race prejudice and superstitions as well as of scanty funds, which is exceedingly gratifying." Annual appropriations grew quickly, reaching $350,000 by 1917. That year, for the first time in more than fifty years, more Indians were born than died: "If this good work continues we may no longer speak of the Indian as a vanishing race." George Kober agreed: "thanks to the progress of medical science and the splendid humanitarian efforts of our Government, a noble race of people has been snatched from the very jaws of death."[3]

World War I gutted these optimistic crusades for Indian health. The war diverted health personnel, reduced medical supplies, and unleashed influenza. Adopting a siege mentality, the Indian medical service made little effort at prevention. As the crises of World War I resolved, the problem of tuberculosis re-emerged. When the National Tuberculosis Association surveyed health conditions on several reservations in 1922, it found tuberculosis mortality rates reaching 1,000/ 100,000. This "undue prevalence of tuberculosis among our North American Indians has been a matter of serious concern for a number of years to all interested in the perpetuation of the aborigines of this country." The Meriam Report, a 1928 Rockefeller Foundation investigation of the "Indian Problem," reviewed all aspects of Indian life and paid particular attention to health: "The health of the Indians as compared with that of the general population is bad." Tuberculosis, "without doubt the most serious disease among the Indians," dominated their concerns. The report, which was extremely critical of existing health services, produced considerable controversy. But tuberculosis persisted. Although mortality had fallen by the 1930s to 41/100,000 among whites, it remained as high as 775/100,000 among tribes in Montana. Tuberculosis mortality remained consistently above 200/100,000 for Indian tribes throughout the 1940s. Recognizing that tuberculosis was "the leading cause of death," BIA physicians concluded that "Tuberculosis control is the major health problem."[4]

Such assessments relied on limited data. Periodic surveys from the 1910s to the 1940s, such as Hrdlicka's studies or the Meriam Report, did collect detailed data, but each captured only a brief moment in time. Several physicians, unable to find adequate official demographic data, reported their own experiences. Researchers had to rely on such incomplete sources, supplemented by sporadic data from state public health reports and federal census data. The resulting estimates had substantial flaws. Some states, lacking reliable statistics, reported estimates of tuberculosis cases that exceeded estimates of Indian population size. Lewis Moorman, who led a 1950 American Medical Association investigation of Navajo tuberculosis, found that the "records are so incomplete, so wanting in content and continuity that they supply no reliable consecutive statistical data on this question." Even such simple tasks as registering births and deaths eluded the BIA into the 1950s: only half of all infants could be matched to birth certificates.[5]

While acknowledging the limits of their data, physicians and researchers believed that the overall message remained painfully clear. Gross disparities in health status existed between the white and Indian populations of the United States. Comparisons of mortality rates made these disparities particularly striking. In 1912, for instance, the commissioner of Indian affairs contrasted mortality between Indians (3,500/100,000) and the general population (1,500/100,000). Such comparisons were clearest when reduced to a simple ratio. Horace DeLien and Arthur Dalhstrom presented the 1925 data on tuberculosis mortality for Indians as seven times the national average, while the Public Health Service (PHS) reported the 1957 Indian tuberculosis case rate as nearly ten times the national average. Historical comparisons were even more dramatic. The PHS, for instance, reported that life expectancy, in 1957 ten years less than among the general population, was "at the level of that for the white population in 1930." The prevalence of tuberculosis "resembles that of the total population 30 years ago."[6]

These two styles of comparison had obvious, and complementary, implications. By showing how the health conditions of current Indian populations resembled those of white populations of decades past, authors appealed to readers' expectations of progress: one population should not be allowed to persist in conditions of a remote, unhealthy, and unacceptable past. By showing how the death rates of current populations differed, authors appealed to readers' sense of equity and justice: one population should not be allowed to suffer while others remained healthy. Such techniques were a response to the challenge that McDermott labeled "statistical compassion," the challenge of evoking "imaginative compassion for people one never knows about except as dots on a graph."[7] Techniques of ethnic and historical comparison made health statistics more tangible, more compelling, and more evocative of an emotional response.

Such comparisons were starkest with the Navajo. As recently as 1905, Hrdlicka had found remarkably good health among the Navajo. While the Sioux suffered tuberculosis mortality at rates as high as 3,080/100,000, the Navajo and Pueblo had little, with rates as low as 60 to 90/100,000. The Navajo were healthier than even the general population, with its tuberculosis mortality of 150 to 550/100,000. This changed quickly; BIA data from 1925 showed that while the general tuberculosis mortality rate was 87/100,000, it was 630/100,000 for all Indians, and 1,510/100,000 for Arizona Indians. In 1947 tuberculosis mortality for Arizona Indians (302.4/100,000) dwarfed both the rate of Indians in general (200/100,000), the general population of Arizona (33/100,000), and the national population (30/100,000). By 1955 disparities in case rates for certain infectious diseases had reached shocking proportions. Incidence among the Navajo exceeded that among the general population by a factor of 15.8 for tuberculosis, 101.6 for pneumonia, and 1,163 for trachoma.[8] Something had gone terribly wrong.

The Navajo, or the Diné, descended from Athabascan migrants who arrived in the southwest sometime around the sixteenth century. Like the Sioux, their culture was strongly influenced by European contact.

Interacting with existing Pueblo groups, and then with Spanish colonists, they reshaped their lives around sheep, horses, and cattle. Pastoral life agreed with them. Their population grew from 2,000 in 1700 to 10,000 in 1850. The arrival of Anglo-Americans in 1846 disrupted this successful adaptation. An army led by Kit Carson burned Navajo crops and killed their herds, starving them into submission. After surrendering at the Canyon de Chelly in 1864, the Navajo were forced to endure four years of captivity on a small reservation along the Pecos River near Fort Sumner, New Mexico. Although General James Carleton hoped to convert them into prosperous agriculturalists, overcrowding, inadequate provisions, and demoralization eroded their health. In 1868 the government declared this effort to civilize the Navajo a failure and allowed them to return to their homelands, now a reduced and well-defined reservation.[9]

These initial contacts brought new diseases to the Navajo. Smallpox, for instance, struck the region in 1853 and 1870. Contact also brought some promising new treatments. Henry Dodge vaccinated 900 Navajo in 1853; government physicians vaccinated many more in 1870. Yet despite occasional successes, government health services on the reservation suffered from low standards, high physician turnover, and a corrupt bureaucracy. The Navajo often had to rely on their traditional healers to overcome these new diseases. Navajo health was preserved only by gradual improvements in economic conditions. Although their houses and crops had been destroyed, the Navajo benefited from sheep provided by the government, and from tourists brought to the southwest by railroads. By 1900 the tribe was prosperous, earning nearly $400,000 each year selling blankets (woven by women) and silver and turquoise jewelry (crafted by men) to eager tourists.

The health and prosperity did not last. The Navajo reservation, roughly the size of West Virginia, straddled the borders of New Mexico, Arizona, and Utah (Figure 1). It did not offer a hospitable climate for their growing population. As one physician described, "It is an alkali-ladened desert with a sprinkling of oases, varicolored mountains, mesas, and valleys—the land of 'painted' deserts. Cyclonic sandstorms during the dry months, torrential rains with little warning in the spring and fall, snowstorms in heavy drifts plus subzero temperatures, are hazards of existence not infrequently encountered." Population growth, expanding herds, overgrazing, and droughts all contributed to soil erosion. Prosperity gave way to desperation. In the 1930s

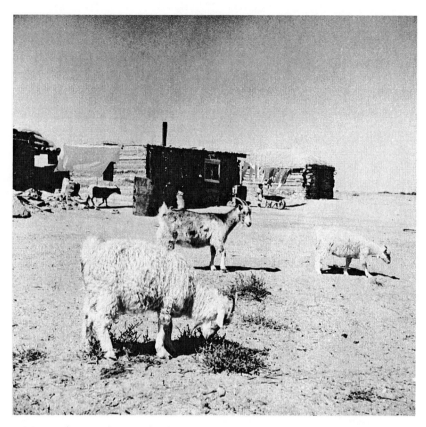

7. Navajo sheep and pastureland ca. 1955. Navajo sheep formed the basis of much of the Navajo economy. Overgrazing, however, was often blamed for the desertification that left the reservation mired in poverty. Neither the traditional log-walled hogan (on the right) nor the more jerry-rigged cabin (center) provided their inhabitants with adequate sanitation. (Courtesy of New York Weill Cornell Medical Center Archives. Photograph Collection, Navajo Project, #2309.)

the federal government intervened. John Collier, President Franklin Roosevelt's New Deal commissioner for Indian affairs, imposed radical transformations on Navajo life. These were well intentioned, and sometimes successful. The overall impact, however, was devastating. Concern with overgrazing led Collier to reduce drastically the number of Navajo sheep. Herd reduction, "perhaps the most traumatic event of recent Navajo history," shattered the Navajo economy. Standards of living on the reservation plummeted (Figure 7).[10]

Job opportunities through the Civilian Conservation Corps initially relieved some of the hardship. Although these ended in the late 1930s, crisis was again averted by employment opportunities during World

War II. When the war ended, crisis finally did strike. During the war, Navajo soldiers and workers became accustomed to steady jobs, money, education, and modern housing. None of these could be found amidst the primitive conditions on the reservation. Many Navajo did not even receive social security payments from Arizona and New Mexico, even though the federal government provided matching funds to those states. With inadequate housing, diet, and social services, many Navajo were reduced to "abject poverty," conditions "incredible to most Americans who have not seen them." Even the considerable income earned from helium deposits, uranium mines, logging, sawmills, and natural gas ($20 million annually) did not improve Navajo lives.[11]

Deteriorating economic and social conditions created terrible health conditions. By 1936 the Navajo had the highest tuberculosis rates of all Indian tribes: 25 percent were infected. During the war, 10 percent to 25 percent of Navajo soldiers and workers had to be sent back to the reservation because of active tuberculosis. Postwar surveys confirmed the epidemic: "Tuberculosis and infant mortality have reached what is believed to be the highest rate in continental United States." Navajo health "lagged almost two generations behind that of the general population."[12]

Physicians had little difficulty explaining this proliferation of tuberculosis among the Navajo. The decades that followed Walker's campaigns against tuberculosis at Pine Ridge brought no fundamental discoveries about the etiology of tuberculosis. Most physicians still accepted the basic model of an interaction between infection with Koch's bacillus and the response by the host's defenses. These defenses, the crucial determinant of the outcome, reflected a mix of genetic, environmental, and behavioral factors. What had changed, however, was the emphasis given to each of these factors.

Observers continued to contest the role of heredity. Many believed that some ill-defined genetic susceptibility left American Indians particularly vulnerable to tuberculosis. This was part of the broader belief that the Indians were a distinct race from whites. Such sentiments appeared in Hrdlicka's physical anthropology of the southwestern tribes. Hundreds of pages of data and analysis led Hrdlicka to conclude that the Indians were "in a large measure a race of their own." The differences could be subtle, ranging from differences in weight, heart rate, and timing of dentition, to decreased frequency of sneezing and hiccoughing. Such physiological changes led Hrdlicka to believe that the Indians responded differently to disease, requiring different medicines. Other physicians and government officials were similarly quick to blame tuberculosis on the "Indian's susceptibility." In 1923 the New Mexico State Department of Health went so far as to assert an ongoing process of natural selection: "Resistant race has not been bred as yet. Now undergoing process of weeding out the nonresistant strains." Faith in this process of natural selection grew from the belief that tuberculosis had only recently been introduced to the Navajo, during their captivity at Fort Sumner. Genetic explanations were deployed just as easily to explain the surprisingly low incidence of noninfectious diseases among the Navajo, including hypertension, cancer, heart disease, and baldness.[13]

Although such genetic explanations of Navajo ill health persisted, most observers discounted them. The National Tuberculosis Association argued in 1923 that "tuberculosis attacks without any racial preference." Physician Herbert Burns agreed: "Heredity exerts no known control over infection." Other studies of Indians with tuberculosis found that "the character of tuberculous lesions, as determined roentgenologically, is not significantly different from that observed among the white population." Many Indians responded well to medical treatments, and others recovered even without medical treatment, suggesting that "the same defense mechanism set up in the body of the white patient to combat the disease is also present in the body of the Indian patient." Even when physicians found a correlation between prevalence of tuberculosis and purity of Indian blood (37.54 percent among one-eighth to two-eighths Indian versus 70.13 percent among five-eighths to seven-eighths Indian), this was attributed to social factors, not genetics. The overall results seemed clear: "Observation and careful study have revealed that it is the same type of tubercle bacillus that causes their disease and that under similar conditions they resist it in the same manner as persons of the white race." While the reservations clearly suffered severely from tuberculosis, "identical" epidemics existed among populations "living under like conditions among people of the Caucasian and Yellow races."[14]

Environmental theories often superseded the debates about genetics. These, however, presented a difficult puzzle. Physicians had long recommended that tuberculosis patients travel to the high deserts of the southwest for convalescence. Microbiologist René Dubos was therefore surprised to find that "despite the blessings of the sunny, warm and dry climate of Arizona," tuberculosis was prevalent among the Navajo. What, if not genetics, overwhelmed the benefits of such a benevolent climate? Like their predecessors among the Sioux in the 1880s, physicians agreed that the real explanation for Navajo tuberculosis could be found in the living conditions of daily life. As Sydney Tillim argued in the 1930s, "Benefits to health from an outdoor life are over-balanced by the ill effects of, overcrowding, lack of sanitary provisions, and the poverty which leads to a poor, inadequate supply of food." Arthur Myers and Virginia Dustin agreed: "Tuberculosis is simply a contagious disease. Wherever it is permitted to exist, it spreads to all races of people." Finding "Ideal conditions" among the Navajo and other "so-called 'primitive' human race," tuberculosis spread easily: "This fact has been largely ignored while tuberculosis workers have ascribed the disease to such poorly understood factors as low resistance, high susceptibility and lack of immunity." The "massive and continuous exposure to tuberculosis" resulted in "approximately a universal infection" (Figure 8).[15]

Report after report rejected arguments based on "racial susceptibility" and argued instead about the decisive role of "provocative environmental influences." Noting that even the poorest whites were well off compared to the Navajo, researchers stressed that the "extreme poverty of the Indians must have a deleterious influence on their health since there seems to be a definite relationship between economic status and incidence of illness." To make matters worse, the epidemic of tuberculosis exacerbated economic conditions. The Navajo were caught in a vicious circle: poverty caused disease which prevented relief of poverty. Many researchers held the government ultimately responsible for the problems. Fred Foard, director of medical services for the BIA, blamed the confinement of 65,000 Navajo on land "which could not possibly adequately support more than 30,000." The "niggardly" appropriations of the BIA, which maintained the reservations as rural slums, did not help.[16]

But as had happened so many times before, physicians and government officials moved seamlessly from tracing disease to the facts of poverty, filthy housing, and inadequate food, to tracing disease to the behaviors that the Navajo adopted in those conditions. They com-

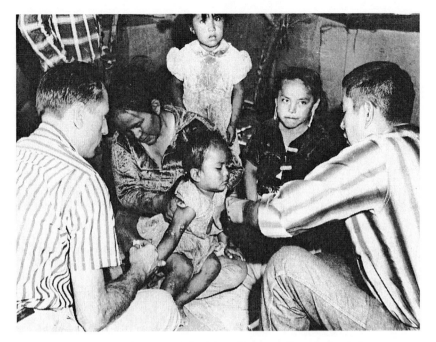

8. House call to a Navajo Hogan. The Many Farms staff worked to bring medicine into the homes of their patients, often struggling against the crowded and impoverished conditions they found. Here, physician David Rabin and health visitor William Crosby examine a young girl with impetigo. (Courtesy of New York Weill Cornell Medical Center Archives, Photograph Collection, Navajo Project #2308.)

plained that the Navajo crowded too many people into unventilated houses. Healthy and sick alike expectorated freely without disinfecting their sputum. Meals were eaten irregularly, and food was poorly prepared. Intemperance, apathy, indolence, and hopelessness all weakened the people. No one sought proper medical attention. Tillim blamed "their lack of intelligence in all things medical." Even Dubos, a critic of the social conditions that spawned tuberculosis, acknowledged that the disease was both "the consequence of gross defects in social organization, and of errors in individual behavior."[17]

The Navajo had different understandings of tuberculosis, something that challenged physicians and health officials. Navajo explanations emerged from traditions that integrated medicine and religion. To protect themselves from the many dangers in their lives, they accepted many prohibitions on their behavior: avoid lightning-struck trees, do not kill bears, do not eat fish, and many others. Disease could be caused by transgressing such taboos, by ghosts, by witchcraft, by animals (including bears, all fish, coyotes, porcupines, snakes, eagles, moths, ants, grasshoppers, and crickets), or by natural phenomena (lightning, whirlwinds). More mundane explanations existed in parallel to these ideas, ranging from old ideas about rapid changes in temperature, to bacon consumed at Fort Sumner, sugar placed in coffee, or "bugs or insects" that consumed Navajo patients. Such ideas puzzled non-Navajo observers. Other explanations, however, rang painfully true. Many Navajo connected tuberculosis to the arrival of white people and to the policies of the federal government. Hoskie Cronemeyer, a member of the Navajo Tribal Council, told Cornell researchers that "It came across the ocean with the white people when they came to this country." Another council member, Annie Wauneka, attributed tuberculosis to New Deal herd reduction and the resulting lack of adequate food.[18] Few physicians would have contested such accusations.

These beliefs shaped Navajo willingness to accept western medicine. When lightning struck a tree near a Tucson sanatorium, the fifty Navajo patients wanted to leave, fearing that the lightning-cursed building would exacerbate their disease. To overcome this, physicians initially tried to dissuade the Navajo from their traditional explanations and convince them of the power of modern medicine. McDermott and his team, for instance, showed the tribal council stained sputum samples that revealed the mycobacteria. He then flew Navajo healers and leaders to New York City to show them how tuberculosis was understood and treated at New York Hospital. Initially McDermott had some success. When Manuelito Begay, a prominent medicine man and council member, saw the tubercle bacillus, he exclaimed, "Today I have met the enemy of the Navajo people." Tribal Chairman Sam Akeah was more impressed by the New York City skyline. Doubts about the bacillus, however, quickly appeared. Begay became skeptical: "They tell me that it is inflicted by a person coughing in your face—that is the way you get tuberculosis in your system. Right away I disagree with it. A person should not be that weak to be susceptible to a man's cough." He reasserted traditional explanations, based on lightning strikes or a failed Wind Chant. He did, at least, praise the value of such dialogue: "Although we do not agree on this, we do recognize one another and that is at least a step forward." Other Navajo also scoffed at medical explanations of tuberculosis. One woman argued that if infected sputum sowed tuberculosis in Navajo homes, then chicken, who constantly pecked at the infected dirt floors, should have been devastated by the disease.[19]

Even as the Navajo resisted medical explanations, they accepted some medical treatments. The Navajo had long exhibited therapeutic opportunism, having incorporated ceremonies from the Pueblo (ritual techniques), Apache (specific ceremonies), Native American Church (peyote), and western medicine. These interactions produced a complex system of diagnosis (hand trembling, star gazing, singing) and treatment (ceremonies, chants, sand painting, body painting, prayer sticks, herbal infusions). Choice of ceremony did depend on the medicine man's understanding of the cause of disease: while the "Shooting Way" was the appropriate ceremony for diseases caused by thunder and lightning, the "Mountain Top Way" was the "treatment par excellence" for illnesses caused by "contact with bears." Despite this Navajo interest in etiology, McDermott's team found the Navajo to be "a very practical-minded people. The way in which results are obtained has less interest for the Navajo than the fact that certain means bring desired ends."[20] The Navajo simply needed to be shown that a given treatment was effective. The problem, of course, was actually achieving efficacy against tuberculosis.

Reforms

If success against a disease followed easily from an understanding of its causes, then the problem of Indian tuberculosis would have been solved. Observers had no difficulty finding many explanations for the increased prevalence of tuberculosis among the Navajo. Overcrowded houses, inadequate food, and ill-advised health behaviors all facilitated the spread of tuberculosis. The Navajo, less impressed with the power of the tubercle bacillus, had their own explanations. Both groups, however, agreed about two things. First, persistent tuberculosis was a symptom of failed economic development. Second, tuberculosis was ultimately the consequence of government efforts to subdue and integrate the Navajo into American society. Like the Sioux, they had been healthy before the arrival of Americans, and they had become sick as a result of specific American policies. As the National Tuberculosis Association noted in 1923, "the advent of the white man created a struggle for existence and subsistence which favored the development of the disease."[21]

The Navajo, however, had at least one major advantage over the Sioux. By the time tuberculosis became the dominant health problem for the Navajo, the federal government had a firmly established tradition of accepting responsibility for the health of American Indians and for providing medical services on the reservations. Enlivened by the enthusiasm of progressive-era reformers, the government quickly increased budgets for Indian health in the early twentieth century. Congress had made the first specific appropriation for Indian health, $40,000, in 1911. In 1921 it passed the Snyder Act, which called on the BIA to fund programs for the "benefit, care, and assistance of the Indians throughout the United States . . . for the relief of distress and conservation of health." Appropriations increased to $596,000 in 1925, $2,980,0000 in 1935, $5,730,000 in 1945, and $17,800,000 by 1955. Although World War I disrupted programs, the BIA succeeded in hiring more medical personnel between 1900 and 1923, growing from eighty-three to two hundred doctors, and from twenty-four nurses to over one hundred. Hospital construction followed suit. The first hospital on the Navajo reservation was built at Fort Wingate in 1889. Many others came in rapid succession: Leupp and Shiprock, 1908; Tuba City, 1911; Fort Defiance, 1912; Crownpoint, 1914; Toadlena and Kayenta, 1926; Tohachi, 1927; and Chinle, 1932. A sanatorium was built at Winslow in 1933. During the 1920s, the Indian Medical Service was formally organized within the BIA. It borrowed professional officers from the PHS, hired public health nurses, and appointed district medical directors. Moving beyond medical treatment, the BIA also pursued disease control, health education, sanitation, and dental services. Tuberculosis was targeted with X-ray surveys and vaccine trials. John Collier encouraged a whole new attitude in the BIA. He insisted that the medical staff not simply impose decisions and practices on the Indians but instead work respectfully and cooperatively with them.[22]

Such efforts were not motivated simply by treaty obligations or humanitarian desires to help a suffering people. Report after report warned of the threat that contagious diseases among American Indians posed to their white neighbors. Indian tuberculosis was an "important reservoir of infection" that threatened both healthy Indians and whites. In 1950 Lewis Moorman warned that "this hotbed of uncontrolled communicable conditions" could not be ignored: "the stage is set for a dangerous seeding of fertile soil with tubercle bacilli from these overfilled reservoirs." James Perkins, managing director of the National Tuberculosis Association, urged Congress to make "extraordinary efforts" against tuberculosis among Arizona Indians, "a health menace to all of the Western States." Federal officials were especially concerned by the large numbers of American Indian migrant farm workers.[23]

Other physicians paid attention to American Indians because of the valuable opportunities they offered for medical research. Herbert Burns wrote that the "Indian, without his knowledge or consent, offers us a human experiment in immunology as well as epidemiology which we can ill afford to ignore." Indians played a crucial role in the evaluation of the Bacille Calmette-Guérin (BCG) vaccine. The vaccine, an attenuated derivative of the tubercle bacillus, had been given to 100,000,000 people worldwide in the 1920s, without any consensus about its value. Researchers needed a large, stable population with a high prevalence of tuberculosis for a long-term field study. American Indians provided the ideal group. Researchers screened 8,240 Pima, Shoshone, Arapaho, Chippewa, Sioux, Thlingit, Haida, and Tsimshian; 1,551 received the vaccine, and 1,457 received saline controls. Twenty-year follow-up showed only 0.84 percent of the vaccinated group had died of tuberculosis, compared to 4.7 percent for the control group.[24]

Many physicians and government officials were pleased with the improving health care they provided to American Indians. The commissioner of Indian affairs in 1920 believed that Indians are "better cared for to-day than at any time in the history of the race." In the 1930s the BIA worked "to better the Indian's health through hospital service, nursing work, immunization programs, clinical work and health education." A tuberculosis program used education, prevention, detection, isolation, and treatment of active cases at sanatoria. Alexander Leighton and Dorothea Leighton, psychiatrist-ethnographers who worked among the Navajo, believed that good health care would be "one of the best means of establishing better collaboration between the Indians and our white society." By 1955, with a health budget of nearly $18 million, BIA officials took pride in their efforts: "The past half century has been one of revolutionary improvement in preventive and curative medicine generally."[25]

Others disagreed. Public health nurse Elinor Gregg found terrible conditions in reservation hospitals in the 1920s. Chinle, for instance, had only "a shabby and derelict hospital which was a boarding-school infirmary with a no-account doctor and a stupid practical nurse." Such complaints had triggered an investigation by the Red Cross in 1924. But when the report documented the overwhelming ineffectiveness of BIA efforts, Commissioner Charles Burke initially suppressed the report, and then simply created a new position for a supervisor of nursing services. Little changed. The 1928 Meriam Report described many problems with hospital facilities on many reservations: Indians had to travel great distances to reach hospitals, they were rarely seen by doctors, and they received poor care. Resultant deaths "cast a shadow over the institution, thus affecting other cases that should come in." Navajo hospitals, in particular, were overwhelmed by the high prevalence of many diseases, especially tuberculosis. The opening of the new Navajo Medical Center at Fort Defiance in 1938 alleviated but did not solve the problems.[26]

By 1950, as a result of the inadequate supply of sanatorium beds, "40% of known active cases of tuberculosis are wandering at large among their own people, each a definite menace to all with whom he comes in contact." This lack was particularly frustrating because the decline of tuberculosis among the general population had left a surplus of sanatorium beds elsewhere. A BIA investigation of Navajo health in 1955 noted "It is ironical that this cesspool of contagion is still unplumbed while tuberculosis sanatoria throughout the country are closing for lack of patients." Because of the lack of beds, "adequate care" was "impossible." Researchers had developed a new treatment, the antibiotic streptomycin, but since this required daily injections, only a "limited number of patients" received it. Preventive services were equally limited. Efforts to identify tuberculosis during the 1930s had turned up thousands of cases each year, but the program collapsed during World War II when half of the BIA medical staff joined the armed forces. Sanitation and other preventive campaigns were also neglected.[27]

Some researchers believed that health programs failed because they did not consider "psychological and cultural factors" among the Navajo. Most, however, felt that even the best, most culturally sensitive health care would have been powerless against the terrible socioeconomic conditions on the reservations. In 1936 PHS officials had argued: "Any great and permanent improvement in health must await some solution of the Indian's economic problem." Inadequate BIA funding only made matters worse. Recognizing these failures, PHS officials in 1957 wrote a scathing critique of past efforts to improve Indian health: "The health facilities are either non-existent in some areas, or for the most part, obsolescent and in need of repair; personnel and housing is lacking and inadequate; and workloads have been such as to test the patience and endurance of professional staff." They had a familiar explanation, tracing past failures "to a gross lack of resources equal to the present load of sickness and accumulated neglect."[28] Regardless of cause, the failure was clear. For nearly fifty years, government physicians and officials had studied the problem of Navajo tuberculosis; funding for the Indian Medical Service had grown dramatically. Yet despite the improvements in health care for American Indians, tuberculosis persisted.

These problems did not go unnoticed. Alarmed by the deteriorating conditions after World War II, three congressional subcommittees visited the reservation in October 1947. They found that lands initially intended for 9,000 Navajo now held over 60,000; per capita income remained below $400. The "alarming degree" of distress and ill health "cries out for immediate relief." William E. Warne, assistant secretary of the interior for Indian affairs, was astonished: "In the United States of today we believe we have mastered these ancient enemies, and generally we have, but not in the Navajo country." This recognition came at a time when most of the country possessed unprecedented optimism and confidence. The United States had created the atom bomb and won the war, it had deployed new antibiotics, and it held two thirds of the world's gold reserves. Empowered by prosperity and faith, the federal government had committed itself to programs for the betterment of populations worldwide. Medical knowledge and technology, mediated by the National Institutes of Health and the World Health Organization, would improve the health of people at home and overseas.[29] These sentiments converged on the Navajo.

Congress and President Harry S Truman acted quickly. In November 1947 a special session of Congress appropriated $2 million for Navajo and Hopi relief. In December Truman described the "emergency situation faced by the Navajos." Congress appropriated another $500,000. A special report on the Navajo situation, the Krug Report, appeared in March 1948. Hearings led to another $1 million in emergency relief. But severe blizzards the following winter led to loss of livestock, hardship, and continued suffering. The Krug Report had argued that improvements in health could only come in parallel with improvements in education and economic conditions. All aspects of Navajo life needed reform: "so long as the Navajos remain on the barren wasteland on which they live, without communities, roads, water, sanitation, or the opportunity to earn a living wage, they must continue to live in squalor and disease." The problems had to be attacked with "a comprehensive plan. The critical conditions now threatening every phase of Navajo life are all interrelated and cannot be successfully dealt with on a piece-meal basis." Such a program could "assist them in becoming healthy, enlightened citizens, capable of enjoying the full benefits of our democracy." The Krug Report called for a $90 million program, of which $4.75 million would be spent on hospitals and health conservation. Congress accepted the demands and passed the Navajo-Hopi Long-Range Rehabilitation Act on 19 April 1950.[30]

Despite this explicit commitment by the BIA to comprehensive, integrated health and economic reform, the ambitions were not realized. Like officials on the Sioux reservations who responded to daunting obstacles by suggesting only superficial reforms, BIA officials implemented the rehabilitation act without vision. Even with the prospect of unprecedented funding focused on the Navajo and Hopi reservations, the BIA pursued traditional programs, especially hospital construction. Of the $4,367,437 appropriated for health services, $1,568,041 (36 percent) was spent on hospital construction, $2,179,073 (50 percent) on off-reservation sanatorium treatments, and only $340,090 (7 percent) on disease control efforts. Although tuberculosis was one of the dominant motivating factors for the congressional appropriations, health care had only received 5 percent of the total funding, and tuberculosis itself received little specific attention. The Krug Report suggested only that "a continuing survey should be maintained, and a central inventory established."[31]

A second attempt to improve health care came in 1955, when Congress transferred the Indian medical services from the BIA, within the Department of the Interior, to the PHS, within the Department of Health, Education, and Welfare, creating the new Indian Health Service (IHS). This was not a new idea. Transfer had been proposed many times during the early twentieth century. Reformers had long argued that it made sense to have all government health services supervised by one agency of dedicated health professionals. Transfer, however, had been opposed by both the BIA and the PHS. In 1923 opponents of transfer argued that Indian medical programs needed to be "closely blended with the educational, social, and industrial problems which concern a race in its critical social and economic transition." Lewis Orme, assistant secretary of the interior, made a nearly identical argument in 1953: "The various service programs for Indians are so closely related that it is deemed inadvisable to separate the administration of the health services from the administration of other services to Indians." Others feared that the transfer would expose American Indians to the vagaries and discrimination of general PHS facilities.[32]

These protests were eventually overwhelmed by officials, physicians, and Indians who had become fed up with the failures of the BIA to improve health conditions. The 1948 Hoover Commission found that the BIA, focused on resource development and not health, "has not yielded a proportionate return on the Government's investment in the Indians as a people." A 1950 American Medical Association report blamed Navajo tuberculosis on both bad living conditions and inadequate medical campaigns, including "inadequate health education, ineffective methods of casefinding, insufficient beds for known cases, haphazard management, plus serious therapeutic deficiencies." This report concluded that "the desired evolution of what amounts to almost a medical miracle cannot be realized under the present administrative methods." Annie Wauneka, testifying to Congress on behalf of the health committee of the Navajo Tribal Council, agreed: "We think there is no real health program. If there is, we haven't heard about it or seen it. And our sick people are paying for it."[33]

Advocates of the transfer believed that the PHS had already proven its value in managing infectious diseases in the general population. The PHS, a professional career service with higher salaries and fully accredited hospitals, could attract better-qualified physicians. It had a long-standing commitment to preventive health programs. Furthermore, as an agency dedicated to health care, it was likely to receive more adequate appropriations than the BIA, which remained mired in political squabbles. The transfer also served other purposes. New Deal activism, especially Collier's efforts to protect American Indians, had angered western conservatives who saw the BIA as an obstacle to land and resource development. Working to assimilate American Indians into mainstream society, congressional leaders in 1953 repealed the special status of Indians with regard to personal property, livestock, firearms, intoxicants, and civil and criminal jurisdiction. Health care came next: transferring the IHS to the PHS. By stripping the BIA of its health care portfolio, which had the greatest public and congressional support, Republicans hoped to diminish the power of the BIA and facilitate their development schemes. The act passed on 5 August 1954 and took effect on 1 July 1955.[34]

Despite the rehabilitation act and the IHS reforms, relief did not come quickly. The 1957 IHS survey found wide disparities between Indians and the general population in both health outcomes and health services. Tuberculosis mortality remained a serious problem: 171.2/100,000 for Navajo and Hopi, versus 10 to 23/100,000 for the general population. Infant mortality, which had fallen to 28/1,000 among the general population, remained 76/1,000 among all Indians and 132/1,000 among the Navajo and Hopi.[35] As had happened for decades, American Indian ill health proved to be a resilient problem. Tuberculosis and poverty persisted despite federal efforts to relieve them.

The struggles by the BIA to improve American Indian health during the first half of the twentieth century left a difficult legacy. The Meriam Report had proposed two standards by which such efforts could be judged: how much the BIA had improved conditions from baseline or how closely the results approached their desired goal.[36] By the first standard, the BIA had done well, improving health conditions in many areas. By the second standard, however, the BIA left much to be desired. American Indian health lagged behind the general population by nearly every measure. Had the BIA done its best, given the very limited funding provided by Congress? Or had it failed in its role as advocate for the Indians to obtain the necessary resources?

The BIA had faced an admittedly difficult task. Many observers, like Dubos, believed that tuberculosis was a "social disease," rooted in Indian poverty and economic nondevelopment. It could only be overcome by "integrating biological wisdom into social technology, into the management of everyday life." He envisioned a new model of medicine, a "hospital without walls" that would manage all aspects of life.[37] However, even as Dubos put forth his vision of social medicine, a new possibility appeared on the horizon: antibiotics. Their emergence in the postwar period renewed hope that a technical, medical intervention might solve the problem of tuberculosis, even in the absence of economic development.

Antibiotics

The rise of medical bacteriology in the late nineteenth century left many legacies for the twentieth century. Two dominant aspects coexisted in tension. On one hand, epidemiologists recognized that social factors determined the patterns of distribution of infectious diseases. This suggested that campaigns against infectious diseases should target key social variables, including poverty, nutrition, and sanitation. On the other hand, bacteriologists identified many of the specific microorganisms that caused infectious disease. This suggested that research efforts should focus on finding specific chemicals that could kill these organisms. Pursuit of such "magic bullets" initially yielded few results. Well into the twentieth century, public health officials had to confine their efforts to social reform. As the experiences of the Sioux and Navajo showed, these officials often struggled in vain against problems rooted in failed economic development. The appearance of new antibiotics after World War II transformed the focus of public health.

The history of antibiotics has been well told. Robert Koch, the discoverer of the tubercle bacillus, proposed one of the first specific remedies, tuberculin, in 1890. Initial enthusiasm quickly gave way to disillusionment as health officials realized that tuberculin could actually cause tuberculosis. More success came with Paul Ehrlich's Salvarsan 606 (arsphenamine), an arsenical compound with some activity against syphilis. Its low potency and high toxicity, however, in the context of the complex social problem of sexually transmitted diseases, limited its impact. Research with therapeutic immunoglobulins had more promise, yielding immunizations against diphtheria and tetanus toxins, and gamma globulins active against streptococcal infections. These were soon overshadowed by antibiotics. In 1932 German researcher Gerhardt Domagk isolated a dye, Prontosil (a sulfa compound), which had impressive activity against a range of bacteria; he reported its first clinical use in 1935. Penicillin, isolated in 1929, was first used in 1941, producing dramatic success against syphilis and many other diseases. None of these drugs, however, demonstrated significant effects against tuberculosis. This changed in 1944 when Selman Waksman published his successful results with streptomycin. Many other compounds followed quickly, culminating with the appearance of isoniazid in 1951. By the late 1950s, physicians had access to powerful medical treatments for tuberculosis. As historians Allan Brandt and Martha Gardner have shown, antibiotics seemed to mark "the fulfillment of 'magic bullet' medicine—the therapeutic cornerstone of the 'golden age.'"[38]

The Navajo, through their collaboration with Walsh McDermott, played a crucial role in this story. McDermott himself had suffered greatly from tuberculosis, after contracting it in 1935 during his residency at New York Hospital. After many months at the Trudeau Sanatorium at Saranac Lake in New York, he returned to his training only to face nine more hospitalizations over nineteen years and the resection of most of his left lung before eventually controlling his own case with isoniazid. This experience had a decisive impact on his career. While at Saranac, McDermott worked in the outpatient clinic, gaining expertise treating syphilis with Salvarsan. On his return to New York City, he chose to specialize in infectious disease and began experiments with Salvarsan and the other new sulfa drugs. His history of tuberculosis barred him from active duty during World War II. Left behind as others went to war, McDermott became head of the infectious disease service at New York Hospital in 1942. This position made him one of the first three civilian physicians given access to the rationed supply of penicillin.[39]

This was an awesome responsibility and a source of tremendous excitement. McDermott had to make daily decisions about which patients would receive the powerful new drug: "I had to go see the patients and decide whether it made sense for the patient to have penicillin or not." The decisions straddled the boundary between treatment and research, between the needs of the patient and the war effort: "the decision was not based on what was good for the patient although that came into it . . . the major portion of the decision had to be what information would we get from this if we give it to this patient. What information will we get which will be of help in our knowledge of penicillin for the [war?] effort."[40]

The experience gave McDermott valuable connections to pharmaceutical companies and to the expanding federal research establishment. The postwar period witnessed a dramatic increase in federal research funding. The budget for the National Institutes of Health grew from $850,000 in 1946 to $12,475,000 in 1948, $81 million in 1955 and $400 million in 1960. Government agencies, especially the National Research Council, began organizing large cooperative trials of new antibiotics, including penicillin and streptomycin. McDermott, exploiting these new opportunities in the late 1940s and early 1950s, conducted laboratory investigations, clinical trials, and field trials with penicillin and many other antibiotics in both New York City and Guadalahara, Mexico.[41]

Tuberculosis remained McDermott's special interest. When streptomycin was introduced in 1945, McDermott's service at New York Hospital was the second group in the United States (after Corwin Hinshaw's group at the Mayo Clinic) given access to the new drug. A second promising antibiotic, para-aminosalicylic acid (PAS), soon appeared. Although streptomycin was clearly an enormous improvement, Hinshaw was concerned that some of its "most dramatic effects have been temporary." By 1951 McDermott could report on five years of experience using streptomycin: it had little power against meningeal tuberculosis (infection of the central nervous system), but it worked well against severe cases of pulmonary and miliary (blood-borne) tuberculosis, where the benefits outweighed the risk of neurotoxicity. As early as 1946, however, researchers recognized that antibiotics bred resistance in bacteria. McDermott's team found that this led to relapse in many patients. Resistance developed especially quickly in cases of miliary tuberculosis, one of the most fatal forms of the disease. Because of the limitations of streptomycin, tuberculosis treatment remained eclectic. McDermott and Hinshaw both endorsed traditional methods, including rest, surgery, and change of environment. McDermott also tested other antibiotics, including PAS, viomycin, and gliotoxin. Charles LeMaistre, working in McDermott's laboratory, led a series of studies with corticosteroids.[42]

Because of concerns with antibiotic resistance, McDermott and other researchers looked for new antibiotics. When allied researchers heard rumors in 1949 that Domagk had developed Conteben (a thiosemicarbazone), a new antituberculous drug, McDermott and Hinshaw were sent to investigate. Evaluating the results of two years of

German experience at 300 hospitals with 7,000 patients, they realized that Conteben had some value, but was too toxic for general use. Its derivatives, however, merited further study. Since the Allies did not acknowledge patent rights for materials produced by German companies during the war, the drugs were brought to the United States for further development. Early results were problematic. One derivative was too toxic for human trials. Another seemed more active and less toxic during in vitro studies; a clinical trial, however, had to be stopped in August 1951 when half of the ten patients developed bone marrow suppression.[43]

New hope came in March 1951 when three companies—Squibb, Hoffman-La Roche, and Bayer—each working independently and in secret, zeroed in on one derivative of Conteben, isoniazid. Hoffman-La Roche began trials in June 1951 at the Seaview Hospital in New York City. Initial results seemed remarkable: patients, filled with energy, danced in hospital corridors. Squibb began trials with McDermott at New York Hospital in November. McDermott became aware of the simultaneous discovery on New Year's Eve Day, 1951, when Hoffman-La Roche approached him to begin further trials. Frustratingly, McDermott and the other researchers lacked an appropriate population of research subjects.[44]

The researchers faced a complicated situation. Studies with sulfa drugs and streptomycin had shown that pulmonary tuberculosis was a poor model for clinical research: its course varied from patient to patient and its clinical criteria, especially chest X-rays, were "highly subjective." One study of X-ray interpretation showed that skilled radiologists and pulmonologists disagreed with each other in nearly one third of cases; individual physicians, examining the same film on two different occasions, disagreed with themselves in over 20 percent of cases. To generate useful data in pulmonary tuberculosis, researchers needed to use the "chance-selection" method to compare new drugs to the existing standard, streptomycin. McDermott believed that two other forms of the disease, miliary and meningeal tuberculosis, provided simpler research models: "Miliary tuberculosis represents the ideal naturally occurring situation for the evaluation of antimicrobial drugs." Its course, fatal if untreated, was "so predictable that its outcome affords an absolute criterion of the success or failure of treatment." McDermott also worried that previous exposure to streptomycin might change the susceptibility of the mycobacteria to the new drug.[45]

Because of these concerns, McDermott sought a very particular research population when he learned of isoniazid: he needed a population with many people suffering from acute military or meningeal tuberculosis, who had not yet received the benefits of antibiotics. Such patients were rare. The recent proliferation of new drugs "had created a serious problem from the standpoint of provision of suitable case material for drug evaluation." Nearly all of the patients on the chest service at New York Hospital were already enrolled in studies. Since the value of streptomycin had already been proven, McDermott believed that he could not ethically withhold it from new patients to evaluate new drugs of unproven value. McDermott anguished over this problem. When he began his first human trial of isoniazid in November 1951, he used only patients already resistant to streptomycin and PAS, knowing that his patients' recent exposure to the effects and side effects of these drugs confounded his evaluation of isoniazid.[46]

Faced with these problems, McDermott complained that "suitable case material on the New York Hospital Service was not available for the immediate large-scale studies." He later described that he had been "looking for an ethnic [ethical?] situation in which we could test the drug."[47] Unbeknownst to McDermott in the autumn of 1951, his ideal research population existed on the Navajo Reservation. Decades of government mismanagement and economic nondevelopment had left the Navajo mired in rural poverty, with an inadequate infrastructure for hygiene, sanitation, or health care. Antibiotics created new opportunities: could this new medical technology defeat the social disease?

Moorman, writing in 1950, had been optimistic: "Considering the acute forms of tuberculosis so often encountered among the Navaho Indians, may we not hope that ultimately chemotherapy will come to our rescue and help reduce the demand for long-continued confinement in sanitarium beds—what a boon to a primitive, undisciplined race accustomed to the chase but not the cure." The Navajo, however, missed out on the initial antibiotics. Health officials had decided that streptomycin, which required daily injections, could not be used widely on the impoverished and sparsely settled reservation. As a result, McDermott found that "large numbers of children and adults with acute forms of tuberculosis were there in circumstances which made the use of streptomycin difficult or impossible." Isoniazid, in contrast, could be given orally. It could be tested, on its own, on patients who had never been exposed to other antibiotics. According to a reporter who covered McDermott's research, the situation "was made to order for the New York Hospital research project."[48]

The Navajo's suitability for antibiotic research, of course, was nothing but a reflection of the disparities in health status and health care that had afflicted their reservation for decades. Although the BIA had long recognized the severe burden of tuberculosis and other diseases suffered by the Navajo, it had been unable to find a solution. The 1950s brought a convergence of new developments, all of which brought new hope to the problem. Congress, finally recognizing the magnitude of the challenges facing the Navajo, had allocated substantial funding for health and economic development. The transfer of the IHS to the PHS brought new expertise to the problem. Isoniazid created new potential for treating tuberculosis, even in the absence of economic development. When McDermott and his team heard about these opportunities, they "rushed out there" and began a ten-year effort to deploy technology against disease, to evaluate the efficacy of antibiotics, and to test the ability of an intensive system of medical care to ensure the "total health" of a population.[49] The outcomes surprised everyone.

8

Experiments at Many Farms

BY THE MIDTWENTIETH CENTURY the Navajo had the highest rates of tuberculosis in the United States. Decades of economic nondevelopment had created a problem that the Indian Health Service (IHS) could not overcome. Many Navajo received no treatment at all. Change, however, would come. Pushed by postwar crises, Congress dramatically increased funding for Navajo relief and development programs in 1950. As government involvement on the reservation increased, the crisis of Navajo health became more visible. The disparities in health status between the Navajo and the general population created a compelling obligation for the government to intervene, and a valuable opportunity for medical researchers.

When Walsh McDermott, a leading tuberculosis researcher, learned of Navajo tuberculosis, he rushed his team to the reservation to begin treatment with isoniazid. Realizing that tuberculosis was but one of many preventable diseases on the reservation, the team set out to create a comprehensive health system, a "hospital without walls" that would take responsibility for the "total health" of the Navajo. McDermott's team sought to bring scientific medicine into a foreign cultural context to help people who died needlessly from disease. The team also planned to use the unique circumstances of the Navajo reservation to demonstrate the efficacy of modern medicine, both the power of antibiotics against tuberculosis, and the power of a medical system against the disease burden of a rural, impoverished society. These ambitious projects became the Health Care Experiment at Many Farms.[1]

The experiments came at a crucial juncture in the history of medical research and medical care. McDermott's faith that medicine could overcome the entrenched health problems of Navajo society reflected the unprecedented optimism of postwar government and science. Inspired by its achievements and empowered by prosperity, the federal government had committed itself to programs for the betterment of populations worldwide. New discoveries, especially of penicillin and DDT, led many Americans to believe that medicine had achieved unprecedented efficacy. The development of oral antibiotics, which allowed outpatient treatment, gave doctors new opportunities, and new challenges, for implementing their confidence. Determined to transform their faith into scientific truth, they committed themselves to demonstrating efficacy through laboratory and clinical research. This pursuit created a new medical world in which every act of treatment simultaneously became an experiment. The results surprised everyone: medical science could not overcome adverse social and economic conditions. As disparities in health status persisted into the 1970s, the Navajo people turned away from their reliance on the government and articulated a new vision of medical self-reliance.

Many Farms

The convergence of interests on Many Farms came unexpectedly. In December 1951 an outbreak of infectious hepatitis struck a Navajo boarding school near Tuba City, Arizona. With 315 of the 417 students sick in bed with fevers and jaundice, the nurse, doctor, and teachers "were wearing themselves to exhaustion caring for the children." They sought aid from the recently established Epidemiological Intelligence Service (EIS) of the Communicable Disease Center (CDC). Created in 1950, the EIS offered expertise and assistance against outbreaks of contagious disease. It sent Charles LeMaistre, one of its first trainees, to investigate. Traveling through blizzards, he arrived on New Year's Day and found "a near panic situation." He conducted careful clinical and laboratory investigations and treated patients with gamma globulin.[2]

Before joining the EIS, LeMaistre had worked in McDermott's laboratory at New York Hospital, studying new treatments for tuberculosis.

During his investigations at Tuba City, he found many adults and children suffering, untreated, with acute forms of the disease. Since the small hospital was full of patients, case-finding efforts had been abandoned. Patients, "luckless individuals," had to be turned away and "sent home to die." When LeMaistre returned to New York to gather supplies for hepatitis, he told McDermott about untreated tuberculosis among the Navajo. McDermott was shocked by the situation. Fortuitously, "unbeknownst" to LeMaistre, McDermott was then in the midst of the secret trials of isoniazid. He had begun trials with Squibb Pharmaceuticals at New York Hospital in November, and had been approached by Hoffman-La Roche that same New Year's weekend. Results were promising, but not definitive. McDermott needed an "ethnic" ("ethical"?) situation to test the drug. He needed patients who had never received antibiotics and could not be treated with streptomycin. The Navajo "provided exactly that situation." As one reporter described, each patient with miliary tuberculosis was "like a human test tube."[3]

McDermott sent LeMaistre back to Tuba City with instructions to work through proper Bureau of Indian Affairs (BIA) channels to arrange an official invitation for McDermott to come to the reservation. The BIA granted McDermott permission to treat a single child with meningeal tuberculosis. He brought a team of researchers from Cornell Medical Center and began working with Charles Clark at the Western Navajo Hospital in Tuba City. They found five patients with meningeal tuberculosis, and two others with miliary (blood-borne) tuberculosis. They treated all of them. Isoniazid gave rapid results: "within a few weeks the new medicines were rescuing desperately sick Navajo youngsters from an otherwise certain death." Their first patient, seven-month old Patty, a feverish, nine-pound "wizened starveling," was afebrile and gaining weight within seventeen days. Elsie and Little Joe were cured and "went to the circus instead of the cemetery."[4]

News of the secret trials in New York and Tuba City reached the media in February. McDermott and other researchers held a news conference that received ecstatic coverage as a victory in the war against tuberculosis. The Navajo "were *immensely* pleased." The tribal council met with McDermott on 3 March. Navajo leaders, "very much interested in expanding the studies," invited McDermott to begin larger studies at the Navajo Medical Center at Fort Defiance, a hundred-bed tuberculosis hospital in eastern Arizona. Working with Carl Muschenheim (chief of the chest service at New York Hospital), Charles Clark, and several others, McDermott began treating patients at Fort Defiance, Tuba City, and the Sage Memorial Presbyterian Mission Hospital in Ganado, Arizona. Squibb provided free isoniazid. On 25 April the council voted unanimously to provide $10,000 to cover expenses. Initially the hospitals were too overcrowded to provide adequate care. In August, however, Fort Defiance received a new medical director, Kurt Deuschle. Deuschle arranged to transfer the healthiest patients to off-reservation sanatoria, allowing him to treat the sickest patients with antibiotics at reservation hospitals. Five patients became twenty-five and then eighty. Isoniazid continued to produce excellent results: "it appears that isoniazid exerts a high degree of anti-tuberculous activity in humans." In 1953 McDermott could tell the Navajo council that the Navajo were among "the first patients in the world" to benefit from isoniazid. The results "have been appreciated around the world." By 1954 Navajo children no longer died from tuberculosis. Doctors "all over the world" looked to the Cornell-Navajo project for the latest information about tuberculosis treatment. Navajo leaders celebrated this "miracle."[5]

Two developments soon pushed McDermott's work in a new direction. First, many patients resisted inpatient treatment of tuberculosis, which required long confinement in hospitals. McDermott and Deuschle responded by enlisting the aid of Navajo leaders and healers. They worked closely with Annie Wauneka, the only woman on the tribal council, who had been appointed to the health committee to convince Navajo patients to accept hospitalization. Educating herself about medical explanations of tuberculosis, she overcame her own skepticism, agreed "to tell my people that only 'white man's medicine' could cure tuberculosis," and traveled to hospitals to convince patients. Such collaboration had many benefits. When Navajo patients fled a Tucson sanatorium after lightning struck a nearby tree, Deuschle had a medicine man from Fort Defiance flown in to sing a purifying ritual: "Anxiety was relieved and peace of mind restored." Although such efforts were successful, McDermott dreamed of an outpatient treatment program, one that could intervene "in the disease process in a typical community, distant from Fort Defiance with its full set of hospital services." He envisioned "a total program for tuberculosis control among the Navajo."[6]

Second, health surveys conducted by McDermott and René Dubos in 1953 and 1954 showed that tuberculosis was the tip of an iceberg. Infant mortality was three to four times the national average. Life expectancy (thirty to forty years) was half the national average. The pattern of disease and mortality was "exactly what one would have expected from the nature of the society": infections caused over 75 percent of all disease; 50 percent of children were infected with tuberculosis by age ten. Health conditions resembled those of the general population "fifty to one hundred years ago," or those found "in less developed countries." McDermott had no difficulty explaining such health conditions: Navajo hogans (their traditional log dwellings) were like "a transfer cabinet in a bacteriology lab—the air of the whole room gets poisoned." To make matters worse, the BIA lacked the focus and expertise needed to solve such health problems. While some physicians were dedicated, others were "poorly trained indifferent misfits." Geographic and cultural barriers limited Navajo access to these services. A "considerable gap" existed between the "advanced knowledge of modern medicine and the application and acceptance of this technology in the community." The "central and most disturbing fact" about Navajo health was that most of their diseases were preventable. McDermott estimated that 97 percent of the Navajo burden of disease could be managed on an outpatient basis. This suggested an "obvious answer": "an adequate field health service" that functioned as the hospital without walls.[7]

The Cornell researchers were not the first to attempt a field health service for an impoverished rural population. Innovative approaches to providing health care to rural communities had been attempted in the American south in the 1910s, in England in the 1920s, in China in the 1930s, and in South Africa and Israel in the 1950s. Instead, the uniqueness of the work at Many Farms came from the self-conscious attempt to tie comprehensive medical treatment to comprehensive medical research. The team hoped to study Navajo diseases and "their possible shaping by Navajo culture." The team wanted to find ways to deliver modern medicine across "formidable cultural and linguistic barriers," while monitoring "the biologic and social consequences of this innovation." They could then apply this information to "people in similar socioeconomic circumstances elsewhere" and to "contemporary U.S. medical problems."[8]

McDermott described his vision at the 1954 tribal council meeting.

The Navajo supported this effort and voted another $10,000 to cover expenses. Sam Akeah, chairman of the tribal council, told how the Navajo were "deeply thankful" for McDermott's efforts and very willing to cooperate. Further assistance came in August 1954 when Congress voted to transfer the IHS from the BIA to the Public Health Service (PHS). The PHS, knowing that it needed small pilot programs to develop innovative new methods for providing health care, supported McDermott's project. Serious planning began in the summer of 1955. McDermott wanted to concentrate all of the effort in an intensive program on a small part of the reservation. With the assistance of Wauneka and John Adair, an anthropologist with long experience among the Navajo, he convinced the council to accept this politically unpopular plan. They chose a small area centered around the communities of Many Farms and Rough Rock.[9]

The Many Farms region provided a microcosm of the challenges facing the reservation. As McDermott explained, "The Navajo stay on their ancestral land and raise sheep, thus overgrazing the land so that it blows away and is subject to flash floods which make the roads impassable so that the children cannot get to school to learn English. Hence, they cannot successfully compete in the world outside the reservation and must of necessity stay home and raise more sheep" (Figure 7) Winter blizzards, summer sandstorms, and inadequate water all made life difficult. Roughly 2,000 people lived in 130 family camps scattered across 800 square miles of mesas and canyons. No villages existed, only clusters of camps around trading posts and missions. Schools provided education through second grade. Sanitary facilities did not exist. Water supplies were often contaminated. Roads were unreliable. Over one third of the Navajo had no private means of transportation, over one third had a horse and wagon, and fewer than 20 percent had a car or pickup truck. With few resources, most depended on government welfare.[10]

McDermott announced his plans on 16 September 1955 at a community meeting in the Many Farms irrigation office, the only building large enough to accommodate many people. Planning and construction proceeded rapidly. Run by a private university, and not by the bureaucracy of the BIA, the clinic was completed in only a few months: "from the local community's point of view, Cornell had produced a building almost by magic." Navajo medicine men purged the building of evil spirits and then, on 7 May 1956, in "a gala affair" attended by

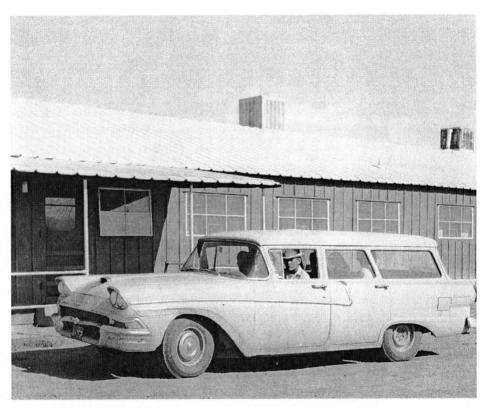

9. The Health care experiment at Many Farms. The Many Farms project provided health visitors with station wagons for house calls and for taking patients to off-reservation hospitals. Here, a health visitor picks up several patients at the project's clinic at Many Farms. (Courtesy of New York Weill Cornell Medical Center Archives. Photograph Collection, Navajo Project, #2305.)

over 1000 Navajo from throughout the Chinle valley, McDermott dedicated the Cornell Clinic at Many Farms.[11]

The small clinic had three examination rooms, a room for basic surgical procedures, an X-ray machine, a fluoroscope, and a clinical laboratory. In 1958 the team added a library, a conference room, and a satellite clinic (in a donated railroad refrigerator car) at Rough Rock, twenty-two miles from the main facility. Daily operations were managed by two resident physicians, three public health nurses, an anthropologist, an office administrator, four Navajo health visitors, two interpreters, and seven other Navajo technicians and assistants (Figure 9). The clinic developed an excellent reputation among the Navajo: "eventually half of the Navaho reservation was pretty well under the care of the Cornell Unit." Operations required "large sums of money," obtained from a variety of public and private sources.[12]

McDermott knew that the project depended on Navajo cooperation. The initial success of the tuberculosis research had made them popular, "we were well known and we were well liked." This enabled Navajo trust and cooperation: "tuberculosis therapy was the entering wedge in setting up a successful medical program in this community." The team worked hard to ensure continuing excellent community relations, working closely with tribal leaders and using former patients as intermediaries. Unlike prior physicians on the reservations, they also took a positive approach towards Navajo medicine men, believing that mutual understanding and cooperation would benefit both groups. McDermott's team met with medicine men in 1953 to educate each other about their health beliefs. McDermott then took a group of Navajo healers and leaders to New York to demonstrate the efforts against tuberculosis on the wards and laboratories of New York Hospital. Such efforts earned their respect and gratitude.[13]

McDermott and Deuschle did worry that supporting medicine men might undermine their own efforts. The opposite happened. Navajo healers came to the clinic with their own health problems. Navajo diagnosticians even referred patients to the clinic for treatment. As one hand-trembler explained, "Sometimes your hand will point where there is a hospital, so you will know that the patient needs to be taken there." Many healers and patients accepted a division of labor, with Navajo medicine men treating the cause of the disease and the Many Farms clinic treating the pain and discomfort.[14] These developments reflected a new strategy against American Indian disease, one in which health programs would be run cooperatively with local groups. Native culture, no longer threatening, could be constructively co-opted.

McDermott did not simply want acceptance. He wanted the health program to be aware of, and involved in, the daily lives of Navajo patients. This would have been impossible without the project's crucial innovation: the health visitor program. The team believed that the reach of understaffed field health projects could be extended by training local assistants. They selected former tuberculosis patients and led them through a four-month curriculum that covered the basic skills and knowledge of medicine and public health, from anatomy to sanitation, dental care, and child health (Figure 10). After a one-year appren-

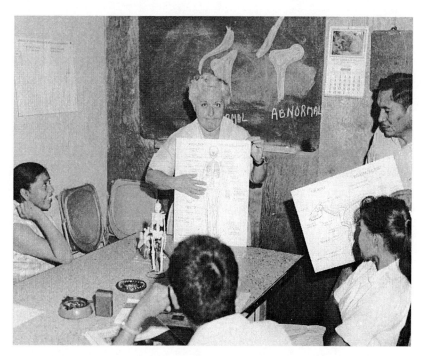

10. Teaching comparative anatomy to Navajo health visitors. To teach medical anatomy to health visitors, clinic staff relied on existing Navajo knowledge of sheep anatomy (obtained from butchering). Since the Navajo traditionally discarded the heart and lungs of sheep, they did not distinguish the two organs with different words. This caused severe problems for medical translation because of the distinct and important roles of the heart and lungs in physiology and pathophysiology. (Courtesy of NewYork Weill Cornell Medical Center Archives. Photograph Collection, Navajo Project, #2303.)

ticeship, health visitors worked independently, but always in close consultation with the clinic staff. Culturally fluent and trusted by the community, they "were invaluable to the clinic staff." They "enabled the medical team to reach out to the home and gather demographic information that could not have been obtained by other means."[15]

McDermott's team also worked to overcome incompatibilities between the Navajo and English languages that had long caused terrible miscommunication. Navajo, for instance, lacked generic words for "color," for short periods of time, or for subtleties and gradations of pain. These linguistic obstacles were exaggerated by what Adair and Deuschle perceived as "the behavior of the stolid and undemonstrative Navajo patient." To overcome this, the Cornell team selected skilled interpreters and trained them in both Navajo and western concepts of disease. They made detailed studies of Navajo descriptions of symptoms, especially pain, even subjecting Navajo volunteers to "a series of painful stimuli" and recording their descriptions. These efforts enabled the physicians to question their patients "with sufficient accuracy to permit the full range of application of modern medicine."[16]

With these arrangements in place, McDermott and his team pursued their many goals. First, they needed information. Researchers had long bemoaned the terrible quality of Navajo demographic data. The BIA's data collection had been confounded by the variability of individuals' names over their lifetimes and the lack of a postal address system on the reservation. An effort to distribute identification numbers had been ignored by most Navajo who were, according to Adair, "not a record-conscious people." To overcome these problems, the team undertook "a constant and prodigious effort to collect this vital statistics data accurately and completely," questioning teachers, missionaries, traders, and community leaders. They developed an innovative patient record system based on clans and family residential camps, which reflected both "the health picture of an individual" and "the health status of the unit as a whole," offering "a compact body of research material based upon social and medical environment." While collecting information about Navajo lives, they also extracted data from Navajo bodies, trying "to acquire complete medical and routine laboratory examinations of all members in the district." They performed physical exams, vision and hearing tests, X-rays, urinalyses, blood counts, syphilis tests, ear, throat, and stool cultures, and electrocardiograms. The team saw this work as a major triumph: they had established a "medical scan" of the Navajo.[17] This success demonstrated the extent to which the Navajo cooperated with the Many Farms researchers.

These efforts "enabled the medical team to carry on sensitive medical research and derive reliable results that would not have been possible otherwise." They published scores of articles on tuberculosis, infant health, Navajo diet, the etiology of diarrhea, cardiac risk factors, accident rates, Navajo income sources, hemolytic anemia, Navajo linguistics, and geographic variations in iron-binding globulins. After the influenza pandemic of 1957 and 1958, the first "within the era of modern virology," they used their access to the Navajo and to Cornell medical students to study the persistence of subclinical infection in rural and urban settings. They also unraveled the puzzle of congenital hip disease. Although the incidence of the disease among the Navajo far exceeded that among the population of New York City (1,000/100,000 as opposed to 3.8/100,000), the Navajo had long resisted conventional surgical treatments. When the doctors tried to study this disease, "our own Navajo staff showed a marked resistance." Anthropologists had more success: "Careful and discreet inquiry" revealed that the Navajo did not consider congenital hip disease a social or physical handicap. They believed that many had actually been made worse by surgery. This demonstrated "the basic principle that what constitutes a 'disease' in one culture does not necessarily constitute a 'disease' in another culture."[18]

This mix of studies, most of which were not therapeutic, highlights a challenge faced by the staff: balancing service and research. McDermott was clearly interested in research, believing that the "actual experiment is fascinating in that it is to take all the capabilities of a university connected medial center and to apply them to the problems of a very poverty-stricken society, to put the two in apposition so to speak, to see what results you get." But he also believed that it "It would not have been ethically appropriate to go in and study the Navahos, so to speak, and then do nothing in return." The "social contract" required a deeper commitment. McDermott also knew that the Navajo would not have cooperated unless "there were clearly visible, immediate benefits." Aware of these tensions, the Cornell team was "entirely candid" about the project's multiple purposes. The Navajo, "in exchange for high quality health services," would be an "instructional medium" for developing "an effective health program under Reservation conditions." The researchers, aided by Navajo leaders, reassured the Navajo that the program was "not an experiment." Wauneka explained that "these methods have been tried elsewhere and shown to be very effective." Deuschle emphasized that "the white man was using the same mode of treatment in his own community as he was using in theirs." Such struggles to justify the balance of treatment and research have occurred wherever modern medicine has encountered the health needs and research opportunities of underserved populations.[19]

Outcomes

Drawn to the Navajo reservation by the opportunities for antibiotic research, McDermott and his team used the wide disparities in health status to justify an elaborate research project. They used Navajo ill health to explore collaboration between medical and social scientists, to develop new approaches to international health assistance, and to test the effectiveness of a comprehensive medical system against the entrenched diseases of rural poverty. These many motivations for the work at Many Farms each generated specific interventions. The outcomes were predictably complex.

The team's work with antibiotics produced the first results, with a promising report published in October 1952. Over the next ten years, they tested the toxicity and efficacy of isoniazid, PAS, pyrazinamide, streptovaricin, and nicotinamide, alone or in multidrug regimens, and published long-term follow-up data. Despite their successes, McDermott remained extremely concerned about the growing problem of antibiotic resistance, weighing the benefits of widespread treatment against the costs of resistance: "since the introduction of isoniazid far more people have died because they did *not* receive the drug than have been seriously affected, one way or another, by isoniazid-resistant tubercle bacilli." Decisions had to be made case by case. He believed that resistance would not become a major problem in New York City, where tuberculosis was declining rapidly. In areas like the Navajo reservation, however, where many infected people lived together, the threat of resistance would be a greater concern. Such fears left McDermott skeptical enough about the power of antibiotics to believe that global eradication of tuberculosis, encouraged by many enthusiasts, remained unlikely.[20]

Some of McDermott's pessimism stemmed from his recognition of a fundamental limitation of the technology of outpatient antibiotics. His team believed that the typical patient "can be assured of a 'cure' if he follows the doctor's instructions." This had been demonstrated with hospitalized patients. But isoniazid, which allowed outpatient treatment, transferred responsibility to the patient. Since "the mere delivery of a therapeutic agent into the hands of the patient is no guarantee that the drug will be taken as prescribed," treatment could be compromised. Although the team had special concerns because they were separated from Navajo patients by language, religion, and understanding of disease, they knew that adherence to prescriptions was a universal problem: "To be faithful in the daily ingestion of a pill appears to be strangely difficult in any society."[21]

McDermott was not alone in this concern. Physicians had doubted the reliability with which patients self-administer medications since the time of the Hippocratic writers. The development of outpatient antibiotics after World War II added new fears to this old problem. Studies among the general population showed that patients rarely finished their prescriptions of penicillin for strep throat. Tuberculosis posed a more serious problem. Since it could be highly contagious, patients who did not complete adequate treatment threatened public health. Furthermore, antibiotics taken irregularly bred resistant bacteria. These concerns justified physicians' anxiety about patient reliability. While McDermott worked at Many Farms, other tuberculosis experts struggled with this problem in London, Hong Kong, and Madras, India. Peter Stradling and Graham Poole found that London patients "left to manage their own drug administration often fail to achieve adequate regular dosage." Wallace Fox, who led the Madras study, identified self-administration as the "major problem of long-term chemotherapy in the treatment of any disease."[22]

These concerns had special significance at Many Farms because of the parallel goals of treatment and research. McDermott had to know whether treatment failure reflected ineffective therapy, the development of resistance, or the failure of patients to take the drug. His team made evaluation of the reliability of self-administration an explicit goal of the project. Tuberculosis treatment, straddling the boundary between medicine and public health, offered a history rich in autocratic precedent. While McDermott worked on the Navajo Reservation, thirty-one states allowed forced isolation and treatment of "recalcitrant" patients. But the Navajo reservation, like much of the world, lacked the resources required for such programs. In some areas, health officials sought a compromise: not incarceration, but directly observed therapy. Stradling and Poole, believed: "Therapy must thus be evolved which, so far as possible, excludes the risk of patient error."[23] McDermott's team, however, did not even have the resources needed for fully supervised therapy.

Since many of the patients were receiving prophylactic treatment, adherence could not be gauged by clinical condition. Some doctors relied on "'clinical intuition,'" hoping to recognize "certain characteristics or personality traits" that revealed "the potentially unreliable patient before treatment is begun." Others estimated isoniazid use by monitoring prescription refills and making spot-checks of pill inventories in patients' homes. All agreed that there was "a pressing need for objective criteria." One solution, "urgently needed," was urine testing. When direct assays for isoniazid proved infeasible on the reservation, the team prepared pills that contained isoniazid and riboflavin, a vitamin that can be detected in urine with a fluorometer. Such preparations "might offer a means whereby the recalcitrant patient who is not accepting medication can be quickly detected." The technique, tested in 1959, successfully differentiated patients who had or had not taken the drug.[24]

The researchers, particularly Thomas Moulding, also developed innovative pill-packaging systems. The simplest placed a one-month supply of pills in a wall calendar. Prominently displayed, the calendar provided both "psychologic gratification" to patients who kept a perfect record, and a reminder to those who forgot. To prevent forgetful patients from discarding forgotten doses, Moulding next developed a clockwork device that "would allow the patient to remove his medication only at the proper time." When this proved too fragile and expensive, he crafted a cylindrical device that patients rotated each day to receive their pills. The regularity of this rotation was recorded in the tracing left on a sheet of film by a radioactive emitter hidden inside. Occasional urine tests revealed the "deception" of patients who removed and discarded pills. These techniques allowed "the physician to know how well his patient has been following instructions and to mobilize that degree of personal or social persuasion needed when it is found that the patient has not taken medication properly."[25]

Such surveillance introduced secrecy, possibly deception, into the patient-doctor relationship. The team feared "a change in the relationship of family and physician from one of trust to one of resentment of a mysterious form of 'inspection.'" Several families, for instance, refused to cooperate with urine testing, afraid that the tests would expose the use of peyote, which had recently been banned by the tribal council. Moulding feared that the "lack of trust" implied by such techniques might "cause sufficient antagonism that patient cooperation would be lost." However, the researchers believed that the only alternatives to surveillance of outpatient treatment were "prolonged hospitalization or running the risk of insufficient therapy." Aware of the dangers, they hoped that the problem could "be managed through careful conduct."

Moulding suggested telling patients that forgetting was inevitable; surveillance simply allowed patients and physicians to be aware of the magnitude of the forgetting.[26]

Forced to rely on the cooperation of outpatients in the campaign against tuberculosis, McDermott's team turned to surveillance and targeted persuasion. Instead of wielding power over hospitalized Navajo bodies, Deuschle and Moulding sought power through acquisition of knowledge about Navajo bodies. They feared, however, that surveillance would erode the trust on which outpatient treatment depended. This dilemma resembles the well-described transitions from autocratic to democratic discipline, from prisons and asylums to mutual community surveillance. In both, progressive desires for community participation gave way to distrust and surveillance.[27]

McDermott's concerns about antibiotic resistance and self-administration did not diminish the magnitude of his team's accomplishments. McDermott believed that the Navajo research made pivotal contributions to tuberculosis treatment. This achievement was widely recognized. In 1955 McDermott and Muschenheim were awarded the prestigious Albert Lasker Award. In 1963 McDermott received the Trudeau Medal of the National Tuberculosis Association, and in 1975 the Kobel Medal of the Association of American Physicians. McDermott and his team were quick to share credit with the Navajo. Accepting the Lasker Award, Muschenheim noted that the "honour of this award is also shared by the Navaho Tribe for contributing from their own funds to the isoniazid study, which was conducted in large part among their people."[28]

The researchers had less success with other aspects of the project. Their small, university-based research program had developed many innovations, which McDermott hoped would be used throughout the IHS. The bureaucratic structures of the IHS, however, resisted these changes. The depth of IHS regulations angered the Many Farms physicians: "Some of the more rigid doctors take on the attitude that 'government' is a mass conspiracy solely invented to keep them from seeing their patients." The health visitor program, invaluable at Many Farms, produced particular outrage among IHS officials. They feared that health visitors, "pseudo-doctors, trained in few weeks" would begin "unlicensed practice of medicine and nursing." At a 1959 meeting in Washington, D.C., one angry IHS nurse argued that the university researchers had failed to make the role compatible with existing IHS structures: "We have thousands of things to consider that you don't; salary levels, tenure, overlap of functions, compatibility of personnel, overall program determinations. Believe me, it isn't easy. In government we have lots of things to consider." Constrained by such pressures, the Many Farms project had little lasting impact on care provided by the IHS.[29]

Similarly mixed results came from their efforts to integrate medical and social science. In the early 1940s, Cornell psychiatrists Alexander and Dorothea Leighton had worked on the Navajo reservation with anthropologist Clyde Kluckhohn, studying the impact of culture on patterns of disease and the provision of medical care. World War II interrupted their work: Alexander Leighton directed the Foreign Morale Analysis Division of the Office of War Information. Joined by Dorothea Leighton, Kluckhohn, Ruth Benedict (who trained Adair), and Tom Sasaki (a sociologist who later worked at Many Farms), this group designed techniques of "psychological warfare" to deploy against the Japanese and joined the United States Strategic Bombing Survey to study "the feelings and attitudes" of Hiroshima survivors. Energized by this work, these researchers saw a broad role for social scientists in the postwar international order. They believed that the turbulence created by globalization created new opportunities: social scientists could help "apply technical knowledge without disrupting the whole fabric of human life."[30]

McDermott and Deuschle, recognizing the importance of such expertise, recruited Adair at an early stage of the project. Although focused on the provision of care at Many Farms, the Cornell team had its eyes on international development. They had studied health assistance programs and realized that many failed because they ignored the local cultures and politics of both donors and recipients. McDermott also knew that physicians and social scientists would have to collaborate to prevent rapid modernization from adversely affecting developing populations: "Unless we can acquire wisdom in this matter, the possibility of actually doing harm through technologic development programs in health is very real." Physicians, nurses, and social scientists would have to "work productively as full partners *from the beginning* of such an enterprise." Social scientists, accustomed to being ignored by physicians, welcomed these overtures.[31]

Some aspects of this collaboration met with success. The Navajo were pleased with the project, especially with their roles in its design and conduct. Adair and Deuschle believed that "from the point of view of the community, we had indeed built a 'Hospital Without Walls.'" Collaboration between medicine and anthropology had "been a basic ingredient in whatever success has been attained." This success served as a model for the growing field of medical anthropology. Tensions, however, did appear. Physicians and anthropologists had to sacrifice their accustomed autonomy to the research goals of the project directors. They debated whether to emphasize treatment (doctors) or prevention (nurses and anthropologists). Since they shared both social and professional lives at their isolated clinic, these tensions had few outlets. This had severe consequences for their mental health: "Anxiety, tension, worry, sometimes augmented by overwork and lack of relaxation resulted in mental stress; a number of the staff had to resort to psychiatric aid to regain their equilibrium." Deuschle and Adair identified these tensions as the largest failure of the program. Despite deliberate efforts, they had failed to pay "sufficient attention to the beliefs, values, and structuring of our own society."[32]

Physicians and anthropologists had been drawn to Many Farms, in part, because of their common interest in international health. The project tapped into the new energy directed towards international health in the postwar period. The creation of the World Health Organization in 1948 inaugurated a period of unprecedented international health activity. Tuberculosis, which had increased dramatically during the war, received special attention: by 1957 the WHO estimated that 60 percent of the world's population was infected. Many officials shared McDermott's excitement that isoniazid would allow outpatient treatment programs. Cold War politics increased the stakes. In his inaugural address in January 1949, President Harry Truman listed health assistance as one of his goals for United States foreign policy. By 1955 the United States participated in health programs in thirty-eight countries. Many concerns motivated these programs, including desire to combat the spread of Soviet influence. The Center for Disease Control (CDC) itself, as well as programs funded by the National Institutes of Health, private universities, and the U.S. military, all grew out of this integration of health care and foreign policy.[33]

McDermott's team, impressed by both the "sheer size of the international technologic development movement," and the "recently developed power to make rapid and truly significant changes in the status of their health," all felt this excitement. The Navajo reservation, "a crude replica in miniature of conditions in many parts of Asia, Africa, and South America," "a Third World country within the United States," provided a convenient model. It "offered a natural, readily accessible laboratory within which to develop procedures and techniques" for international health. McDermott believed that there was "no limit to the use such projects can be put to."[34] His team could study the Navajo to improve the health of similar populations worldwide. Seen in this perspective, the Many Farms project worked the cutting edge of postwar global political development, of a new conception of the United States as an international power. The lessons of American Indian health, once an issue on the periphery of new colonies, became newly relevant as the United States extended its power in a new era of postmodern colonialism.

Many of these hopes were fulfilled. International health planners watched Many Farms closely. Some of the project materials, "some of the designs, etc.—were sent to other places, such as down in Mexico." Many cited Many Farms as a model for tuberculosis control and international health. On the basis of their work, project participants became influential international health advisors. McDermott "became sought after as a world health consultant." Deuschle advised programs in the Dominican Republic, Nigeria, Vietnam, Turkey, Colombia, Jamaica, Mexico, and China. For the rest of his career, McDermott remained committed to broad outreach, "the deliberate extension of a tangible benefit to a larger public, beyond the constituency that is normally served." But he was not naïve. He knew that international health programs faced many challenges: "Any knowledgeable person who is soberly honest with himself knows that international development both at home and abroad has to operate in a dismal swamp of human selfishness, avarice, ignorance, laziness, self-delusive verbosity, and cheap politics of the most undemocratic sort."[35]

Amid these dreams of international health, the basic motivation of the researchers' work among the Navajo had been the desire to treat disease. Their clinical work brought many successes. The Cornell clinic operated from 1956 to 1962. According to the researchers, the clinic and its collaboration between physicians, social scientists, tribal leaders, medicine men, interpreters, and health visitors, "operated harmoniously and productively throughout the term of its existence." Adair and Deuschle believed that the team "enjoyed a splendid reputation among the Navajo." Sixty percent of the population was seen each year. Over ninety percent of the population (2,079 of 2,299) was seen at least once. This high level of utilization made marked impacts in several areas, especially tuberculosis. While the Many Farms clinic operated, there were no deaths from that disease, and its incidence among children declined from 50 percent to 6 percent. This data supported claims that tuberculosis "has, in the past few years, been brought under a considerable degree of control."[36]

The Many Farms team, however, had targeted the full burden of Navajo disease, not just tuberculosis. They knew that the many diseases arose from poverty that created a host of susceptibilities, including malnutrition, overcrowding, and inadequate sanitation. But infused with the confidence of postwar medicine, they had hoped that medical technology would allow them to prevent and treat disease even in the context of rural poverty. The overall data, however, were not encouraging. The incidence of the most common diseases (pneumonia, diarrhea, otitis media, measles, and impetigo) remained essentially constant between 1956 and 1961. Fewer than one third of children received adequate immunizations. Only 54 percent of women had even a single prenatal visit, only 59 percent of births were attended by physicians, and only 23 percent received postpartum care. Since no accurate mortality data existed before the project, it was impossible to determine whether overall mortality rates had changed. However, the incidence of the leading causes of death, childhood pneumonia and diarrhea, had not changed. These failures surprised the researchers: "When one considers our pre-experiment expectations, soundly grounded in the conventional wisdom, these results were clearly disappointing."[37]

McDermott faced a crisis. He had rushed to Tuba City for two reasons: to relieve the suffering of patients who died needlessly and to demonstrate the power of isoniazid. In these he was successful, winning both lasting gratitude from the Navajo and international recognition from medicine and the media. These initial successes inspired the more ambitious project, the implementation of a field health service that would treat the full burden of Navajo disease and test the full scope of medicine's power. McDermott had been confident that the experimental method would validate the efficacy of modern medicine and its power to improve health conditions of even an impoverished society. In this the Many Farms clinic was unsuccessful.

The researchers were not defeated by the outcome. Instead, they reformulated their results to salvage positive lessons from their work among the Navajo. First, they declared that the failure to improve overall health conditions did not indict modern medicine; it simply represented the "gross misfit between our modern medicine and the disease pattern of overly traditional societies." McDermott reminded his readers that medicine made many demands on patient behavior and took certain things for granted, "that somebody has windows in the house and water in the room—things like that." While some diseases, like tuberculosis, could be managed with antibiotics in "slum conditions," others, like infant mortality, required fundamental changes in household conditions and practices. Mothers caring for infants, with dirt floors, no windows, no tap water, and no toilets could only do so much: "It's a little hard say for a twenty-year old mother with three small children and it's 17 below outside and snowing, to apply rules of adequate ventilation, etc. That's the setup, you know. Education isn't a cure-all here." Since living conditions did not improve during the project, the disappointing outcomes could have been predicted. Medical technology might, in theory, be able to reproduce the health benefits of "150 years of dramatic social change," but this would require a *"tour de force,"* with more money, more personnel, and more facilities.[38]

Second, McDermott argued that important aspects of the power of physicians remained untested. Their work among the Navajo gave the Many Farms researchers new appreciation of the complexity of patient-doctor relationships. Armed with the authority of science, doctors had unmatched power to reassure patients who did not have serious disease and to provide hope for those who did. They could provide care in a way that no one else could: "who can measure the value obtained by those Many Farms parents who could see obviously expert professionals hovering over their child, desperately ill with pneumonia caused by respiratory syncitial virus? They see someone making a fight. To point out that, in the particular circumstances, the penicillin the child is receiving happens to be valueless, in a technological sense, would seem a petty, if not callous, irrelevancy." This intangible aspect of medical care, which McDermott labeled "samaritanism," was "extraordinarily difficult to analyze and measure." The Many Farms project had never intended to evaluate this form of care, focusing instead on the evaluation of medical technology.[39]

These attempts to rationalize the failures at Many Farms left fundamental tensions unaddressed. The results led McDermott to proclaim the power of intangible aspects of the patient-doctor relationship. But the surveillance required to ensure adequate self-administration of outpatient antibiotics placed this relationship at risk, introducing distrust between patients and doctors. Physicians faced a potentially difficult choice. They could assist patients with technology and with expert reassurance, but these two aspects of physician power sometimes existed in tension. Even as medical technology provided new tools for diagnosing and treating patients, thereby improving physicians' ability to provide reassurance, technology eroded the intimacy of patient-doctor relationships. By reducing the importance of physical exams, or by requiring systems of surveillance, new technologies erected barriers between patients and doctors.

McDermott's many dreams for Many Farms remained elusive throughout the remainder of his career. He never doubted the fundamental power of medical technologies, always maintaining a "profound sense of wonder" at the power of antibiotics. As he described so compellingly, antibiotics had transformed once-fatal diseases, notably pneumonia and tuberculosis, into treatable, outpatient conditions. He believed that physicians could take these antibiotics into the most challenging conditions of urban slums and rural poverty and cure once-formidable infections. But instead of defining a central role for physicians in international health, the research at Many Farms showed that physicians and their technologies were actually ill-suited for the health needs of most of the world's populations. In settings of extreme poverty, where basic standards of hygiene and sanitation did not exist, public health and skilled nursing could provide more appropriate, and realistic, care. An intensive and powerful system of medical care, taken for granted by most people in the United States, remained an unattainable and inappropriate luxury for others.[40]

Taken together, the health care experiments at Many Farms revealed the power and limitations of postwar medicine. Physicians had developed great confidence in their many new treatments and had committed themselves to rigorous analyses of efficacy. Every medical act became an experiment, from a physician optimizing a patient's antibiotic regimen, to the formal structures of clinical trials. But nearly every time that clinical studies validated the efficacy of therapies, clinical experience showed that substantial obstacles hindered their deployment. Postwar medicine had also witnessed the proliferation of new health care needs and resources: new expectations of expanded access to health care in the United States and new excitement about improved international health were matched by increased health care funding, through Medicare, Medicaid, and international development programs. These new demands and new opportunities left physicians obligated to subject their medical systems to trials of their efficacy. But even as thousands of studies combined to create a vision of conglomerated power, lingering questions remained about the contribution of medicine to the health of societies.[41]

Aftermath

Although McDermott and his collaborators reduced some of the disparities in health status and were immensely productive with their research, they did not meet their own expectations for relieving the Navajo burden of disease. One central aspect of the Many Farms project limited its potential success: although McDermott's team had accepted responsibility for the "total health" of the Navajo, they did so for only six years. While the Cornell Clinic operated, it shouldered the federal government's obligation to provide health care. When the experiment and its clinic ended, this responsibility reverted to the government.

The Many Farms team did not pack up and leave abruptly. The project had planned to operate from 1956 to 1960; a two-year extension lasted until 1962. Clinical services were gradually transferred to a new clinic at Chinle. Only fourteen miles away, with three doctors, dentists, and public health nurses, the Chinle clinic "provided good health care." Starting in the fall of 1960, the Many Farms clinic closed one day each week. In 1961, with the road to Chinle newly paved, the clinic closed two days each week. When the Many Farms clinic closed permanently in 1962, it marked the end of a careful transition. As McDermott remembered, "there were many community meetings so that the people knew exactly when we were going, how we were going, why we were going, etc., and what was taking our place. There was no 'pulling the rug out from under them' or anything like that. They knew to the full what was happening and appreciated it, so that as far as I know our reputation is still good in those parts."[42] The team had relinquished its responsibility for Navajo health.

No simple summary can do justice to the project's many outcomes. The Many Farms team defined the challenges of providing health care on the reservation and proposed many innovative solutions, but few of them outlived the project. They took credit for the decline of tuberculosis, but admitted that they had minimal impact against other leading causes of morbidity and mortality. They claimed success at collaborative research, but knew that they had not adequately managed many tensions. They believed that health care systems could be customized to the socioeconomic and disease substrates of specific populations, but they suspected that their methods of surveillance and persuasion threatened patient-doctor relationships.

Although these lessons had little direct impact on the IHS, they had a lasting impact on the researchers. McDermott remembered his time at Many Farms as "one of the truly important events of my life." It redirected his interests from laboratory and clinical research to local, national, and international public health. It established his reputation as an expert on health policy, earning him influential positions in academic medicine and government. As he later reflected, "I always say that the Navaho studies was like Henry Thoreau who went to Walden Pond and generalized about the world and we went to many ponds and I find myself telling the Republic of India how to handle its affairs or something on the basis of what went on there with the Navaho." He also continued his interest in American Indian health long after the project ended, chairing President Lyndon Johnson's Task Force on American Indians and reviewing health programs for the Association of American Indian Affairs.[43]

Many Farms had similar influences on other participants. Deuschle became a pioneer in the new field of community medicine. Chairing departments at the University of Kentucky and then at Mt. Sinai School of Medicine, he implemented the lessons of Many Farms in the impoverished Appalachian highlands and the urban ghettos of New York City. Moulding continued his campaign against noncompliance, advocating urine testing, pill calendars, and radioactive pill dispensers in domestic and international settings. Muschenheim, "outraged" by the health conditions of American Indians, worked as an advocate for Indian health for twenty-five years. René Dubos used the Navajo to illustrate the impact of social change on the health of societies. Abdel Omran, who led studies of accident rates at Many Farms, became a leading theorist of the "epidemiological transition" from underdeveloped to developed societies. Adair continued to work among the Navajo and Zuni long after the project ended, returning to the reservation "in his frail old age" to receive a Navajo blessing ceremony.[44] The postproject successes of the researchers made lessons learned in the local community of Many Farms widely influential in the medical and public health campaigns of the United States.

The Navajo did not reap similar benefits from their participation at Many Farms. Initial outcomes looked promising: a satisfactory health care system had been created for the first time. Its success against tuberculosis fueled excitement that the disease might be eradicated, even from American Indians. Other diseases decreased as well, with reduced disparities for infant mortality, maternal mortality, and gastrointestinal diseases. Observers credited much of this improvement to the revamped IHS: during its first decade under PHS control, it expanded from 125 to 300 physicians, assisted by more nurses and better hospitals. McDermott saw other explanations. Returning to the reservation for a reunion in November 1977, he found it "just unrecognizable." He was most impressed by overall improvements in reservation infrastructure, especially the success, made possible by plastic pipes, of bringing water into Navajo homes.[45]

Despite such changes, American Indian health remained poor. Parity with national standards had not been reached. Age-adjusted mortality exceeded the national average for pneumonia, influenza, and tuberculosis. There had been little progress against diabetes, cancer, or alcoholism. The fundamental causes of ill health, it turned out, had not changed. As described by IHS director Everett Rhoades in 1990, "Indians are poorer, less educated, and live in less satisfactory surroundings" than the general population.[46] Health disparities would persist as long as underlying inequities continued.

The Navajo responded to the continuing disparities by attempting to take matters into their own hands. In July 1970 President Richard Nixon had articulated a new vision of Indian self-determination: "The time has come to break decisively with the past and to create the conditions for a new era in which the Indian future is determined by Indian acts and Indian decisions." Motivated by Nixon's call for self-determination, the Navajo Tribal Council voted in June 1971 to create an American Indian medical school. They petitioned Elliot Richardson, secretary of the Department of Health, Education, and Welfare (HEW), to conduct a feasibility study. As Annie Wauneka wrote, "we call on your Department to help us obtain a full commitment of the Federal Government to provide us with an American Indian Medical School which will give our people the necessary training at all professional levels and the essential tools and facilities to accomplish the paramount objective—the care by Indians of our peoples' health." In March 1972 Richardson's commission endorsed these plans. The tribal council established the Navajo Health Authority in June.[47]

To support its call for an American Indian medical school, the Navajo Health Authority issued a press release that documented the persistent disparities in health status. The "health status of the Indian today is comparable to that of the U.S. as a whole 20 to 25 years ago." Life expectancy among the Navajo was only two thirds the national average (forty-seven versus seventy-one years); infant mortality one and a half times the national average; diabetes two times; suicide three times; accidents four times; tuberculosis fourteen times; gastrointestinal infections twenty-seven times; dysentery forty times; and rheumatic fever sixty times. Eighty percent of the Navajo had no running water or flush toilets. Sixty percent had no electricity. Meanwhile, from a population of over one million American Indians, there were only two full-blooded Indian physicians and thirty-six physicians of Indian descent. These conditions were unacceptable: "For too long, American Indians have lived in shockingly poor health." All other aspects of Indian life had been neglected: "On practically every scale of measurement and according to most social indicators—income, education, housing, health, employment—the Indian is at the bottom." Although the United States had signed the charter of the World Health Organization in 1948, which declared that "good health is a fundamental right of every person," the government "had failed in its many attempts to apply this principle to benefit its own American Indian citizens."[48]

The Navajo believed that the terrible health conditions had been exacerbated by poor health care, especially *the inability of practically all medical personnel to relate their knowledge and skills as health professionals in a manner which would be received by Indian patients.* The message was clear: "It is obvious that *the old methods have failed* to meet the needs of Native Americans." The Navajo Tribal Council moved quickly with its plans to build its own medical school. With approval from HEW, it set aside land and money for the school and searched for a dean. The $30 million center would provide undergraduate clinical medical education, residency programs, continuing education, and training for other health personnel.[49]

The medical school was part of the tribal council's broad vision of Indian autonomy: "the day will soon arrive when more than just 2.4% of HEW's Indian health programs will be run by Indians. The day will arrive when a more effective health-care delivery system utilizing Indian professionals will replace the current system. The day will arrive when the American Indian will determine what his own health standards and services should be." For nearly five centuries, American Indians had faced the diseases and health care of Europeans and their descendants. Indians had survived both: "Indian history has proven to be more than a record of being oppressed, brutalized and exploited; more than a record of prolonged failures, broken treaties and promises, deprecation and deprivation. The Indian record is one of having overcome these obstacles, of endurance and of survival. With this in mind, all Indian tribes, together and as a united group, can meet their own health needs in a manner which will be consistent with their desires."[50]

These ambitious plans reflected Navajo frustration with decades of failed attempts to improve health care and relieve ill-health. For nearly a century, researchers had documented and explained the increased morbidity and mortality experienced by American Indians. The twentieth century had brought a remarkable expansion of government involvement in health care, funding medical services, medical research, and international health. Yet even the remarkable convergence of motivations and resources at Many Farms had failed to reduce the dominant causes of morbidity and mortality. Although the IHS gradually reduced absolute levels of disease on reservations, disparities between the health of the American Indians and the general population persisted. This left the Navajo unsatisfied: persistent disparities in health status stood as proof of the lack of efficacy of the government and its physicians. Self-reliance seemed a better option. Emboldened by the movements for American Indian self-determination in the 1970s, they set out in pursuit of their own effective health care.

Epilogue and Conclusions

IN THE EARLY YEARS of colonization, many American Indians interpreted their relative vulnerability to epidemics as evidence of European control over epidemics. They asked the English to unleash epidemics against their own enemies. For centuries they continued to believe that European and American physicians had considerable power over diseases and welcomed their efforts to provide medical care. But by the late twentieth century the persistent disparity inspired opposite conclusions about medical power over disease. Despite decades of effort by the federal government, Indian ill health continued. Frustrated by continuing disparities, the Navajo Tribal Council reached a new understanding: *"the old methods have failed."*[1]

In the 1970s the Navajo responded with a dream of medical autonomy. They believed that Navajo health problems would only be solved by Navajo action: the Navajo needed their own training program for their own doctors. They "resolved to create their own health professionals in their own medical schools." Preliminary efforts began quickly. The Navajo Health Authority established an Area Health Education Center, funded by the National Institutes of Health, in cooperation with the University of New Mexico College of Medicine. It offered a range of undergraduate and graduate training programs in medicine, nursing, and other health sciences. These programs received funding from the W. K. Kellogg Foundation and the Macy Foundation.[2]

221

The Health Authority's greatest ambition remained a medical school. A pan-Indian medical school would serve "as *a model for the American Indian community*" and finally provide "equal health rights to all." The Authority hoped to build the $30,000,000 center by 1977. But self-reliance had its limits: since the tribal council could provide only $50,000 each year, the Health Authority needed substantial additional funding. It sought aid from its old friend Walsh McDermott. Since 1972 McDermott had worked as the special advisor to David Rogers, president of the new Robert Wood Johnson Foundation (Rogers had worked in McDermott's lab at New York Hospital and collaborated on Indian health projects). Though sympathetic to Navajo concerns, the foundation chose not to provide funding. The medical school was never built. Despite the failure of its greatest ambition, the Navajo Health Authority did succeed in establishing collaborative training programs with many institutions that prepared American Indian students for careers in medicine and trained non-Indian health professionals to provide care to Indian populations.[3]

Although the dream of self-sufficiency went unfulfilled, it represented a crucial development in the history of American Indian health care. When Europeans arrived in America, they found populations long accustomed to taking care of themselves and their diseases. In 1633 Paul Le Jeune had mocked a Montagnais sorcerer's treatment of a feverish boy, suggesting that the boy "must be left to rest, and not be killed by this great noise which makes him worse." The sorcerer disagreed: "'That is very good for you people; but, for us, it is thus that we cure our sick.'"[4] Nearly four hundred years later the Navajo Tribal Council asserted a similar ideal of self-reliance. Had American Indian health come full circle? Not at all.

Every aspect of American Indian life had been transformed by the arrival of Europeans. The Navajo vision of health care in the late twentieth century bore little resemblance to its initial condition when Spanish soldiers and missionaries first arrived in the southwest. The Navajo sought to organize their own medical school, but this medical school would not have been based on traditional Navajo medicine. Instead, it would have taught a curriculum of scientific biomedicine that resembled the curriculum of any medical school in the United States. The curriculum, however, would adapt biomedicine to Navajo needs, incorporating Navajo values and medical practices: "It will be fully accredited and will include both modern medical education and native healing practices."[5] The trajectory of Navajo health care was not a full circle, but rather a spiral, returning toward initial conditions but with irreversible historical changes.

Other spirals characterize many aspects of American Indian health and health care. By the year 2000, American Indian populations had survived a cycle of demographic collapse and recovery. Over four million Americans claimed Indian ancestry, a population arguably larger than had existed before Columbus. But while the size of the populations had been restored, they had undergone crucial changes. Most American Indians now have a mix of Indian, African-American, and European-American heritage.[6] Identities, both genetic and cultural, have been fractured. Lives and societies, now being reconstructed, will always bear evidence of this history.

Patterns of disease have undergone similar transformations. Pre-contact populations suffered from a variety of degenerative and parasitic diseases that reflected their hunter-gatherer and early agricultural life. When Europeans arrived, they brought with them a series of acute infections that had thrived in the urban centers of Europe: smallpox, measles, influenza, and many others. These epidemics spread through American Indian populations as the frontier of European contact and influence spread throughout the Americas.[7] Over time these epidemics faded away, only to be replaced by tuberculosis and other diseases that thrived in the squalor of reservation life. Tuberculosis, in turn, passed as well. By the late twentieth century, the populations again faced chronic diseases that reflected their modes of living: heart disease, diabetes, obesity, and the other so-called diseases of civilization. Whatever the prevailing disease, American Indians suffered more severely than their European and American observers. This persistent disparity stands as stark testimony, not to the inherent susceptibility of Indians to specific diseases, but to the ability of disparities of wealth and power to generate disparities in health regardless of disease substrate.

Changing patterns of disease demanded changing patterns of explanation. Century after century colonists and their descendants tried to understand the etiology of epidemics and their patterns of distribution. They always struggled to rationalize the suffering they observed. Some themes held constant. Observers assigned disease to intrinsic characteristics, individual choices, and extrinsic forces. The details, however, changed, from concern with religious practices and stolen blankets, to emphasis on socioeconomic conditions and genetic susceptibilities. Whatever the specific hypotheses, observers always generated an over-abundance of explanations of Indian demise. They could then pick and choose, emphasizing whichever explanations had the greatest meaning and utility.

The disparities in death and disease between American Indians and other groups required specific explanations. If God sent disease against both colonists and Indians, then God seemed to play favorites. If the misbehaviors of all people left them susceptible to disease, then Indians made particularly poor choices. While all individuals had constitutional susceptibilities to disease, Indians were peculiarly vulnerable because of their history of gentler natural selection. Whether explanations emphasized religion, behavior, or evolution, American Indians always suffered more, and were always deemed responsible for their suffering.

Efforts to provide medical care endured just as persistently as the disparities themselves. Edward Winslow treated Massasoit's constipation, James Kenny bled Delaware patients, and Kurt Deuschle brought isoniazid to the Navajo. The meanings and associations of these efforts, however, always changed. Early colonists acted out of compassion and Christian duty. Nineteenth-century government officials worked to meet treaty obligations. By the twentieth century health officials began to fear the consequences of untreated disease among American Indians, a "reservoir of infection" that threatened everyone. As parallels between the plights of American Indians and developing peoples worldwide became increasingly clear, health care on the reservations became a model for international aid. Provision of health care served the needs of patients, public health, and international development.

Persistent disparities in health status also allowed use of American Indian disease for medical experiment. Curious investigators from Thomas Jefferson to Walsh McDermott co-opted Indian ill health and vulnerability. As the desire to experiment persisted, its meanings and expectations evolved, from incidental observations of medical treatments, to sustained efforts to design and improve whole systems of medical care. The meanings of such research also changed and remain difficult to assess. Research populations have often suffered in the name of science, but some likely benefited, from Miami chief Little Turtle to Navajo child Little Joe.[8]

As diseases and motivations changed, so did the capacities and claims of medical intervention. Inoculation instrumentalized disease: small-pox, once the domain of providence, became a tool for medicine or the military. New understandings produced new treatments, from vaccination to antibiotics. New technologies, in turn, required new and more complicated medical systems. These appeared slowly among the villages and reservations of Indian country where physicians often struggled unsuccessfully against Indian diseases. As late as 1960 McDermott admitted defeat, acknowledging the "gross misfit" between modern medicine and Indian medical needs. But by 1989 the United States Public Health Service claimed great success against disease, arguing that its efforts since 1955 had reduced tuberculosis by 96 percent, infant mortality by 92 percent, pulmonary infections by 92 percent, and gastrointestinal infections by 93 percent. Although parity with the general population had been not achieved, the gap continued to narrow.[9]

Efforts to relieve these disparities have been but one part of the changing relationships between American Indians and the colonial and federal governments. Colonists and their descendants have tried to annihilate, extrude, contain, preserve, incorporate, and assimilate Indians. Provision of health services for American Indians has changed from a treaty obligation, to gratuity appropriations, to a fiercely contested item on the federal budget. After 1970 federal ideology moved from termination of the special status of Indians to empowerment and self-determination. Policies sought to preserve their autonomy, while increasing their social and economic connections to general society. Meanwhile, the realities of shrinking budgets in the 1990s threatened to turn self-determination into self-reliance. Confronting this mixed legacy, the Bureau of Indian Affairs (BIA) acknowledged that the American Indians had many reasons to distrust the federal government. In September 2000, on the 175th anniversary of the BIA, Kevin Gover, assistant secretary of the interior for Indian affairs, admitted that "the works of this agency have at various times profoundly harmed the communities it was meant to serve." He realized that he could not ask for forgiveness, and instead asked only that "we allow the healing to begin": "Together, we will face a challenging world with confidence and trust."[10] He wanted the legacies of past failures to inform work in the future, not prevent it.

Persistent health disparities, contested funding, and calls for renewed trust all reflected unfulfilled needs. American Indians continued to experience the worst health outcomes of any population in the

United States. The median age at death among some populations was as low as 44. Infant mortality on some reservations remained 2.6 times the national average. As American Indians moved into cities, they faced deteriorating health conditions. Infant mortality in some urban groups actually increased during the 1980s. Rural Indians remained the most disadvantaged of all, suffering elevated rates of mortality from heart disease, diabetes, injuries, and cancer. The federal government, meanwhile, struggled to provide an adequate supply of physicians, making special efforts to recruit American Indian health professionals.[11] But these efforts simply raised deeper discontents. Health disparities have never yielded to the provision of more doctors and more medical services. American Indians have remained the least healthy population, just as they have remained the least wealthy. Meanwhile, the quest to provide Indian doctors for Indian patients reflected old and conflicted ideologies about the value of incorporating American Indians into the general population or preserving them as a distinct minority.

American Indian discontent and federal dreams of self-determination and self-reliance converged to motivate American Indian desires to take their health into their own hands. The Navajo Health Authority failed in its dream to establish its own medical school. But in 1975 Congress passed Public Law 63–638, the Indian Self-Determination and Education Assistance Act, which allowed American Indians to manage and operate their own health care programs through block grants and subcontracting. Instead of relying on the Indian Health Service (IHS), tribes could take their share of federal money and spend it on their own health as they saw fit, hiring their own doctors, running their own clinics, or contracting with private health care providers. By 2001 50 percent of all IHS appropriations were administered by individual tribes. Other laws provided more money for scholarships, research, and health care, hoping to bring Indian health into parity with the general population. But funding quickly stagnated. In 2001 per capita health spending for American Indians was only $1,351, compared to $3,766 for the general population. Meanwhile persistent economic non-development kept most Indians living in either rural or urban poverty.[12]

The advent of American Indian casinos has further destabilized the politics of American Indian health. Indian gaming emerged as the unanticipated convergence of diverse political interests: old legal precedents of tribal sovereignty, federal interest in reducing Indian dependency, state needs for new tax revenues, ill-defined BIA standards for conferring tribal status, loopholes in state gambling laws, and the tremendous political power of lobbying and advertising made possible by vast casino profits. Legalized by the 1988 Indian Gaming Regulatory Act, Indian casinos grew quickly, from 14 in 1990 to 290 in 2002. Casinos have been an economic windfall: income has increased from $100 million in 1988 to $12.7 billion in 2002. Foxwoods, the largest casino in the world, produced $1.5 billion each year for the 635 members of the Mashantucket Pequot tribe. Each member of the Skakopee Mdewakanton Dakota in Minnesota reportedly earned $1 million each year; unemployment on their reservation fell from 70 percent to 4 percent. These profits were often funneled into improved schools and health services. Such successes, however, were rare. Most profits came only to the handful of casinos situated near population centers: 13 percent of casinos accounted for 66 percent of the take. Typically 40 percent of all profits went to non-Indian investors. Since many casino jobs went to non-Indians, overall unemployment on reservations with casinos actually increased, from 54.0 percent in 1991 to 54.4 percent in 1997. Poverty in counties with casinos only decreased slightly, from 17.7 percent to 15.5 percent. Despite even the extraordinary profits of Foxwoods, the Mashantucket Pequot faced enormous debts. Meanwhile half of all tribes chose not to open casinos.[13]

Although many tribes have benefited, the development of American Indian gaming could prove a catastrophe for American Indian health. Public perception of American Indians as gambling moguls might dissolve the obligation felt by Congress to provide care for them. This could end the support crucially needed by the majority of tribes that have not shared in the casino windfall. This threat comes at a time of increasing pressure on state Medicare and Medicaid budgets.[14] If misperception of Indian self-reliance on casino revenues leads Congress to decrease support for American Indian health care, while most reservations remain in poverty, then the future of Indian health could be bleak.

The connections between economic nondevelopment, political disadvantage, and health disparities have not been unique to American Indians: similar problems have afflicted indigenous populations worldwide. Stephen Kunitz has shown that wherever indigenous people (and health data) exist, they have less money, worse health, and shorter lives

than their nonindigenous compatriots. These disparities are the legacies of specific policies that have undermined the health of indigenous
populations. Australia, for instance, long left aboriginal affairs to local
governments, where mining and property interests won out over humanitarian concern for aboriginal health and welfare. Since 1967 the
Commonwealth government has taken increasing responsibility for aboriginal affairs, but this has simply led to overlapping jurisdictions, dif-
fused responsibility, and lost funding. South African populations face
the legacy of apartheid health policies that, compounded by poverty
and malnutrition, produced a 1990 infant mortality rate of 48.3/1,000
among blacks compared to 7.4/1,000 among whites. Efforts to relieve
these disparities, initiated in the new South Africa by Nelson Mandela,
have been hamstrung by shrinking budgets and the growing burden of
HIV.[15]

Faced with widening disparities in health status in the decades after
decolonization in the 1950s and 1960s, the World Health Organization (WHO) produced the Declaration of Alma Ata in 1978. Defining
health as a "fundamental human right," the WHO protested health
disparities: "The existing gross inequality in the health status of the
people particularly between developed and developing countries as well
as within countries is politically, socially and economically unacceptable." The declaration articulated a vision of universal primary care
(health education, nutrition, sanitation, immunization, maternal and
child health, treatment of common diseases) and community participation: "people have the right and duty to participate individually and
collectively in the planning and implementation of their health care."
This began the campaign for "Health for All by 2000."[16]

Such idealism contributed to considerable success at improving health
status worldwide. Infant mortality decreased from 124/1,000 in 1960 to
59/1,000 in 1997. Life expectancy increased from 48 years in 1955 to
65 in 1998. Kerala, a province in southwestern India, produced remarkable gains despite having one of the world's lowest per capita in-
comes (1/100 that of the United States): infant mortality fell to 13/
1,000, while life expectancy reached 69 for men and 74 for women.
This was achieved through land reform, redistribution of wealth and
political power, public food distribution, large-scale public health programs, accessible medical care, and widespread literacy. Yet stark disparities persisted. Infant mortality in the world's fifty poorest countries

in 2000 was 171/1,000 and life expectancy only 52 years. The WHO responded by articulating a new vision, "Health for All in the 21st Century." But this will be elusive while poverty remains entrenched and poor countries spend as little as five dollars per person per year on health services. Even where health services have been provided, they have often become mired in local economic, military, and political interests.[17]

The successes and failures of international health cast an interesting light on health disparities that persist in the United States. Despite continuing reductions in overall mortality in all ethnic and socioeconomic groups, many disparities in health status between rich and poor and between white and minority populations have increased over recent decades. African Americans and American Indians have worse health outcomes than poorer people in China, Costa Rica, or Kerala. Much of this can be attributed to an inequitable distribution of economic resources. The persistence and growth of these health disparities led Surgeon General David Satcher to make health disparities a major focus of federal health policy. The "Healthy People 2010" initiative of the Department of Health and Human Services, launched in January 2000, had two stated goals: first, to improve "quality and years of healthy life," and second, "to eliminate health disparities among segments of the population, including differences that occur by gender, race or ethnicity, education or income, disability, geographic location, or sexual orientation." It planned to pursue these goals through health education, advocacy of healthy behaviors, and provision of helpful health care services.[18] These modest measures fell far short of the efforts needed to achieve success in Kerala.

Successful efforts to improve health conditions have shown that substantial political will and social activism can overcome serious economic obstacles and produce good health.[19] The ability of the IHS to improve health conditions on the Indian reservations over the past fifty years, despite continuing economic nondevelopment, is an impressive accomplishment. But the disparities in health status persist. Will continuing political and social action, such as the "Healthy People 2010" initiative, bring equity to health conditions in the United States? Past experience in the United States, especially with minority health and health care, has shown that the needed political will and social activism seldom exist. Will economic development eventually bring improved health conditions to American Indians? The prospect at present seems bleak. Casinos may bring wealth to some tribes, improving socioeconomic conditions, but they are far from a cure-all. They may end up extracting a greater cost by undermining political will to intervene on behalf of American Indians.

Casinos are but the latest in the long series of developments that have been used by everyone from colonists to congressmen to reduce their obligations to cure American Indian ill health. Ever since their earliest contacts with Europeans, American Indians have been relatively disadvantaged in many crucial respects. This has been reflected in worse health outcomes, from smallpox to diabetes. These disparities in health status have been observed and recognized, in the journals of bewildered colonists and the demographic reports of government officials. They have been rationalized as the consequence of divine wrath, natural selection, or adverse socioeconomic conditions. Such explanations have always suggested possible interventions, both opportunistic and therapeutic. The implementation of such interventions has always depended on the motivation of those who have observed health disparities, on the obligation that they have felt for those who suffer.

Motivation and obligation have been extremely fragile. Any local context that makes the ill health of others an asset, from the need to acquire new land to the need for research subjects, can undermine the desire to intervene. Any explanation that attributes disease or disparity to the misbehavior of its victims creates moral distance between those who could help and those who need help. Even such progressive ideology as the call for American Indian self-determination and self-reliance will allow the general population to relinquish its responsibility for the burden of morbidity and mortality still suffered by American Indians. All of these mechanisms rationalize inequality. In the absence of fundamental economic development, disparities will persist. American Indians will continue to live in rural or urban poverty, suffering worse health outcomes than the general population. Other members of society will continue to respond to the challenge of the disparities, finding new ways to rationalize both the disparities and their interventions. As long as inequality remains tolerable, observers will be able to respond with surprising creativity.

Notes

Index

Notes

Abbreviations

AJPH	*American Journal of Public Health*
ARCIA [year]	*Annual Report of the Commissioner of Indian Affairs* (Washington, D.C.: Government Printing Office).
Audubon, *Journals*	Maria R. Audubon, ed., *Audubon and his Journals*, with notes by Elliot Coues, 2 vols. (New York: Charles Scribner's Sons, 1897).
Bouquet Papers	Henry Bouquet, *The Papers of Henry Bouquet*, ed. S. K. Stevens, Donald H. Kent, Autumn L. Leonard, and Louis M. Waddell, 6 vols. (Harrisburg: Pennsylvania Historical and Museum Commission, 1972–1994).
Bouquet Papers (1940–1942)	Henry Bouquet, *The Papers of Col. Henry Bouquet*, ed. Sylvester K. Stevens and Donald H. Kent, series 21631–21655 (Harrisburg: Pennsylvania Historical Commission, 1940–1942).
Bradford, *Plymouth Plantation*	William Bradford, *Of Plymouth Plantation, 1620–1647*, ed. Samuel Eliot Morison (New York: Alfred A. Knopf, 1979).
Chardon, *Journal*	Francis Chardon, *Chardon's Journal at Fort Clark, 1834–1839: Descriptive of Life on the Upper Missouri; of a Fur Trader's Experiences Among the Mandans, Gros Ventres, and Their Neighbors; of the Ravages of the Small-Pox Epidemic of 1837*, ed. Annie Heloise Abel (Pierre, South Dakota: Department of History, State of South Dakota, 1932).

CMHS	Collections of the Massachusetts Historical Society.
CMP	Carl Muschenheim Papers, NewYork Weill Cornell Medical Center Archives, 89F, 3 boxes.
DRCHNY	E. B. O'Callaghan, ed., *Documents Relative to the Colonial History of the State of New York; procured in Holland, England, and France*, 15 vols. (Albany: Weed, Parsons, and Company, 1853–1887).
DSP	Doris Schwartz Papers, NewYork Weill Cornell Medical Center Archives, 18E, 3 boxes.
Early Western Travels	Reuben Gold Thwaites, *Early Western Travels, 1748–1846: A Series of Annotated Reprints of some of the best and rarest contemporary volumes of travel, descriptive of the Aborigines and Social and Economic Conditions in the Middle and Far West, during the Period of Early American Settlement*, 32 vols. (Cleveland: Arthur H. Clark Company, 1904–1906).
Jesuit Relations	Reuben Gold Thwaites, ed., *The Jesuit Relations and Allied Documents: Travels and Explorations of the Jesuit Missionaries in New France, 1610–1791*, 73 vols. (Cleveland: The Burrows Brothers Company, 1896–1901).
LRBIA	Letters Received, 1881–1907, Bureau of Indian Affairs, Record Group 75, National Archives and Records Administration, Washington, D.C.
NCFHPP	Navajo-Cornell Field Health Project Papers, NewYork Weill Cornell Medical Center Archives, D16/8, 49C, 2 boxes.
OHT	Oral History Transcripts, NewYork Weill Cornell Medical Center Archives, 54 F Box 2.
Smith, *Works*	Philip L. Barbour, ed., *The Complete Works of Captain John Smith (1580–1631)* (Chapel Hill: University of North Carolina Press, 1986).
The People's Health	John Adair and Kurt W. Deuschle, with a chapter by Clifford R. Barnett and David L. Rabin, *The People's Health: Medicine and Anthropology in a Navajo Community* (New York: Meredith Corporation, 1970).
The People's Health (1988)	John Adair, Kurt Deuschle, and Clifford Barnett, with a chapter by Barnett and David L. Rabin, *The People's Health: Medicine and Anthropology in a Navajo Community*, 2nd ed. (Albuquerque: University of New Mexico Press, 1988).
Winthrop, *Journal*	John Winthrop, *The Journal of John Winthrop, 1630–1649*, ed. Richard S. Dunn, James Savage, and Laetitia Yeandle (Cambridge: Harvard University Press, 1996).

| *Winthrop Papers* | Malcolm Freiberg, ed., *Winthrop Papers*, vols. 2 & 3 (Boston: Massachusetts Historical Society, 1931, 1943). |
| *WMP* | Walsh McDermott Papers, New York Weill Cornell Medical Center Archives, 106A-G, 50 boxes. |

Introduction

1. F. A. Chardon to P. D. Papin, 28 Nov. 1837, in *Papers of the St. Louis Fur Trade*, part 1; *The Chouteau Collection, 1752–1925*, microfilm (Bethesda: University Publications of America, 1991), reel 25, p. 185; Jacob Halsey to Pratte Chouteau & Co., 2 Nov. 1837, ibid., reel 25, p. 140; [James H. Bradley and Andrew Culbertson], "Affairs at Fort Benton, from 1831 to 1869; from Lieutenant Bradley's Journal," *Contributions to the Historical Society of Montana* 3 (1909): 226.

2. John Winthrop to Simonds D'Ewes, 21 July 1634, *Winthrop Papers*, 3:172; V. T. McGillycuddy, Agent, Pine Ridge, *ARCIA 1885*, 33; Walsh McDermott, "Conversation with Jane K. Zaidi (CUMC Archivist)," 7 Feb. 1972, *WMP*/11/5, p. 1; *The People's Health*, 95.

3. Whenever possible, I refer to specific groups by specific tribal identities (Massachusett, Mandan, Sioux, Navajo). For more general reference, I follow common usage and use "American Indian," "Native American," or simply "Indian" (the term commonly used by American Indians). While some activists have advocated the less biased term "First Nations," this has not yet come into wide usage. See Michael Yellow Bird, "What We Want To Be Called: Indigenous Peoples' Perspectives on Racial and Ethnic Identity Labels," *American Indian Quarterly* 23 (Spring 1999): 1–21. In the colonial period, I identify colonists by their nation of origin (English, French), in general as European, or simply as colonists. After the American Revolution, I refer to the descendants of these European colonists as "settlers," "Americans," or occasionally "whites."

4. Thomas Mayhew to [Henry Whitfield?], ca. 1650, in *The Light Appearing More and More towards the Perfect Day*, ed. Henry Whitfield (1651), in *CMHS*, 3rd ser., vol. 4 (Cambridge: Charles Folsom, 1834), 110; W. F. Wagner, "Introduction," in *Leonard's Narrative: Adventures of Zenas Leonard, Fur Trader and Trapper, 1831–1836* (Cleveland: Burrows Brothers, 1904), 40; Z. T. Daniel, Physician, Cheyenne River, *ARCIA 1891*, 392.

5. See E. Wagner Stearn and Allen E. Stearn, *The Effect of Smallpox on the Destiny of the Amerindian* (Boston: Bruce Humphries, 1945); Henry F. Dobyns, *Their Numbers Become Thinned: Native American Population Dynamics in Eastern North America* (Knoxville: University of Tennessee Press, 1983); Noble David Cook, *Born to Die: Disease and New World Conquest, 1492–1650* (Cambridge: Cambridge University Press, 1998). For virgin soil theory, see Alfred W. Crosby, "Virgin Soil Epidemics as a Factor in the Aboriginal Depopulation in America," *William and Mary Quarterly* 33 (April 1976): 289–299; David S. Jones, "Virgin Soils Revisited," *William and Mary Quarterly*, 60 (October 2003): 703–742. For the impact of social conditions, see Abdel R. Omran, "The Epidemiologic Transition: A Theory of the Epidemiology of Population Change," *Milbank Memorial Fund Quarterly* 49 (October 1971): 509–538; Linda A. Newson, "Indian Population Patterns in Colo-

nial Spanish America," *Latin American Research Review* 20 (1985): 41–74; John W. Verano and Douglas H. Ubelaker, eds., *Disease and Demography in the Americas* (Washington: Smithsonian Institution Press, 1992); Stephen J. Kunitz, *Disease and Social Diversity: The European Impact on the Health of Non-Europeans* (New York: Oxford University Press, 1994).

6. See Charles E. Rosenberg, *The Cholera Years: The United States in 1832, 1849, 1866* (1962; Chicago: University of Chicago Press, 1987); William H. McNeill, *Plagues and Peoples* (New York: Doubleday, 1977); Allan M. Brandt, *No Magic Bullet: A Social History of Venereal Disease in the United States since 1880* (New York: Oxford University Press, 1987); Rosenberg, "What Is an Epidemic? AIDS in Historical Perspective," in *Explaining Epidemics and Other Studies in the History of Medicine* (Cambridge: Cambridge University Press, 1992), 278–292.

7. Charles Rosenberg, "Disease and Social Order in America: Perceptions and Expectations," in *Explaining Epidemics*, 260.

8. Many examples can be found. *Behavior:* John H. Knowles, "The Responsibility of the Individual," *Daedalus* (Winter 1977): 57–80. *Social environments:* Gregory Pappas, "Elucidating the Relationships between Race, Socioeconomic Status, and Health," *AJPH* 84 (June 1994): 892–893. *Race:* Thomas W. Wilson and Clarence E. Grim, "Biohistory of Slavery and Blood Pressure Differences in Blacks Today: A Hypothesis," *Hypertension* 17 supp. 1 (January 1991): 122–132. *Race as a reflection of other factors:* Philip D. Curtin, "The Slavery Hypothesis for Hypertension among African Americans: The Historical Evidence," *AJPH* 82 (December 1992): 1681–1686; R. J. David and J. W. Collins, "Differing Birth Weights among Infants of U.S.-Born Blacks, African-Born Blacks, and U.S.-Born Whites," *New England Journal of Medicine* 337 (23 October 1997): 1209–1214. *Health and social structures:* "Health and Wealth," *Daedalus* 123 (Fall 1994): 1–216; Richard Wilkinson, *Unhealthy Societies: The Afflictions of Inequality* (London: Routledge, 1996); Norman Daniels, Bruce Kennedy, and Ichiro Kawachi, eds., *Is Inequality Bad for Our Health?* (Boston: Beacon Press, 2000).

9. Jared Diamond, *Guns, Germs, and Steel: The Fates of Human Societies* (New York: Norton, 1997); David S. Landes, *The Wealth and Poverty of Nations: Why Some Are so Rich and Some so Poor* (New York: Norton, 1998); Amartya Sen, *Poverty and Famines: An Essay on Entitlement and Deprivation* (Oxford: Oxford University Press, 1981); Sen, *Development as Freedom* (New York: Anchor Books, 1999). For examples of critical anthropology, see Nancy Scheper-Hughes, *Death without Weeping: The Violence of Everyday Life in Brazil* (Berkeley: University of California Press, 1992); Paul Farmer, *Infections and Inequalities: The Modern Plagues* (Berkeley: University of California Press, 1999).

10. Bradford, *Plymouth Plantation*, 62.

11. See Francis Paul Prucha, *The Great Father: The United States Government and the American Indians* (Lincoln: University of Nebraska Press, 1984).

12. On paternalism in Indian policy, see Prucha, *The Great Father;* Ronald N. Satz, *American Indian Policy in the Jacksonian Era* (Lincoln: University of Nebraska Press, 1975); Stephen Kunitz, "The Social Philosophy of John Collier," *Ethnohistory* 18 (Summer 1971): 213–229; Kunitz, "The History and Politics of US Health Care Policy for American Indians and Alaskan Natives," *AJPH* 86 (October 1996): 1464–1473. On Turner, see Gregory Nobles, *American Frontiers: Cultural Encounters and Continental Conquest* (New York: Hill and Wang, 1997), 8–14.

13. Richard White's work epitomizes this approach: White, *The Middle Ground: Indians, Empires, and Republics in the Great Lakes Region, 1650–1815* (Cambridge: Cambridge University Press, 1991). For the development of such "new Indian histories," see Daniel Richter, "Whose Indian History?" *William and Mary Quarterly* 50 (April 1993): 379–393; David R. Edmunds, "Native Americans, New Voices: American Indian History, 1895–1995," *American Historical Review* 100 (June 1995): 717–740; Donald L. Fixico, "Ethics and Responsibilities in Writing American Indian History," *American Indian Quarterly* 20 (Winter 1996): 29–39; Donald L. Fixico, ed., *Rethinking American Indian History* (Albuquerque: University of New Mexico Press, 1997).

14. For discussions of depopulation, see David E. Stannard, "Disease and Infertility: A New Look at the Demographic Collapse of Native Populations in the Wake of Western Contact," *Journal of American Studies* 24 (1990): 325–350; Richard S. Steckel and Jerome C. Rose, *The Backbone of History: Health and Nutrition in the Western Hemisphere* (Cambridge: Cambridge University Press, 2002). For reservations as palliative care, see Dobyns, *Their Numbers Become Thinned*, 343.

15. James Kenny, "Journal, 1761–1763," ed. John W. Jordan, *Pennsylvania Magazine of History and Biography* 37 (1913): 46; George Croghan, "Journal, 1759–1763," ed. Nicholas B. Wainwright, *Pennsylvania Magazine of History and Biography* 71 (October 1947): 395. The other examples are discussed in later chapters.

16. For Delaware faith in bloodletting, see Jane T. Merritt, "Dreaming of the Savior's Blood: Moravians and the Indian Great Awakening in Pennsylvania," *William and Mary Quarterly* 54 (October 1997): 744. For efficacy in the twentieth century, see Walsh McDermott, "Evaluating the Physician and His Technology," *Daedalus* (Winter 1977): 135–157; Harry M. Marks, *The Progress of Experiment: Science and Therapeutic Reform in the United States, 1900–1990* (Cambridge: Cambridge University Press, 1997); David S. Jones, "Visions of a Cure: Visualization, Clinical Trials, and Controversies in Cardiac Therapeutics, 1968–1998," *Isis* 91 (September 2000): 504–541. On the changing nature of efficacy, see Charles Rosenberg, "The Therapeutic Revolution: Medicine, Meaning, and Social Change in Nineteenth-century America," in *Explaining Epidemics*, 9–31; John H. Warner, *The Therapeutic Perspective: Medical Practice, Knowledge, and Identity in America, 1820–1885* (Cambridge, Mass.: Harvard University Press, 1986).

17. For the impact of medicine on the health of societies, see Thomas McKeown, *The Role of Medicine: Dream, Mirage, or Nemesis?* (Princeton: Princeton University Press, 1979); John B. McKinlay and Sonja M. McKinlay, "The Questionable Contribution of Medical Measures to the Decline of Mortality in the United States in the Twentieth Century," *Milbank Memorial Fund Quarterly* (Summer 1977): 405–428; Amy L. Fairchild and Gerald M. Oppenheimer, "Public Health Nihilism vs. Pragmatism: History, Politics, and the Control of Tuberculosis," *AJPH* 88 (July 1998): 1105–1117.

18. See Joel D. Howell, *Technology in the Hospital: Transforming Patient Care in the Early Twentieth Century* (Baltimore: Johns Hopkins University Press, 1995); Allan M. Brandt and Martha Gardner, "The Golden Age of Medicine?" in *Medicine in the Twentieth Century*, ed. Roger Cooter and John Pickstone (Amsterdam: Harwood Academic, 2000), 24.

19. On the ethical complications of medical research on captive populations, see Allan M. Brandt, "Racism and Research: The Case of the Tuskegee Syphilis

Study," *Hastings Center Report* 8 (1978): 21–29; Susan E. Lederer, *Subjected to Science: Human Experimentation in America before the Second World War* (Baltimore: Johns Hopkins University Press, 1995); Marcia Angell, "The Ethics of Clinical Research in the Third World," *New England Journal of Medicine* 337 (September 18, 1997): 847–849; David J. Rothman, "The Shame of Medical Research," *New York Review of Books* (30 November 2000): 60–64.

20. Norbert Elias outlined his theory of the civilizing process in 1939: as societies become more elaborate, with tighter webs of interaction between individuals, individuals must increasingly conform their behavior to acceptable standards. See Elias, *The Civilizing Process: The History of Manners and State Formation and Civilization*, trans. Edmund Jephcott (1939; Cambridge: Blackwell, 1994). See also Johan Goudsblom, "Public Health and the Civilizing Process," *Milbank Quarterly* 64 (June 1986): 161–188; Patrice Pinell, "Modern Medicine and the Civilising Process," *Sociology of Health and Illness* 18 (1996): 1–16; Michel Foucault, *The History of Sexuality*, vol. I; *An Introduction*, trans. Robert Hurley (1976; New York: Vintage Books, 1990).

21. Winthrop, "General Observations for the Plantations of New England," 1629, *Winthrop Papers*, 2:117; Chardon, *Journal*, 18.

22. Arthur Kleinman, *Writing at the Margin: Discourse between Anthropology and Medicine* (Berkeley: University of California Press, 1995), 97.

23. Many ethnographic examples are provided in Clifford Geertz, *The Interpretation of Cultures, Selected Essays* (New York: Basic Books, 1973). For attempts at understanding local meaning in historical sources, see Robert Darnton, *The Great Cat Massacre and Other Episodes in French Cultural History* (New York: Vintage, 1984). An effort to integrate ethnographic and historical methods in the study of American Indians produced the field of ethnohistory: Bruce G. Trigger, *The Children of Aataentsic: A History of the Huron People to 1660* (1976; Montreal: McGill-Queen's University Press, 1987); Neal Salisbury, *Manitou and Providence: Indians, Europeans, and the Making of New England, 1500–1643* (New York: Oxford University Press, 1982); James Axtell, *After Columbus: Essays in the Ethnohistory of Colonial North America* (New York: Oxford University Press, 1988); Colin G. Calloway, *The American Revolution in Indian Country: Crisis and Diversity in Native American Communities* (Cambridge: Cambridge University Press, 1995); Peter C. Mancall, *Deadly Medicine: Indians and Alcohol in Early America* (Ithaca: Cornell University Press, 1995); Karen Ordahl Kupperman, *Indians and English: Facing Off in Early America* (Ithaca: Cornell University Press, 2000).

24. William J. Bouwsma, "Intellectual History in the 1980s: From History of Ideas to History of Meaning," *Journal of Interdisciplinary History* 12 (Autumn 1981): 287–288. See also Robert Nozick, *Philosophical Explanations* (Cambridge, Mass.: Harvard University Press, 1981), 574–575.

25. Debates about the history of psychiatric asylums reveal the difficulty of studying motivation: Gerald Grob, *Mental Illness and American Society, 1875–1940* (Princeton: Princeton University Press, 1983); David Rothman, *Conscience and Convenience: The Asylum and Its Alternatives in Progressive America* (Boston: Scott, Foresman, 1980). For other examples of the elusiveness of altruism and motivation in the history of medicine, see Richard M. Titmuss, *The Gift Relationship: From Human Blood to Social Policy* (New York: Random House, 1971); Harry Cleaver, "Malaria and the Political Economy of Public Health," *International Journal of Health*

Services 7 (1977): 557–579; Lynn Morgan, *Community Participation in Health: The Politics of Primary Care in Costa Rica* (Cambridge: Cambridge University Press, 1993); Robert L. Martensen and David S. Jones, "When US Medicine Became Imperial," *JAMA* 277 (25 June 1997): 1917.

26. David B. Morris, "About Suffering: Voice, Genre, and Moral Community," *Daedalus* 125 (Winter 1996): 40.

27. "Social suffering results from what political, economic, and institutional power does to people, and, reciprocally, how these forms of power themselves influence responses to social problems": Arthur Kleinman, Veena Das, and Margaret Lock, "Introduction: Social Suffering," *Daedalus* 125 (winter 1996): xi.

28. For the parallel problem of black-white disparities in health status, see W. Michael Byrd and Linda A. Clayton, *Race and Health An American Health Dilemma: A Medical History of African Americans and the Problem of Race—Beginnings to 1900* (New York: Routledge, 2000).

29. Pursuit of American Indian perspectives on health disparities would be an extremely valuable undertaking, but one that would require a different research project with different sources. Similar studies could also be made of different epidemics among different tribes, or of responses by other groups in North America (Spanish, French, Russian, Asian), or of health disparities of indigenous populations in other parts of the world (Canada, Latin America, Africa, Australia, Russia).

1. Expecting Providence

1. Bradford, *Plymouth Plantation*, 62, 26 n.8.

2. Roger Williams, *A Key into the Language of America* (1643), ed. John J. Teunissen and Evelyn J. Hinz (Detroit: Wayne State University Press, 1973), 84; Neal Salisbury, *Manitou and Providence: Indians, Europeans, and the Making of New England, 1500–1643* (New York: Oxford University Press, 1982); William Cronon, *Changes in the Land: Indians, Colonists, and the Ecology of New England* (New York: Hill and Wang, 1983); Dane Morrison, *A Praying People: Massachusett Acculturation and the Failure of the Puritan Mission, 1600–1690* (New York: Peter Lang, 1995); Kathleen J. Bragdon, *Native People of Southern New England, 1500–1650* (Norman: University of Oklahoma Press, 1996).

3. Giovanni de Verrazano, "Letter to the King of France," January 1524, in George Parker Winship, ed., *Sailors Narratives of Voyages along the New England Coast, 1524–1624* (New York: Burt Franklin, 1905), 21. See Catherine C. Carlson, George J. Armelagos, and Ann L. Magennis, "Impact of Disease on the Precontact and Early Historic Populations of New England and the Maritimes," in *Disease and Demography in the Americas*, ed. John W. Verano and Douglas H. Ubelaker (Washington D.C.: Smithsonian Institution Press, 1992), 146–147; Laurier Turgeon, "French Fishers, Fur Traders, and Amerindians during the Sixteenth Century: History and Archeology," *William and Mary Quarterly* 55 (October 1998): 585–610.

4. Salisbury, *Manitou and Providence*, 72, 81–82; Oliver A. Rink, *Holland on the Hudson: An Economic and Social History of Dutch New York* (Ithaca: Cornell University Press, 1986), 13–85.

5. John Brereton, *A Briefe and True Relation* (1602; New York: Dodd, Mead, 1903) [Gosnold]; Martin Pring, "A Voyage set out from the Citie of *Bristoll*"

(1603), in Winship, *Sailors Narratives;* James Rosier, *A True Relation of the Most Prosperous Voyage* (1605; Portland, Me.: Gorges Society, 1887) [Waymouth]; James Phinney Baxter, ed., *Sir Ferdinando Gorges and his Province of Maine* (1890; New York: Burt Franklin, 1967) [Smith, Vines, Dermer].

6. Brereton, *Relation,* 6, 11; Samuel de Champlain, "Discovery of the Coast of the Almouchiquious" (1605), in Winship, *Sailors Narratives,* 80; John Smith, *A Description of New England* (1616), in Smith, *Works,* 1:310, 1:340.

7. See the narratives by Arthur Barlowe, Ralph Lane, and John White in David B. Quinn and Alison M. Quinn, ed., *Virginia Voyages from Hakluyt* (New York: Oxford University Press, 1973).

8. Smith, *A True Relation of Such Occurrences and Accidents* (1608), in Smith, *Works,* 1:29–35; Thomas Dermer to Samuel Purchas, 1619, in *Hakluytus Posthumus, or Purchas His Pilgrimes,* ed. Samuel Purchas (1625; Glasgow: James MacLehose and Sons, 1906), 19:133; Karen Ordahl Kupperman, "Apathy and Death in Early Jamestown," *Journal of American History* 66 (June 1979): 24–40.

9. Peter Martyr, *The Decades of the Newe Worlde* (1516), trans. Richard Eden (1555), in *The First Three English Books on America,* ed. Edward Arber (Birmingham, 1885), 199, 172; Bradford, *Plymouth Plantation,* 122.

10. David S. Jones, "Virgin Soils Revisited," *William and Mary Quarterly* 60 (October 2003): 703–742.

11. Thomas Hariot, *A Briefe and True Report of the New Found Land of Virginia* (1588; Ann Arbor: Edward Brothers, 1931), F–F2.

12. Gorges, *Briefe Narration,* in Baxter, *Sir Ferdinando Gorges,* 19:19; Dermer to Purchas, in *Hakluytus Posthumus,* 19:129.

13. Bradford, *Plymouth Plantation,* 25. For the patent, see Gorges, *Briefe Narration,* 19:25–26n315.

14. John Winthrop, "General Observations for the Plantations of New England" (1629), *Winthrop Papers,* 2:117.

15. Bradford, *Plymouth Plantation,* 58; Winthrop, *Journal,* 8 April 1630, p. 5.

16. Bradford, *Plymouth Plantation,* 64, 65.

17. Ibid., 72; [Bradford], "A Relation or Journall of the Proceedings of the Plantation setled at Plimoth in New England," in George Morton, ed., *Mourt's Relation, or Journal of the Plymouth Plantation* (1622), ed. Henry Martyn Dexter (Boston: John Kimball Wiggin, 1865), 15–22, 47–55, 61, 84–85.

18. Edward Winslow, "A Journey to Packanokik, The Habitation of the Great King Massasoit," in *Mourt's Relation,* 103, 130; Bradford, *Plymouth Plantation,* 87; Robert Cushman, "Of the State of the Colony, and the need of public spirit in the Colonists," 12 Dec. 1621, in *Chronicles of the Pilgrim Fathers of the Colony of Plymouth, from 1602 to 1625,* ed. Alexander Young, 2nd ed. (Boston: Charles C. Little and James Brown, 1844), 258.

19. The impact of disease in the northeast before 1600 remains fiercely debated. For competing assessments, compare Ann F. Ramenofsky, *Vectors of Death: The Archeology of European Contact* (Albuquerque: University of New Mexico Press, 1987); Dean R. Snow, "Microchronology and Demographic Evidence Relating to the Size of Pre-Columbian North American Indian Populations," *Science* 268 (16 June 1995): 1601–1604. For Micmac mortality, see Salisbury, *Manitou and Providence,* 56–59. For the 1612–1613 epidemic (misdating the 1616 epidemic?), see Daniel Gookin, *Historical Collections of the Indians in New England* (ca. 1680) (1792; Towtaid: 1970), 9. For the epidemic's diagnosis, Timothy L. Bratton, "The Iden-

tity of the New England Indian Epidemic of 1616–19," *Bulletin of the History of Medicine* 62 (Fall 1988): 351–383.

20. Bradford, *Plymouth Plantation*, 114; Edward Winslow, *Good Newes from New England* (1624), in Young, *Chronicles of the Pilgrim Fathers*, 302, 305; Thomas Morton, *New English Canaan* (1632), in *Tracts and Other Papers*, ed. Peter Force, (1836; New York: Peter Smith, 1947), 2:18–19.

21. Edmund S. Morgan, *The Puritan Dilemma: The Story of John Winthrop* (Boston: Little, Brown, 1958), 32–68; Salisbury, *Manitou and Providence*, 159–202; Richard S. Dunn, "Introduction," in Winthrop, *Journal*, xvii.

22. John White, *The Planters Plea* (1630), in Force, ed., *Tracts and Other Papers*, 2:14; William Wood, *New Englands Prospect* (1634), ed. Alden T. Vaughan (Amherst: University of Massachusetts Press, 1977), 38; Francis Higginson, *New Englands Plantation* (1630), in *New Englands Plantation, with the Sea Journal and Other Writings* (Salem, Mass.: Essex Book and Print Club, 1908), 34. Wood, perplexingly, also described remarkable good health and long lives among the Indians: *New Englands Prospect*, 110–111.

23. John Josselyn (who did not arrive until 1636) lists the 1628 epidemic, which he might have heard about from Samuel Maverick, who was at Winnemisset in 1628. No other colonial writer (including Maverick) mentioned this epidemic. See Josselyn, *An Account of Two Voyages to New-England* (1674), in *John Josselyn, Colonial Traveler: A Critical Edition of Two Voyages to New-England*, ed. Paul J. Lindholdt (Hanover: University Press of New England, 1988), 89, 93. For the 1630–1631 epidemic, see [John Pond] to William Pond, 15 March 1631, *Winthrop Papers*, 3:17.

24. Bradford, *Plymouth Plantation*, 260; Winthrop, *Journal*, 24 July 1633, p. 92; *Early Records of Charlestown* (1664), in *Chronicles of the First Planters of the Colony of Massachusetts Bay, from 1623 to 1636*, ed. Alexander Young (Boston: Charles C. Little and James Brown, 1846), 386. For mortality estimates, see Sherburne F. Cook, "The Significance of Disease in the Extinction of the New England Indians," *Human Biology* 45 (September 1973): 485–508.

25. Winthrop, *Journal*, Nov. 1633, p. 101; 5 Dec. 1633, p. 105; 21 Jan., pp. 108–109. Bradford, *Plymouth Plantation*, 270–271. But as late as November 1634, Winthrop described Connecticut as "full of Indians": *Journal*, 5 Nov. 1634, p. 133.

26. Thomas Mayhew to [Henry Whitfield?], ca. 1650, in *The Light Appearing More and More towards the Perfect Day*, ed. Henry Whitfield (1651), in *CMHS*, 3rd ser., vol. 4. (Cambridge, Mass.: Charles Folsom, 1834), 110; Mayhew to [Edward Winslow?], 18 Nov. 1648, in *The Glorious Progress of the Gospel, amongst the Indians in New England*, ed. Edward Winslow (1649), ibid., p. 77; Mayhew, "To the much Honored Corporation in London," 22 Oct. 1652, in *Tears of Repentance*, ed. [Henry Whitfield] (1653), ibid., p. 259; Winthrop, *Journal*, June 1647, p. 690; John Josselyn, *New-Englands Rarities Discovered* (1672), ed. Edward Tuckerman (Boston: William Veazie, 1865) pp. 43–116.

27. Smith, *New Englands Trials* (1622), in Smith, *Works*, 1:428; Smith, *Advertisements For the Unexperienced Planters of New England, or any where* (1631), ibid., 3:275; Cushman, "Of the State of the Colony," 258; White, *Planters Plea*, 14; Bradford, *Plymouth Plantation*, 270.

28. Dean R. Snow and Kim M. Lanphear, "European Contact and Indian Depopulation in the Northeast: The Timing of the First Epidemics," *Ethnohistory* 35

(Winter 1988): 15–33; David E. Stannard, "Disease and Infertility: a New Look at the Demographic Collapse of Native Populations in the Wake of Western Contact," *Journal of American Studies* 24 (1990): 325–350; Verano and Ubelaker, eds., *Disease and Demography in the Americas.*

29. Bradford to Thomas Weston, 1621, in Bradford, *Plymouth Plantation,* 95; Bradford, *Plymouth Plantation,* 77, 130; Cushman, "The Sin and Danger of Self-Love" (1621), in Young, *Chronicles of the Pilgrim Fathers,* 263. The colony produced its first surplus food in 1623. See Bradford, *Plymouth Plantation,* 120–121; Salisbury, *Manitou and Providence,* 111–122.

30. Christopher Levett, *A Voyage into New England* (1628), in *Collections of the Maine Historical Society* (Portland, 1847), 2:101; Nathaniel Morton, *New-Englands Memorial* (1669; Boston: Club of Odd Volumes, 1903), 41; Phineas Pratt, *A Declaration of the Affairs of the English People That First Inhabited New England* (1662), in *CMHS,* 4th ser. (Boston: Little, Brown, 1858), 4:478–486; Samuel Maverick, *A Briefe Description of New England* (1660) (Boston: David Clapp and Son, 1885); Morgan, *Puritan Dilemma,* 58–59; Salisbury, *Manitou and Providence,* 125–133, 153–157.

31. Higginson, "A True Relacon of ye last voyage to *new England*" (1629), in *New Englands Plantation, with the Sea Journal and Other Writings,* 67–71; [John Pond] to William Pond, *Winthrop Papers:* 3:18–19; Bradford, *Plymouth Plantation,* 223; Thomas Dudley to Bridget, Countess of Lincoln, 12 March 1631, in Young, *Chronicles of the First Planters,* 311–325.

32. Winslow and Samuel Fuller to Bradford, 26 July 1630, in Bradford, *Plymouth Plantation,* 235; Winthrop to Margaret Winthrop, 9 Sept. 1630, *Winthrop Papers,* 2:312; Winthrop, *Journal,* 10 Feb. 1631, p. 45; Bradford, *Plymouth Plantation,* 260.

33. Bradford, *Plymouth Plantation,* 87; Winslow, *Good Newes from New England,* 281; Winthrop, *Journal,* 12 July 1633, p. 92; ibid., 5 Nov. 1634, p. 133.

34. *Early Records of Charlestown,* 386; Winthrop, *Journal,* 12 June, p. 35, 23–26 March, p. 47, 4 April, p. 49, 13 July, p. 54, 6 Sept., p. 56.

35. Winslow, *Good Newes from New England,* 346, 313–323; Cushman, "Of the State of the Colony," 259–260.

36. Winthrop, *Journal,* Nov. 1633, p. 101, 5 Dec. 1633, p. 105. Samuel Maverick's book and letters make no mention of this episode. See Maverick, *Briefe Description of New England;* Maverick, "Letters, 1640–1669," *CMHS,* 4th ser., vol. 7, 307–320. For the Plymouth Traders, see Bradford, *Plymouth Plantation,* 271.

37. *Early Records of Charlestown,* 386. Joyce Chaplin believes that these are the only two episodes of colonists aiding Indians during epidemics. See Chaplin, *Subject Matter: Technology, the Body, and Science on the Anglo-American Frontier, 1500–1676* (Cambridge, Mass.: Harvard University Press, 2001), 180–181. There could, however, have been other examples that simply were not described.

38. Winslow, *Good Newes from New England,* 301; Cushman, "Of the State of the Colony," 258; Morton, *New English Canaan,* 18; Smith, *New Englands Trials* (1622), in Smith, *Works,* 1:428.

39. Bradford, *Plymouth Plantation,* 270; Winthrop to Simonds D'Ewes, 21 July 1634, *Winthrop Papers,* 3:171–172; Winthrop to John Endecott, 3 Jan. 1634, *Winthrop Papers,* 3:149; *Early Records of Charlestown,* 387; William Hubbard, *A General History of New England from the Discovery to MDCLXXX* (1680), 2nd ed. (Boston:

Charles C. Little and James Brown, 1878), 210; Thomas Gorges to Ferdinando Gorges, 22 June 1642, in *The Letters of Thomas Gorges, Deputy Governor of the Province of Maine, 1640–1643*, ed. Robert E. Moody (Portland: Maine Historical Society, 1978), 110; *New England's First Fruits*, 26 Sept. 1642, in *Old South Leaflets*, vol. 3, #51 (Boston: Directors of the Old South Work, 1894), 9.

40. Herbert U. Williams, "The Epidemic of the Indians of New England, 1616–1620," *Johns Hopkins Hospital Bulletin* 20 (1909): 342; John J. Heagerty, *Four Centuries of Medical History in Canada* (London: Simpkin, Marshall, Hamilton, Kent, 1928), 1:57; Alden T. Vaughan, *New England Frontier: Puritans and Indians, 1620–1675* 3rd ed. (1965; Norman: University of Oklahoma Press, 1995), 104. For other prominent examples, see Alfred W. Crosby, "'God . . . Would Destroy Them, and Give Their Country to Another People,'" *American Heritage* 29 (October/November 1978): 40; Cronon, *Changes in the Land*, 90; James Axtell, *Beyond 1492: Encounters in Colonial North America* (New York: Oxford University Press, 1992), 284–285; Noble David Cook, *Born to Die: Disease and New World Conquest, 1492–1650* (Cambridge: Cambridge University Press, 1998), 200.

41. Ronald Takaki, "*The Tempest* in the Wilderness: The Racialization of Savagery," *Journal of American History* 79 (December 1992): 908; Russell Thornton, *American Indian Holocaust and Survival: A Population History Since 1492* (Norman: University of Oklahoma Press, 1987), 75; David E. Stannard, *American Holocaust: Columbus and the Conquest of the New World* (New York: Oxford University Press, 1992), 109.

42. Karen Ordahl Kupperman, *Indians and English: Facing Off in Early America* (Ithaca: Cornell University Press, 2000), x.

43. Philip Vincent, *A True Relation of The late Batell fought in New-England, between the English and the Pequet Salvages* (1638), in *CMHS*, 3rd ser., vol. 6 (Boston: American Stationers' Company, 1837), 34; Williams, *Key into the Language of America*, 133.

44. Morton, *New English Canaan*, 24; Wood, *New Englands Prospect*, 83. Kupperman, *Indians and English*, 2, 58–59, 75. Joyce Chaplin, "Natural Philosophy and an Early Racial Idiom in North America: Comparing English and Indian Bodies," *William and Mary Quarterly* 54 (January 1997): 244, 230; also Chaplin, *Subject Matter*, 8–9, 22–23, 158–197, 244–276, 319–323. Chaplin argues that English observations of the remarkable mortality of Indians provided the seeds for later arguments of Indian racial inferiority. I think she exaggerates the early role of ideas of racial difference: the starkest accounts of epidemic disparities emphasize providence, not bodily difference. Even as racial explanations appeared more frequently in the eighteenth and nineteenth centuries, nonbiological accounts of disparity dominated the discourse (see Chapters 3 and 5).

45. Eric H. Christianson, "Medicine in New England," in *Medicine in the New World: New Spain, New France, and New England*, ed. Ronald L. Numbers (Knoxville: University of Tennessee Press, 1987).

46. Wood, *New Englands Prospect*, 32; Higginson, *New Englands Plantation*, 29, 30; White, *Planters Plea*, 13; Williams, *Key into the Language of America*, 170.

47. Bradford, "Journall of the Proceedings of the Plantation," 27, 28, 39, 68; Wood, *New Englands Prospect*, 28; *Early Records of Charlestown*, 378–379; Winthrop, *Journal*, 10 Feb. 1631, p. 45.

48. Dudley to Bridget, Countess of Lincoln, in Young, *Chronicles of the First*

Planters, 325; Hubbard, *General History of New England*, 324. See also Karen Ordahl Kupperman, "Fear of Hot Climates in the Anglo-American Colonial Experience," *William and Mary Quarterly* 41 (1984): 213–240.

49. *Frostbite:* Winthrop, *Journal*, 28 Dec. 1630, p. 44; Wood, *New Englands Prospect*, 29. *Exhaustion:* Edward Johnson, *A History of New-England* (1654), ed. J. Franklin Jameson (New York: Charles Scribner's Sons, 1910), 115. *Mussels:* Bradford, "Journall of the Proceedings of the Plantation," 4–5. *Leprosy:* Edward Howes to John Winthrop Jr., 18 March 1633, *Winthrop Papers*, 3:113. *Fruit and scurvy:* Winthrop, *Journal*, 8 March 1636, p. 171; Josselyn, *New-Englands Rarities Discovered*, 120. *Contagion:* Robert Ryece to John Winthrop, 9 Sept. 1636, *Winthrop Papers*, 3:305–306. Midwives: Thomas Shepard, "Autobiography," in *God's Plot: Puritan Spirituality in Thomas Shepard's Cambridge*, ed. Michael McGiffert (Amherst: University of Massachusetts Press, 1994), 57. *Women reading:* Winthrop, *Journal*, 13 April 1645, p. 570. *Suckling:* Winthrop, *Journal*, May 1646, p. 620–621. *Pessimism:* Winthrop, *Journal*, 10 Feb. 1631, p. 45; Morison, in Bradford, *Plymouth Plantation*, xxiv. *Bradford's summary:* Bradford, *Plymouth Plantation*, 328–329.

50. Gorges, *Briefe Narration*, 19:76–77; Winslow, *Good Newes from New England*, 345–346, 322; Williams, *Key into the Language of America*, 242.

51. Winslow, *Good Newes from New England*, 313, 317; Williams, *Key into the Language of America*, 243–244; Thomas Mayhew to [Henry Whitfield?], 16 Oct. 1651, in *Strength out of Weaknesse*, ed. Henry Whitfield (1652), in *CMHS*, 3rd ser., vol. 4, p. 167; Josselyn, *Account of Two Voyages*, 94.

52. Thomas Gorges to Henry Gorges, 19 May 1642 (second letter), in *Letters of Thomas Gorges*, 96; Roger Williams to John Winthrop, June 1638, in *The Correspondence of Roger Williams*, ed. Glenn W. LaFantasie (Hanover: University Press of New England, 1988), 1:160.

53. Wood, *New Englands Prospect*, 82; Mayhew to [Whitfield], in *Light Appearing More and More*, 110; Gookin, *Historical Collections of the Indians in New England*, 53–54, 17; Williams to John Throckmorton, 30 July 1672, in *Correspondence*, ed. LaFantasie, 2:675. See Peter C. Mancall, *Deadly Medicine: Indians and Alcohol in Early America* (Ithaca: Cornell University Press, 1995).

54. See David S. Jones, "Rationalizing Epidemics: Historical Accounts of American Indian Health Disparities" (Ph.D. diss., Harvard University, 2001), 135–154. For the Guatemala example, see W. George Lovell, "Disease and Depopulation in Early Colonial Guatemala," in *"Secret Judgments of God": Old World Disease in Colonial Spanish America*, ed. Noble David Cook and Lovell (Norman: University of Oklahoma Press, 1991), 77.

55. For the Jesuit mission, see W. J. Eccles, *France in America*, rev. ed. (East Lansing: Michigan State University Press, 1990); Bruce G. Trigger, *The Children of Aataentsic: A History of the Huron People to 1660* (1976; Montreal: McGill-Queen's University Press, 1987). For Huron questioning, see Paul le Jeune, *Relation of What Occurred in New France in 1637*, 31 Aug. 1637 (1638), *Jesuit Relations*, 11:193.

56. *Rain:* Jean de Brebeuf, "Relation of what occurred in the Country of the Hurons in the year 1636," 16 July 1636, *Jesuit Relations*, 10:41. *Health:* de Brebeuf to the Praepositor General of the Society of Jesus, 20 May 1637, ibid., 11:13. *Sorcerer:* le Jeune, *Relation of What Occurred in New France in 1635*, 28 Aug. 1635, ibid., 7:301.

57. *Hardships:* Pierre Biard, "Relation of New France" (1616), *Jesuit Relations*, 3:109; le Jeune, *Relation of 1637*, 11:195. *Habits:* le Jeune, *Relation of 1634*, 6:263.

Sorcerers: le Jeune, "Relation of What Occurred in New France in 1633" (1634), ibid., 5:235. *Contagion:* Hierosme Lalemant, "Relation of what occurred in the Mission of the Hurons, from the month of June in the year 1639, until the month of June in the year 1640," 27 May 1640, ibid., 19:89.

58. *Mortality:* le Jeune, *Relation of 1637*, 11:195. *Diets:* Biard to the Provincial of Paris, 10 June 1610, *Jesuit Relations*, 1:177; Biard, "Relation of New France," 3:107. *Alcohol:* le Jeune, *Relation of 1637*, 11:195; le Jeune, *Relation of 1634*, 6:239.

59. *Micmac accusations:* Biard, "Relation of New France," 3:105. *Huron accusations:* Lalemant, "Relation of 1640," 19:93, 19:97; le Jeune, *Relation of 1637*, 12:86; le Jeune to the Father Pronvincial, 1637, *Jesuit Relations*, 12:237; le Jeune, *Relation of 1636*, 9:207. *Huron concessions:* Lalemant, "Relation of 1641," 21:235. See also Shepard Krech, ed., *Indians, Animals, and the Fur Trade: A Critique of* Keepers of the Game (Athens: University of Georgia Press, 1981).

60. Lalemant, "Relation of the most remarkable things," 19 May 1641, in *Jesuit Relations*, 21:91–93.

61. Trigger, *Children of Aataentsic*, 595–601. For the classic analysis of how economic policy shaped etiologic theory, see Erwin H. Ackerknecht, "Anti-contagionism Between 1821 and 1867," *Bulletin of the History of Medicine* 22 (September–October 1948): 562–593.

62. Chaplin, "Natural Philosophy and an Early Racial Idiom," 245; Chaplin, *Subject Matter*, 123–124.

2. Meanings of Depopulation

1. *Early Records of Charlestown* (1664), in *Chronicles of the First Planters of the Colony of Massachusetts Bay, from 1623 to 1636*, ed. Alexander Young (Boston: Charles C. Little and James Brown, 1846), 387.

2. Karen Ordahl Kupperman, *Indians and English: Facing Off in Early America* (Ithaca: Cornell University Press, 2000), 11.

3. Perry Miller, *The New England Mind: The Seventeenth Century* (New York: Macmillan, 1939), vii, 8; David D. Hall, *Worlds of Wonder, Days of Judgment: Popular Religious Belief in Early New England* (New York: Knopf, 1989), 20, 243.

4. Thomas Beard, quoted in Hall, *Worlds of Wonder*, 77; Cotton Mather, "Of Providence," in *Magnalia Christi Americana* (1702; Hartford: Silas Andrus and Son, 1853), 2:186. Mather did admit that God, all-powerful, could still ignore natural causes, to "work without, above and against them at his pleasure." Id.

5. Miller, *New England Mind*, 228, 230; Mather, *Magnalia*, 1:54; Nathaniel Morton, *New-Englands Memorial* (1669; Boston: Club of Odd Volumes, 1903), 163.

6. Charles Lloyd Cohen, *God's Caress: The Psychology of Puritan Religious Experience* (New York: Oxford University Press, 1986), 93, 133.

7. Michael P. Winship, *Seers of God: Puritan Providentialism in the Restoration and Early Enlightenment* (Baltimore: Johns Hopkins University Press, 1996), 1, 11; Thomas Shepard, "Autobiography," in *God's Plot: Puritan Spirituality in Thomas Shepard's Cambridge*, ed. Michael McGiffert (Amherst: University of Massachusetts Press, 1994), 63.

8. Winship, *Seers of God*, 2; Miller, *New England Mind*, 229.

9. Shepard, "Journal," 1 Jan. 1642, in *God's Plot*, ed. McGiffert, 107–108.

10. John Eliot, *The Day-Breaking, if not The Sun-Rising of the Gospell With the*

Indians in New-England (1647), in *CMHS*, 3rd ser., vol. 4 (Cambridge: Charles Folsom, 1834), 11. John Smith, *The Generall History of Virginia, New-England, the Summer Iles* (1624), in Smith, *Works*, 2:367–368. Smith examined a variety of natural mechanisms for the rats' demise—a cold winter, loss of food, colonists' attempts to exterminate them with cats, dogs, fire, traps, and ratsbane—and found all inadequate.

11. Bradford, *Plymouth Plantation*, 303; William Hubbard, *A General History of New England from the Discovery to MDCLXXX* (1680), 2nd ed. (Boston: Charles C. Little and James Brown, 1878), 324; Winthrop, *Journal*, 17 Nov. 1636, p. 199; Edmund Browne to Simonds D'Ewes, 7 Sept. 1638, in *Letters from New England: The Massachusetts Bay Colony, 1629–1638*, ed. Everett Emerson (Amherst: University of Massachusetts Press, 1976), 226.

12. Edward Winslow, *Good Newes from New England* (1624), in *Chronicles of the Pilgrim Fathers of the Colony of Plymouth, from 1602 to 1625*, ed. Alexander Young, 2nd ed. (Boston: Charles C. Little and James Brown, 1844), 346; Bradford, *Plymouth Plantation*, 303; Winthrop, *Journal*, May 1646, p. 621. See also Hall, *Worlds of Wonder*, 202.

13. Thomas Dudley to Bridget, Countess of Lincoln, 12 March 1631, in Young, *Chronicles of the First Planters*, 325–326; Daniel Gookin, *Historical Collections of the Indians in New England* (ca. 1680) (1792; n.p.: Towtaid, 1972), 53–54.

14. John Winthrop, "General Observations for the Plantations of New England" (1629), *Winthrop Papers*, 2:117; Winthrop to Nathaniel Rich, 22 May 1634, ibid., 3:167; Winthrop to Simonds D'Ewes, 21 July 1634, ibid., 3:172; Winthrop to John Endecott, 3 Jan. 1634, ibid., 3:149.

15. Ferdinando Gorges, *Briefe Narration*, in James Phinney Baxter, ed., *Sir Ferdinando Gorges and his Province of Maine* (1890; New York: Burt Franklin, 1967), 19:19; John White, *The Planters Plea* (1630), in *Tracts and Other Papers*, ed. Peter Force, vol. 2 (1836; New York: Peter Smith, 1947), 2:14; John Smith, *Advertisements For the Unexperienced Planters of New England, or any where* (1631), in Smith, *Works*, 3:275; Bradford, *Plymouth Plantation*, 271; Winthrop, *Journal*, 5 Dec. 1633, p. 105; *Early Records of Charlestown*, 386.

16. Bradford, *Plymouth Plantation*, 83–84; Phineas Pratt, *A Declaration of the Affairs of the English People That First Inhabited New England*, 1662, in *CMHS*, 4th ser. (Boston: Little, Brown, 1858), 4:479.

17. Smith, *Advertisements For the Unexperienced Planters*, 3:275; Thomas Morton, *New English Canaan* (1632), in Force, *Tracts and Other Papers*, 2:18–19. See also Nathaniel Morton, *New-Englands Memorial*, 27; Hubbard, *General History of New England*, 54–55; Mather, *Magnalia*, 1:51.

18. Winthrop, *Journal*, 5 Dec. 1633, p. 105. See also Edward Johnson, *A History of New-England* (1654), ed. J. Franklin Jameson (New York: Scribner, 1910), 79–80; Hubbard, *General History of New England*, 650–651; Mather, *Magnalia*, 1:78. This use of disease to facilitate conversion has long been highlighted by historians: William A. Starna, "The Biological Encounter: Disease and the Ideological Domain," *American Indian Quarterly* 16 (Fall 1992): 514; Joyce E. Chaplin, *Subject Matter: Technology, the Body, and Science on the Anglo-American Frontier, 1500–1676* (Cambridge, Mass.: Harvard University Press, 2001), 301–302, 315.

19. Thomas Mayhew, "To the much Honored Corporation in London," 22 Oct. 1652, in *Tears of Repentance*, ed. [Henry Whitfield] (1653), in *CMHS*, 3rd ser., vol. 4, pp. 257–259.

20. John Eliot to [Henry Whitfield?], 18 April 1650, in *The Light Appearing More and More towards the Perfect Day*, ed. Henry Whitfield (1651), in *CMHS*, 3rd ser., vol. 4, pp. 133, 134. The messages of providence, however, were not always so clear. In 1650 and 1651 smallpox did not spare converted Indians so thoroughly: "it hath pleased God to make less difference." See Eliot to [Henry Whitfield?], 28 April 1651, in *Strength out of Weaknesse*, ed. Henry Whitfield (1652), in *CMHS*, 3rd ser., vol. 4, p. 165. See also Matthew Mayhew, *A Brief Narrative of the Success which the Gospel hath had, among the Indians, of Martha's Vineyard* (Boston: Bartholomew Green, 1694), 28.

21. Bradford, *Plymouth Plantation*, 271; Winthrop, *Journal*, 5 Dec. 1633, p. 105; Mather, *Magnalia*, 1:78.

22. Winship, *Seers of God*, 1–28.

23. Alfred W. Crosby, "Virgin Soil Epidemics as a Factor in the Aboriginal Depopulation in America," *William and Mary Quarterly* 33 (April 1976): 290; J. S. Cummins, "Pox and Paranoia in Renaissance Europe," *History Today* (August 1988): 28; Noble David Cook and W. George Lovell, "Introduction," in Cook and Lovell, *"Secret Judgments of God": Old World Disease in Colonial Spanish America* (Norman: University of Oklahoma Press, 1991), xv; William H. McNeill, *Plagues and Peoples* (New York: Doubleday, 1977), 180; Jared Diamond, *Guns, Germs, and Steel: The Fates of Human Societies* (New York: Norton, 1997), 211–212. For a discussion, see David S. Jones, "Virgin Soils Revisited," *William and Mary Quarterly*, 60 (October 2003): 703–742.

24. Roger Williams, "Testimony of Roger Williams Relative to the Purchase of Lands at Seekonk and Providence," 13 Dec. 1661, in *The Complete Writings of Roger Williams*, ed. John Russell Bartlett (New York: Russell and Russell, 1963), 6:317; Glenn W. LaFantasie, ed., *The Correspondence of Roger Williams* (Hanover: University Press of New England, 1988), 2:620–621 n.7.

25. Winslow, *Good Newes from New England*, 291–292; Bradford, *Plymouth Plantation*, 99; Smith, *Generall History of Virginia*, 2:451. Increase Mather added that the Indians were just as frightened to hear that the English God controlled disease: "Consideration of that also was some terror to those Indians." Mather, *A Relation Of the Troubles which have hapned in New-England, By reason of the Indians there* (Boston: John Foster, 1677), 8. Many historians have discussed this episode, e.g., Noble David Cook, *Born to Die: Disease and New World Conquest, 1492–1650* (Cambridge: Cambridge University Press, 1998), 210; Kupperman, *Indians and English*, 191.

26. Morton, *New English Canaan*, 71.

27. Williams to Henry Vane and John Winthrop, 1 May 1637, in *Correspondence of Roger Williams*, ed. LaFantasie, 1:72.

28. Browne to D'Ewes, 1638, in *Letters from New England*, 228; Mather, *Magnalia*, 1:85.

29. Compare Samuel Clarke, *A True, and Faithful Account of the Four Chiefest Plantations of the English in America* (London, 1670), 8, 22, 30, 43; and William Wood, *New Englands Prospect* (1634), ed. Alden T. Vaughan (Amherst: University of Massachusetts Press, 1977), 38, 58, 75, 110–111. Compare Hubbard, *General History of New England*, 194–195, 531–532; and Winthrop, *Journal*, 5 Dec. 1633, p. 105; ibid. June 1647, p. 690. Compare Mather, *Relation Of the Troubles*, 7, to [Bradford], "A Relation or Journall of the Proceedings of the Plantation setled at Plimoth in New England," in George Morton, ed. *Mourt's Relation, or Journal of*

the Plymouth Plantation (1622), ed. Henry Martyn Dexter (Boston: John Kimball Wiggin, 1865), 84–85; Gookin, *Historical Collections of the Indians in New England,* 9; Johnson, *History of New-England,* 79; Mather, *Magnalia,* 1:51.

30. Hubbard, *General History of New England,* 57; Hubbard, "Narrative of the Discovery and First Planting of the Massachusetts" (ca. 1680), in *Chronicles of the First Planters of the Colony of Massachusetts Bay,* ed. Young, 32. Mather, *Magnalia,* 78; Mather, *The Angel of Bethesda: An Essay upon the Common Maladies of Mankind* (ca. 1724), ed. Gordon W. Jones (Barre, Mass.: American Antiquarian Society, 1972), 93–94.

31. Johnson, *History of New-England,* 84, 154, 41, 79. Johnson did note that some people disagreed with this providential interpretation, instead attributing climate change to "the cutting downe the woods, and breaking up the Land" (84). Mather, *Magnalia,* 1:54, 1:51; Increase Mather, *A Brief History of the War with the Indians in New-England* (London: Richard Chiswell, 1676), 39, 49, 51, postscript p. 8; Gookin, *Historical Collections,* 9–10; Hubbard, *General History of New England,* 55, 195.

32. *French shipwreck:* Nathaniel Morton, *New-Englands Memorial,* 27; Hubbard, *General History of New England,* 54–55; Mather, *Magnalia,* 1:51. *Nursing care:* Johnson, *History of New-England,* 79; Mather, *Magnalia,* 1:78. *John Sagamore's conversion:* Johnson, *History of New-England,* 79–80; Mather, *Magnalia,* 1:78; Hubbard, *General History of New England,* 650. *Prayers and their limits:* Mather, *Magnalia,* 2:442–43.

33. Smith to Frances Bacon, 1618, in Smith, *Works,* 1: 377–383; Smith, *New Englands Trials* (1620), ibid., 1:391–406; Smith, *New Englands Trials* (1622), ibid., 1:428.

34. [Bradford], "Journall of the Proceedings of the Plantation," 84–85; Bradford, *Plymouth Plantation,* 87, 270, 296. For the savagery of the Pequot War, see - Alfred A. Cave, *The Pequot War* (Amherst: University of Massachusetts Press, 1996).

35. Hall, *Worlds of Wonder,* 139–143, 171–172.

36. Nathaniel Morton, *New-Englands Memorial,* 179; Increase Mather, *Brief History of the War with the Indians,* 32, 39; Joshua Scottow, *A Narrative of the Planting of the Massachusetts Bay Colony Anno 1628. With the Lords Signal Present the First Thirty Years* (1694), in *Collections of the Massachusetts Historical Society,* 4th ser., vol. 4 (Boston: Little, Brown, 1858), 302, 309.

37. John Josselyn, *New-Englands Rarities Discovered* (1672), ed. Edward Tuckerman (Boston: William Veazie, 1865), 165; Josselyn, *An Account of Two Voyages to New-England* (1674), in *John Josselyn, Colonial Traveler: A Critical Edition of Two Voyages to New-England,* ed. Paul J. Lindholdt (Hanover: University Press of New England, 1988), 89; Josselyn, *Chronological Observations of America* (1674), ibid., 174; Gookin, *Historical Collections,* 9–12; Hubbard, *General History of New England,* 51; Mather, *Magnalia,* 1:51.

38. Sherburne F. Cook, "Interracial Warfare and Population Decline among the New England Indians," *Ethnohistory* 20 (Winter 1973): 1–24; Cook, "The Significance of Disease in the Extinction of the New England Indians," *Human Biology* 45 (September 1973): 485–508. Evidence of population reduction observed by colonists (abandoned villages, overgrown fields) might have reflected migrations of Indians away from the coast (away from both the epidemics and the colonists): Morton, *New English Canaan,* 19; Roger Williams, *A Key into the Language of Amer-*

ica (1643), ed. John J. Teunissen and Evelyn J. Hinz (Detroit: Wayne State University Press, 1973), 128.

39. Johnson, *History of New-England*, 48–49; Mr. Moor to the Secretary of the Society for the Propagation of the Gospel in Foreign Parts, 13 Nov. 1705, quoted in John Duffy, "Smallpox and the Indians in the American Colonies," *Bulletin of the History of Medicine* 25 (July–August 1951): 326.

40. Joyce E. Chaplin, "Natural Philosophy and an Early Racial Idiom in North America: Comparing English and Indian Bodies," *William and Mary Quarterly* 54 (January 1997): 245; Chaplin, *Subject Matter*, 174–175.

41. Wood, *New Englands Prospect*, 82; Thomas Mayhew to [Henry Whitfield?], ca. 1650, in *The Light Appearing More and More towards the Perfect Day*, ed. Henry Whitfield (1651), in *CMHS*, 3rd ser., vol. 4. (Cambridge: Charles Folsom, 1834), 110; Williams to John Throckmorton, 30 July 1672, in *Correspondence*, ed. LaFantasie, 2:675.

42. Gookin, *Historical Collections of the Indians in New England*, 8–10, 53–54. Gookin was appointed superintendent of the Indians of Massachusetts in 1656, a position he held, more or less, until 1687. His support for the Indians made him very unpopular during King Philip's War: angry colonists supposedly threatened the lives of both Gookin and missionary John Eliot. See "Introduction," in Gookin, *Historical Collections*, ix.

43. James D. Drake, *King Philip's War: Civil War in New England, 1675–1676* (Amherst: University of Massachusetts Press, 1999), 14, 1, 174; LaFantasie, "Introduction," in *The Correspondence of Roger Williams*, xliii.

44. Drake, *King Philip's War*, 169–174; Jill Lepore, *The Name of War: King Philip's War and the Origins of American Identity* (New York: Knopf, 1998), xiii, 174, 185.

45. Drake, *King Philip's War*, 194.

3. Frontiers of Smallpox

1. Roger Williams to Henry Vane and John Winthrop, 1 May 1637, in *The Correspondence of Roger Williams*, ed. Glenn W. LaFantasie (Hanover: University Press of New England, 1988), 1:72

2. Gregory Nobles, *American Frontiers: Cultural Encounters and Continental Conquest* (New York: Hill and Wang, 1997), ix–xv, 3–16; Richard White, *The Middle Ground: Indians, Empires, and Republics in the Great Lakes Region, 1650–1815* (Cambridge: Cambridge University Press, 1991).

3. Indians held nearly all the lands west of the Appalachians in 1790; less than 3 percent of white Americans lived in the west. This percentage had increased to 28 percent by 1830. In 1820 there were 125,000 Indians east of the Mississippi; by 1844, only 30,000 (and most of these lived around Lake Superior). Michael Paul Rogin, *Fathers and Children: Andrew Jackson and the Subjugation of the American Indian* (1975; New Brunswick: Transaction, 1991), 4.

4. Charles E. Rosenberg, *The Cholera Years* (1962; Chicago: University of Chicago Press, 1987); Paul Starr, *The Social Transformation of American Medicine* (New York: Basic Books, 1982); John H. Warner, *The Therapeutic Perspective: Medical Practice, Knowledge, and Identity in America 1820–1885* (Cambridge: Harvard University Press, 1986).

5. Alexander Philip Maximilian, *Travels in the Interior of North America*, trans. Hannibal Evans Lloyd (1843), in *Early Western Travels*, 22:40, 22:43, 22:138, 22:217, 22:251–252. See also Harry Liebersohn, *Aristocratic Encounters: European Travelers and North American Indians* (Cambridge: Cambridge University Press, 1998), 135–163.

6. Simeon Ecuyer to Henry Bouquet, 11 Mar. 1763, *Bouquet Papers*, 6:167; Ecuyer to Bouquet, 23 April 1763, ibid., 6:178; Ecuyer to Bouquet, 8 Jan. 1763, ibid., 6:142; Ecuyer to Bouquet, 19 March 1763, in *Fort Pitt and Letters from the Frontier*, ed. Mary Carson Darlington (Pittsburgh: J. R. Weldin & Co., 1892), 117. See also Francis Parkman, *The Conspiracy of Pontiac and the Indian War after the Conquest of Canada* (1870; Boston: Little, Brown, 1898), 2:6; A. T. Volwiler, "Introduction" to William Trent, "Journal at Fort Pitt, 1763," in *Mississippi Valley Historical Review* 11 (Dec. 1924): 392; C. Hale Sipe, *The Indian Wars of Pennsylvania*, 2nd ed. (Harrisburg: Telegraph Press, 1931), 418.

7. Chardon, *Journal*, 51–65, 7, 193, 18; Edward T. Denig, "Description of Fort Union, 30 July 1843," in Audubon, *Journals*, 2:180; Bernard De Voto, *Across the Wide Missouri* (Boston: Houghton Mifflin, 1947), 119; George Catlin, *North American Indians* (1841), ed. Peter Matthiessen (New York: Penguin, 1989), 73; Henry A. Boller, *Among the Indians: Eight Years in the Far West, 1858–1866* (1868), ed. Milo Milton Quaife (Chicago: Lakeside Press, 1959), 28–29; Hiram Martin Chittenden, *The American Fur Trade of the Far West* (New York: Francis P. Harper, 1902), 98–106; Chittenden, *History of Early Steamboat Navigation on the Missouri River* (New York: Francis P. Harper, 1903), 139 n.

8. Francis Jennings, *Empire of Fortune: Crowns, Colonies, and Tribes in the Seven Years War in America* (New York: Norton, 1988), 21; White, *Middle Ground*, x.

9. *Mandan:* George Catlin, *Illustrations of the Manners, Customs, and Condition of the North American Indians*, 10th ed. (London: Henry G. Bohn, 1866), 1:80; Henry R. Schoolcraft, *Information Respecting the History, Condition and Prospects of the Indian Tribes of the United States*, (Philadelphia: Lippincott, Grambo, 1851–1857), 3:249. *Population:* C. A. Harris, "Report from the Commissioner of Indian Affairs," 1 Dec. 1836, 24th Cong., 2d sess., 301 H. Doc. 2, p. 403; Harris, "Report from the Office of Indian Affairs," 1 Dec. 1837, 25th Cong., 2d sess., 321 H. Doc. 3, p. 642; T. Hartley Crawford, "Report of the Commissioner of Indian Affairs," 25 Nov. 1838, 25th Cong., 3d sess., 344 H. Doc. 2, p. 474; Russell Thornton, *American Indian Holocaust and Survival: A Population History since 1492* (Norman: University of Oklahoma Press, 1987), 95–96. *Contrasting visions:* Catlin, *Manners, Customs, and Condition*, letters #11–22, and Audubon, *Journals*, 2:10, 13, 27.

10. John C. Ewers, *The Blackfeet: Raiders on the Northwestern Plains* (Norman: University of Oklahoma Press, 1958), 23–60; Stephen E. Ambrose, *Undaunted Courage: Meriwether Lewis, Thomas Jefferson, and the Opening of the American West* (New York: Simon and Schuster, 1996), 387–392; Theodore Binnema, *Common and Contested Ground: A Human and Environmental History of the Northwestern Plains* (Norman: University of Oklahoma Press, 2001).

11. See Rogin, *Fathers and Children*; Ronald N. Satz, *American Indian Policy in the Jacksonian Era* (Lincoln: University of Nebraska Press, 1975); Satz, "Rhetoric Versus Reality: The Indian Policy of Andrew Jackson," in *Cherokee Removal: Before and After*, ed. William L. Anderson (Athens: University of Georgia Press, 1991), 29–54.

12. John Duffy, "Smallpox and the Indians in the American Colonies," *Bulletin of the History of Medicine* 25 (July–August 1951): 324–341; Ewers, *The Blackfeet*, 28–29; Thornton, *American Indian Holocaust and Survival*, 91–94.

13. John Dougherty to William Clark, 29 Oct. 1831, in Lewis Cass, "Small Pox Among the Indians: Letter from the Secretary of War, Upon the subject of the Small Pox among the Indian tribes," 30 March 1832, 22d Cong., 1st sess., 220 H. Doc. 190, pp. 1–2; Catlin, *Manners, Customs, and Condition*, 2:24–25, 43–44; Maximilian, *Travels in the Interior*, 22:271.

14. Thornton, *American Indian Holocaust and Survival*, 94–95; Chardon, in Audubon, *Journals*, 2:47; Schoolcraft, *Information Respecting the History*, 1:257.

15. Mr. Moor to the Secretary of the Society for the Propagation of the Gospel in Foreign Parts, 13 Nov. 1705, quoted in Duffy, "Smallpox and the Indians," 326; Thomas Hutchinson, *The History of the Colony of Massachusetts-Bay, 1628–1691* (Boston: Thomas and John Fleet, 1764), 35 n.

16. Moor to the Secretary of the Society, 326; Edward Winslow, *Good Newes from New England* (1624), in *Chronicles of the Pilgrim Fathers of the Colony of Plymouth, from 1602 to 1625*, ed. Alexander Young, 2d ed. (Boston: Charles C. Little and James Brown, 1844), 350; Catlin, *Illustrations of the Manners, Customs, and Condition*, 1:137, 1:143.

17. Maximilian, *Travels in the Interior*, 23:237, 24:132; Catlin, *Manners, Customs, and Condition*, 2:258; [James H. Bradley and Andrew Culbertson], "Affairs at Fort Benton, from 1831 to 1869; from Lieutenant Bradley's Journal," *Contributions to the Historical Society of Montana* 3 (1909): 265–266; Chittenden, *Early Steamboat Navigation*, 32–36, 238 n.

18. James Kenny, "Journal, 1761–1763," ed. John W. Jordan, *Pennsylvania Magazine of History and Biography* 37 (1913): 15, 152; Chardon, *Journal*, 45. *Dodge Expedition:* Catlin, *Manners, Customs, and Condition*, 2:53, 2:77 2:81–82; De Voto, *Across the Wide Missouri*, 349. For theories of health and environment on the frontier, see Conevery Bolton Valencius, *The Health of the Country: How American Settlers Understood Themselves and Their Land* (New York: Basic Books, 2002).

19. David Zeisberger, *History of the Northern American Indians* (1779–1780), ed. Archer Butler Hulbert and William Nathaniel Schwarze (Columbus: Ohio State Archeological and Historical Society, 1910), 23; John Heckewelder, *An Account of the History, Manners, and Customs of the Indian Nations who once Inhabited Pennsylvania and the Neighbouring States* (1819), rev. ed. (Philadelphia: Historical Society of Pennsylvania, 1876), 222; Catlin, *Illustrations of the Manners, Customs, and Condition*, 2:257; Edwin James, *Account of an Expedition from Pittsburg to the Rocky Mountains, performed in the years 1819–1820* (1823), in *Early Western Travels*, 15:46, 15:118–119, 16:117; Maximilian, *Travels in the Interior*, 23:236, 23:359.

20. Hutchinson, *History of the Colony of Massachusetts-Bay, 1628–1691*, 1:34–35 n; Zeisberger, *Northern American Indians*, 149; Heckewelder, *History, Manners, and Customs*, 220–226; Catlin, *Manners, Customs, and Condition*, 2:258.

21. Chardon, *Journal*, 37. *Indian skill:* John Lawson, *History of North Carolina* (1714; Richmond: Garrett and Massie: 1951), 231; Heckewelder, *History, Manners, and Customs*, 224–229; Catlin, *Manners, Customs, and Condition*, 1:39; David G. Burnet, "Comanches and other Tribes of Texas, and the Policy to be pursued respecting them," 29 Sept. 1847, in *Information Respecting the History*, ed. Schoolcraft, 1:233; Josiah Gregg, *Commerce of the Prairies*, 2nd ed. (1845), in *Early Western*

Travels, 19:334. *Overdoses*: Zeisberger, *Northern American Indians*, 56; Maximilian, *Travels in the Interior*, 23:119–120. *Religious aspects*: Lawson, *History of North Carolina*, 227; Heckewelder, *History, Manners, and Customs*, 231–243; Burnet, "Comanches and other Tribes," 1:233; Catlin, *Manners, Customs, and Condition*, 1:39.

22. Zeisberger, *Northern American Indians*, 159 n.34; Maximilian, *Travels in the Interior*, 23:290, 23:359; Catlin, *Manners, Customs, and Condition*, 1:99. Adario, quoted in E. Wagner Stearn and Allen E. Stearn, *The Effect of Smallpox on the Destiny of the Amerindian* (Boston: Bruce Humphries, 1945), 30. *Harms of sweat baths*: Lawson, *History of North Carolina*, 5; Adair, quoted in Stearn and Stearn, *Effect of Smallpox*, 39; Catlin, *Manners, Customs, and Condition*, 2:257–258; Burnet, "Comanches and other Tribes," 1:234; Gregg, *Commerce of the Prairies*, 19:334; Audubon, *Journals*, 2:46–47; P. J. De Smet, *Letters and Sketches: With a Narrative of a Year's Residence among the Indian Tribes of the Rocky Mountains* (1843), in *Early Western Travels*, 27:265. For historians, see Thornton, *American Indian Holocaust and Survival*, 102; Robert Boyd, *The Coming of the Spirit of Pestilence: Introduced Infectious Diseases and Population Decline among Northwest Coast Indians, 1774–1874* (Seattle: University of Washington Press, 1999), 19; Adrienne Mayor, "The Nessus Shirt in the New World: Smallpox Blankets in History and Legend," *Journal of American Folklore* 108 (Winter 1995): 68–69.

23. M. de Montcalm to Marquis de Paulmy, 18 April 1758, in *DRCHNY*, 10:700. See John J. Heagerty, *Four Centuries of Medical History in Canada* (London: Simpkin, Marshall, Hamilton, Kent, 1928), 1:41; Jennings, *Empire of Fortune*, 316–317; Ian K. Steele, *Warpaths: Invasions of North America* (New York: Oxford University Press, 1994), 204–205; Elizabeth A. Fenn, "Biological Warfare in Eighteenth-Century North America: Beyond Jeffrey Amherst," *Journal of American History* 86 (March 2000): 1566. For the Piegan episode, see Heagerty, *Four Centuries*, 35; Ewers, *The Blackfeet*, 28–29.

24. Zeisberger, *Northern American Indians*, 24, 131; Heckewelder, *History, Manners, and Customs*, 221–223; Elbert Herring, "Report of the Commissioner of Indian Affairs," 29 Nov. 1833, 23d Cong., 1st sess., 254 H. Doc. 1, p. 171; James, *Expedition from Pittsburg to the Rocky Mountains*, 15:44; Maximilian, *Travels in the Interior of North America*, 23:359. See also Peter C. Mancall, *Deadly Medicine: Indians and Alcohol in Early America* (Ithaca: Cornell University Press, 1995).

25. Heckewelder, *History, Manners, and Customs*, 221.

26. Joel N. Shurkin, *The Invisible Fire: The Story of Mankind's Victory over the Ancient Scourge of Smallpox* (New York: G.P. Putnam's Sons, 1979), 114; Kenny, "Journal, 1761–1763," 178; "Conference Between Governor Hunter and the Indians," 13 to 17 June 1717, in *DRCHNY*, 5:485–487; George Catlin, *Catlin's Notes of Eight Years Travel and Residence in Europe* (London: Published by the author, 1848), 2:41.

27. Heckewelder, *History, Manners, and Customs*, 220–221; James, *Expedition from Pittsburg*, 15:19; Burnet, "Comanches and Other Tribes of Texas," 1:231; Maximilian, *Travels in the Interior*, 23:120; Catlin, *Manners, Customs, and Condition*, 2:228, 2:258.

28. Zeisberger, *Northern American Indians*, 79–80, 149; Heckewelder, *History, Manners, and Customs*, 223, 261; Timothy Flint, Letter #18, 26 June 1820, in *Flint's Letters from America, 1818–1820*, in *Early Western Travels*, 9:249; Catlin, *Manners, Customs, and Condition*, 1:99, 2:256.

29. "Conference Between Governor Hunter and the Indians," 5:485–487; William Cosby, "Propositions made by his Excellency," 8 Sept. 1733, in *DRCHNY,* 5:963; "Answer made by the Sachims of the Six Nations to His Excellcy Wm Cosby Esqre," 11 Sept. 1733, ibid., 5:965.

30. "Conference between M. de Vaudreuil and the Senecas," 1–3 Oct. 1755, in *DRCHNY,* 10:345–346; Montcalm to De Paulmy, 18 April 1758, ibid. 10:700.

31. Jonthan Belcher to the Penobscot Indians, 28 July 1733, in *CMHS,* 6th ser., vol. 6, (1893), 344; Belcher to David Dunbar, 17 Sept. 1733, ibid., 367; Colonel [William] Johnson to Governor Clinton, 7 May 1747, in *DRCHNY,* 6:362; Paul Kelton, "Avoiding the Smallpox Spirits: Colonial Epidemics and Southeastern Indian Survival," *Ethnohistory* 51 (Winter 2004).

32. Kelton, "Avoiding the Smallpox Spirits"; *Minutes of the Provincial Council of Pennsylvania,* vol. 29, *29 January 1756–11 January 1758* (Harrisburg: Theo. Fenn, 1851), 199, 517, 546, 550; Duffy, "Smallpox and the Indians," 337; D. Peter MacLeod, "Microbes and Muskets: Smallpox and the Participation of the Amerindian Allies of New France in the Seven Years' War," *Ethnohistory* 39 (Winter 1992): 42–64; Thomas Hutchinson, *The History of the Province of Massachusetts-Bay, from 1749 to 1774,* ed. John Hutchinson (London: John Murray, 1828), 52.

33. Herring, "Report of the Commissioner of Indian Affairs," 25 Nov. 1834, 23rd Cong., 2d sess., 271 H. Doc. 2, p. 242; Herring, "Report of the Commissioner of Indian Affairs," 24 Nov. 1835, 24th Cong., 1st sess., 286 H. Doc. 2, p. 290.

34. Thomas Jefferson, quoted in N. Barquet and P. Domingo, "Smallpox: The Triumph over the Most Terrible of the Ministers of Death," *Annals of Internal Medicine* 127 (1997): 640; Benjamin Waterhouse to Matthias Spalding, 15 April 1802, quoted in Walter C. Alvarez, "Some Correspondence Relating to the Introduction of Vaccination into America," *California and Western Medicine* 23 (May 1925): 583. See Bernard W. Sheehan, *Seeds of Extinction: Jeffersonian Philanthropy and the American Indian* (Chapel Hill: University of North Carolina Press, 1973), 230.

35. Cotton Mather, *The Angel of Bethesda: An Essay upon the Common Maladies of Mankind* (c. 1724), ed. Gordon W. Jones (Barre, Mass.: American Antiquarian Society, 1972), 107–116; Michael K. Trimble, "The 1837–1838 Smallpox Epidemic on the Upper Missouri," in *Skeletal Biology in the Great Plains: Migration, Warfare, Health, and Subsistence,* ed. Douglas W. Owsley and Richard L. Jantz (Washington, D.C.: Smithsonian Institution Press, 1994), 85.

36. John B. Blake, "The Inoculation Controversy in Boston, 1721–1722" (1952), in *Sickness and Health in America: Readings in the History of Medicine and Public Health,* 2nd ed., ed. Judith Walzer Leavitt and Ronald L. Numbers (Madison: University of Wisconsin Press, 1985), 347–355; I. Bernard Cohen, ed., *Cotton Mather and American Science and Medicine: With Studies and Documents Concerning the Introduction of Inoculation or Variolation,* 2 vols. (New York: Arno, 1980).

37. Mather, *Diary of Cotton Mather,* vol. 2, *1709–1724* (New York: Frederick Ungar, 1974), Jul. through Nov. 1721, pp. 631–661; Thomas Hutchinson, *The History of the Province of Massachusetts-Bay, 1691–1750* (Boston: Thomas and John Fleet, 1767), 273–275; Perry Miller, "The Judgment of Smallpox," in *The New England Mind: The Seventeenth Century* (New York: Macmillan, 1939); Blake, "Inoculation Controversy in Boston," 350–352; Patricia Cline Cohen, *A Calculating*

People: The Spread of Numeracy in Early America (Chicago: University of Chicago Press, 1982).

38. Duffy, "Smallpox and the Indians," 337–338; Mary C. Gillett, *The Army Medical Department, 1775–1818* (Washington: Government Printing Office, 1981), 14; Elizabeth A. Fenn, *Pox Americana: The Great Smallpox Epidemic of 1775–82* (New York: Hill and Wang, 2001), 31–43.

39. Fenn, *Pox Americana*, 44–103.

40. Heagerty, *Four Centuries*, 1:43; Sherburne F. Cook, "Smallpox in Spanish and Mexican California, 1770–1845," *Bulletin of the History of Medicine* 7 (February 1939): 154–166; Duffy, "Smallpox and the Indians," 333; Stearn and Stearn, *Effect of Smallpox*, 36, 41, 51–55; Donald R. Hopkins, *Princes and Peasants: Smallpox in History* (Chicago: University of Chicago Press, 1983), 219–220.

41. Gillett, *Army Medical Department, 1775–1818*, 14; Hopkins, *Princes and Peasants*, 81.

42. Alvarez, "Correspondence Relating to the Introduction of Vaccination," 583; Eldon G. Chuinard, *Only One Man Died: The Medical Aspects of the Lewis and Clark Expedition* (Glendale, Calif.: Arthur H. Clarke, 1979), 104–105, 142–143; Barquet and Domingo, "Smallpox: the Triumph," 640.

43. Gillett, *Army Medical Department, 1775–1818*, 14; Mary C. Gillett, *The Army Medical Department, 1818–1865* (Washington: Government Printing Office, 1987), 15; "An Act to Encourage Vaccination," 27 Feb. 1813, *Laws of the United States, from the 4th of March, 1789, to the 4th of March, 1815*, vol. 4 (Philadelphia: John Biorent and W. John Dunae, 1815–1845), 508–509; Robert Thomas, *A Treatise on Domestic Medicine*, 1st Am. ed. (New York: Collins, 1822), 121–125.

44. Jefferson, "Instructions to Lewis and Clark," 20 June 1803, in *Original Journals of the Lewis and Clark Expedition, 1804–1806*, ed. Reuben Gold Thwaites (New York: Dodd, Mead, 1904–1905), 7:250; Chuinard, *Only One Man Died*, 101–111, 177–186.

45. Philip King Brown, "A Review of the Early Vaccination Controversy with an Original Letter by Jenner Referring to it, and to the Spread of Vaccination to the Spanish Possessions of America, the Philippines, and other European Settlements in the Orient," *California State Journal of Medicine* 12 (May 1914): 176–177; Stearn and Stearn, *Effect of Smallpox*, 61; Samuel M. Wilson, "On the Matter of Smallpox," *Natural History* 103 (September 1994): 64–65. Heagerty, *Four Centuries*, 48–49.

46. Lewis to Jefferson, 3 Oct. 1803, in *Original Journals of the Lewis and Clark Expedition*, 7:278; Chuinard, *Only One Man Died*, 178–179, 183–184n, 206–212.

47. Charles Larpenteur, *Forty years a Fur Trader on the Upper Missouri*, ed. Milo Milton Quaife (1933; Lincoln: University of Nebraska Press, 1989), 109; Thomas, *Domestic Medicine*, 27, 66–69, 119–121; Maximilian, *Travels in the Interior*, 24:18–19, 24:81–82.

48. Thomas, *Domestic Medicine*, 121–124.

4. Using Smallpox

1. Thomas Hutchinson, *The History of the Province of Massachusetts-Bay, 1691–1750* (Boston: Thomas and John Fleet, 1767), 275.

2. Henry Bouquet to Jeffrey Amherst, 23 June 1763, in *Bouquet Papers*, 6:251.

The original manuscripts can be found in the Henry Bouquet Papers in the British Library, London.

3. Bouquet to Amherst, 25 June 1763, in *Bouquet Papers*, 6:256; Amherst to Bouquet, 29 June 1763, ibid., 6:277; Bouquet to Amherst, 3 July 1763, ibid., 6:288–289; Amherst to Bouquet, 7 July 1763, ibid., 6:299–300; [Amherst], Postscript [to Bouquet], [7 July 1763], ibid., 6:301; Bouquet to Amherst, 13 July 1763, in *Bouquet Papers (1940–1942)*, ser. 21634, p. 215; [Amherst], Postscript [to Bouquet], [16 July 1763], in *Bouquet Papers*, 6:315. Amherst's statements are undated and signed only "JA." Circumstantial evidence and handwriting analysis place them in the above sequence. See Bernhard Knollenberg, "General Amherst and Germ Warfare," *Mississippi Valley Historical Review* 41 (December 1954): 492–493; Louis M. Waddell, in *Bouquet Papers*, 6:301.

4. Knollenberg, "Amherst and Germ Warfare," 494.

5. Simeon Ecuyer to Bouquet, 16 June 1763, in *Bouquet Papers*, 6:231; Ecuyer to Bouquet, 26 June 1763, ibid., 6:259–260; Alexander McKee, "Discourse between Delawares and Ecuyer at Fort Pitt," 24 June 1763, enclosure of Ecuyer to Bouquet, 26 June 1763, ibid., 6:262; William Trent, "Journal at Fort Pitt, 1763," ed. A. T. Volwiler, *Mississippi Valley Historical Review* 11 (December 1924): 400.

6. Ecuyer to Bouquet, 26 June 1763, 6:259–260; McKee, "Discourse between Delawares and Ecuyer," 6:261–263; William Trent, "Dr The Crown to Levy, Trent & Company, for Sundries had by Order of Capt. Simon Ecuyer Commandt" (1763), in *Bouquet Papers (1940–1942)*, ser. 21654, pp. 218–219.

7. Francis Parkman, *The Conspiracy of Pontiac and the Indian War after the Conquest of Canada* (1870; Boston: Little, Brown, 1898), 1:vii–viii, 42–47; C. Hale Sipe, *The Indian Wars of Pennsylvania*, 2nd ed. (Harrisburg: Telegraph Press, 1931), 423–424; Knollenberg, "Amherst and Germ Warfare," 489–494; Knollenberg and Kent, "Communications," *Mississippi Valley Historical Review* 41 (March 1955): 762–763. *Biological warfare:* Ward Churchill, *Indians Are Us? Culture and Genocide in Native North America* (Toronto: Between The Lines, 1994), 34, 343 n.52. Also Francis Jennings, *Empire of Fortune: Crowns, Colonies, and Tribes in the Seven Years War in America* (New York: Norton, 1988), 447–448; Adrienne Mayor, "The Nessus Shirt in the New World: Smallpox Blankets in History and Legend," *Journal of American Folklore* 108 (Winter 1995): 54–77; George W. Christopher, Theodore J. Cieslak, Julie Pavlin, and Edward Eitzen, "Biological Warfare: A Historical Perspective," *JAMA* 278 (6 August 1997): 412; Elizabeth A. Fenn, "Biological Warfare in Eighteenth-Century North America: Beyond Jeffrey Amherst," *Journal of American History* 86 (March 2000): 1552–1580.

8. Jennings, *Empire of Fortune*; Fred Anderson, *Crucible of War: The Seven Years' War and the Fate of Empire in British North America, 1754–1766* (New York: Knopf, 2000).

9. George Croghan, "Journal, 1759–1763," ed. Nicholas B. Wainwright, in *Pennsylvania Magazine of History and Biography* 71 (October 1947), 394–395, 311, 403 n, 423–424, 432–434; McKee, "Report Written at Lower Shawnese Town," 8 Nov. 1762, forwarded from Ecuyer to Bouquet, 22 Nov. 1762, in *Bouquet Papers*, 6:133. For the course of the war, see Howard H. Peckham, *Pontiac and the Indian Uprising* (Princeton: Princeton University Press, 1947); Jennings, *Empire of Fortune*, 439–442; Anderson, *Crucible of War*, 469–471.

10. Amherst to Bouquet, 6 June 1763, in *Bouquet Papers*, 6:209; Amherst to

Bouquet, 16 July 1763 (2nd letter), in *Bouquet Papers (1940–1942)*, ser. 21634, p. 219; Amherst to Bouquet, 7 Aug. 1763, *Bouquet Papers*, 6:352; Amherst to Bouquet, 11 Jan. 1763, ibid., 6:147; Bouquet to Amherst, 25 June 1763, 6:255.

11. John E. Ferling, *A Wilderness of Miseries: War and Warriors in Early America* (Westport, Conn.: Greenwood, 1980), 22, 28; Don Higginbotham, "The Early American Way of War: Reconnaissance and Appraisal," *William and Mary Quarterly* 44 (April 1987): 233; Patrick M. Malone, *The Skulking Way of War: Technology and Tactics among the New England Indians* (Baltimore: Johns Hopkins University Press, 1991), 105.

12. Ecuyer to Bouquet, 30 May 1763, in *Bouquet Papers*, 6:195; Ecuyer to Bouquet, 16 June 1763, 6:231–232; Bouquet to Amherst, 13 July 1763, in *Bouquet Papers (1940–1942)*, p. 215; [Amherst], Postscript [to Bouquet], [16 July 1763], in *Bouquet Papers*, p. 315. See Mark A. Mastromarino, "Teaching Old Dogs New Tricks: The English Mastiff and the Anglo-American Experience," *Historian* 49 (November 1986): 10–25.

13. *Smallpox and war:* John Duffy, "Smallpox and the Indians in the American Colonies," *Bulletin of the History of Medicine* 25 (July–August 1951): 331; D. Peter MacLeod, "Microbes and Muskets: Smallpox and the Participation of the Amerindian Allies of New France in the Seven Years' War," *Ethnohistory* 39 (Winter 1992): 42–64. *Smallpox and Bouquet's soldiers: Minutes of the Provincial Council of Pennsylvania*, vol. 29, *29 January 1756–11 January 1758* (Harrisburg: Theo. Fenn, 1851), 358; Adam Stephen to Bouquet, 29 June 1762, in *Bouquet Papers*, 6:99. *Backwoods traditions:* Michael N. McConnell, *A Country Between: The Upper Ohio and Its Peoples, 1724–1774* (Lincoln: University of Nebraska Press, 1992), 194; Francis Jennings, *The Founders of America* (New York: Norton, 1993), 298–299 (quotation). *Accusations:* Paul Kelton, "Avoiding the Smallpox Spirits: Colonial Epidemics and Southeastern Indian Survival," *Ethnohistory* 51 (Winter 2004); Cornelius J. Jaenen, *The French Relationship with the Native Peoples of New France and Acadia* (Ottawa: Minister of Indian Affairs and Northern Development, 1984), 181–182; Fenn, "Biological Warfare," 1565–1567.

14. Trent, "Dr The Crown to Levy, Trent & Company," 218–219; Bouquet to Amherst, 11 Aug. 1763, in *Bouquet Papers*, 6:361.

15. *Motivated by Indian weakness:* Bernard W. Sheehan, *Seeds of Extinction: Jeffersonian Philanthropy and the American Indian* (Chapel Hill: University of North Carolina Press, 1973), 228. Bouquet to Amherst, 13 July 1763, p. 215.

16. Higginbotham, "Early American Way of War," 234; McConnell, *Country Between*, 195; Anderson, *Crucible of War*, 543; Fenn, "Biological Warfare," 1567–1573, 1577–1578; Fenn, *Pox Americana: The Great Smallpox Epidemic of 1775–82* (New York: Hill and Wang, 2001).

17. Alfred T. Goodman, "Biographical Sketch of William Trent," in *Journal of Captain William Trent: From Logstown to Pickawillany* (1752), ed. Goodman (Cincinnati: Robert Clarke & Co., 1871), 57–67; Trent, "Journal at Fort Pitt, 1763," 394; Trent, "List of Indian Traders and Servants Killed or Captured," enclosure in Bouquet to Amherst, 30 Sept. 1763, in *Bouquet Papers*, 6:412–413; Ecuyer to Bouquet, 2 June 1763, ibid., 6:202; Ecuyer to Bouquet, 16 June 1763, 6:232; *Bouquet Papers (1940–1942)*, ser. 21654, pp. 218, 222, 223, 227.

18. *Reports of smallpox:* William Grant, "Deposition of Gershom Hicks," 15 April 1764, in Grant to Bouquet, 15 April 1764, in *Bouquet Papers*, 6:515; "News

from Colonel McNeill," in Andrew Lewis to Bouquet, 10 Sept. 1764, in *Bouquet Papers (1940–1942)*, ser. 21650, part 1, p. 127; Bouquet to Johnson, 25 Jan. 1765, in *Bouquet Papers*, 6:750. *Cause and effect:* Jennings, *Founders of America*, 298–299; Fenn, "Biological Warfare," 1557. *Endemicity:* McConnell, *Country Between*, 195. *Other routes:* Fenn, "Biological Warfare," 1557. *July attack:* "Indian speeches at Fort Pitt," 26 July 1763, in Ecuyer to Bouquet, 2 Aug. 1763, in *Bouquet Papers*, 6:333–336; Ecuyer to Bouquet, 2 Aug. 1763, 6:332. For later accusations and possible attempts, see Mayor, "Nessus Shirt in the New World," 54–77; Duncan McDougall, quoted in Hubert Howe Bancroft, *History of the Northwest Coast*, vol. 2, *1800–1846*, vol. 28 in *The Works of Hubert Howe Bancroft*, 39 vols. (San Francisco: A. L. Bancroft, 1884), 2:176; Isaac McCoy, *History of Baptist Indian Missions* (1840), ed. Robert F. Berkhofer (New York: Johnson Reprint, 1970), 441–442.

19. Thomas Hariot, *A Briefe and True Report of the New Found Land of Virginia* (1588; Ann Arbor: Edward Brothers, 1931), F verso.

20. Clyde D. Dollar, "The High Plains Smallpox Epidemic of 1837–38," *Western Historical Quarterly* 8 (Jan. 1977): 18–21; Chardon, *Journal*, 118.

21. Charles Larpenteur, *Forty Years a Fur Trader on the Upper Missouri*, ed. Milo Milton Quaife (1933; Lincoln: University of Nebraska Press, 1989), 109; Jacob Halsey to Pratte Chouteau & Co., 2 Nov. 1837, in *Papers of the St. Louis Fur Trade*, part 1, *The Chouteau Collection, 1752–1925*, ed. William R. Swagerty, reel #25 (Bethesda: University Publications of America, 1991), pp. 139–140 [also in Chardon, *Journal*, 394–396]; [James H. Bradley and Andrew Culbertson], "Affairs at Fort Benton, from 1831 to 1869; from Lieutenant Bradley's Journal," *Contributions to the Historical Society of Montana* 3 (1909): 222.

22. Dollar, "High Plains Smallpox Epidemic," 34–37. Chardon, *Journal*, 121–161; Audubon, *Journals*, 2:42–47; George Catlin, *Illustrations of the Manners, Customs, and Condition of the North American Indians*, 10th ed. (London: Henry G. Bohn, 1866), 2:257–259.

23. [Bradley and Culbertson], "Affairs at Fort Benton," 221–227; P. J. De Smet, *Letters and Sketches: with a Narrative of a Year's Residence among the Indian Tribes of the Rocky Mountains* (1843), in *Early Western Travels*, 27:265.

24. "New Orleans, *June* 6, 1838," in Hannibal Evans Lloyd, "Translator's Preface," in Alexander Philip Maximilian, *Travels in the Interior of North America*, in *Early Western Travels*, 22:34–35; Audubon, *Journals*, 2:43–46; Catlin, *Manners, Customs, and Condition*, 2:257. See also [Bradley and Culbertson], "Affairs at Fort Benton," 224–226; Chardon, *Journal*, 123–133; Audubon, 2:44; Larpenteur, *Forty Years a Fur Trader*, 110–115.

25. "New Orleans, *June* 6, 1838," 22:33, 22:35. *Mortality estimates:* Mitchell, in Audubon, *Journals*, 2:47; Catlin, *Manners, Customs, and Condition*, 2:258; Henry R. Schoolcraft, *Information Respecting the History, Condition and Prospects of the Indian Tribes of the United States*, 6 vols. (Philadelphia: Lippincott, Grambo, 1851–1857), 1:257–258, 1:486.

26. "New Orleans, *June* 6, 1838," 22:33–36.

27. Dollar, "High Plains Smallpox Epidemic," 27–29, 38; [Bradley and Culbertson], "Affairs at Fort Benton," 226. C. A. Harris, "Report from the Office of Indian Affairs," 1 Dec. 1837, 25th Cong., 2d sess., 321 H. Doc. 3, p. 596; Chardon, *Journal*, 96, 122; Schoolcraft, *Information Respecting the History*, 6:486. See also Michael K. Trimble, "The 1837–1838 Smallpox Epidemic on the Upper

Missouri," in *Skeletal Biology in the Great Plains: Migration, Warfare, Health, and Subsistence*, ed. Douglas W. Owsley and Richard L. Jantz (Washington: Smithsonian Institution Press, 1994), 85–87.

28. T. Hartley Crawford, "Report of the Commissioner of Indian Affairs," 25 Nov. 1838, 25th Cong., 3d sess., 344 H. Doc. 2, p. 424.

29. *Tobacco:* Chardon, *Journal*, 129. *Fort Union:* Halsey to Pratte Chouteau & Co., 2 Nov. 1837, reel 25, p. 139; Larpenteur, *Forty Years a Fur Trader*, 110–111. *Fort McKenzie:* [Bradley and Culbertson], "Affairs at Fort Benton," 222–223; "New Orleans, *June* 6, 1838," 22:34. See also Arthur Ray, "Smallpox: The Epidemic of 1837–38," *Beaver: Magazine of the North* 306 (Autumn 1975): 9.

30. Chardon, *Journal*, 132. *Hospital:* "New Orleans, *June* 6, 1838," 22:34. *Inoculation:* Larpenteur, *Forty Years a Fur Trader*, 109–110; [Bradley and Culbertson], "Affairs at Fort Benton," 224. Halsey, who did not mention inoculation, reported only four deaths at Fort Union: Halsey to Pratte Chouteau & Co., 2 Nov. 1837, reel 25, p. 139; David L. Ferch, "Fighting the Smallpox Epidemic of 1837–38: The Response of the American Fur Company Traders—Conclusion," *Museum of the Fur Trade Quarterly* 20 (Spring 1984): 4–6.

31. The reliability of some accounts is suspect. When Chardon described the epidemic to Audubon in 1843, he added details that did not appear in his daily journal: blanket theft by a Mandan chief, a reward for the return of the blanket, and attempts to keep the Arikara and Mandan away from the fort. See Audubon, *Journals*, 2:42–43; Bernard De Voto, *Across the Wide Missouri* (Boston: Houghton Mifflin, 1947), 281; Dollar, "High Plains Smallpox Epidemic," 33–38. Other accounts, written even later, must also be suspect, especially the narratives of Larpenteur and Culbertson, which provide the crucial examples of inoculation. The details of Larpenteur's account (such as the traders' use of Thomas's *Domestic Medicine*), however, do lend credibility. For the Indian responses, see Chardon, *Journal*, 127–133.

32. John C. Ewers, *The Blackfeet: Raiders on the Northwestern Plains* (Norman: University of Oklahoma Press, 1958), 65; W. F. Wagner, "Introduction," in *Leonard's Narrative: Adventures of Zenas Leonard, Fur Trader and Trapper, 1831–1836* (Cleveland: Burrows Brothers, 1904), 40; Hiram Martin Chittenden, *The American Fur Trade of the Far West* (New York: Francis P. Harper, 1902), 624; Henry F. Dobyns, "Native American Trade Centers as Contagious Disease Foci," in *Disease and Demography in the Americas*, ed. John W. Verano and Douglas H. Ubelaker (Washington, D.C.: Smithsonian Institution Press, 1992), 216; Dollar, "High Plains Smallpox Epidemic," 38; D. L. Ferch, "Fighting the Smallpox Epidemic of 1837–38: The Response of the American Fur Company," *Museum of the Fur Trade Quarterly* 19 (1983): 2; Ferch, "Fighting the Smallpox Epidemic of 1837–38—Conclusion," 8.

33. Wagner, "Introduction," in *Leonard's Narrative*, 8; Chittenden, *American Fur Trade of the Far West*; Annie Heloise Abel, "Historical Introduction," to Chardon, *Journal*, xv–xlvi, xlii; De Voto, *Across the Wide Missouri*.

34. Catlin, *Manners, Customs, and Condition*, 2:258; [Bradley and Culbertson], "Affairs at Fort Benton," 222.

35. *Theft:* Chardon, in Audubon, *Journals*, 2:42–43; [Bradley and Culberston], "Affairs at Fort Benton," 222; De Smet, *Letters and Sketches*, 27:26. *Publication opportunism:* Maximilian, "Author's Introduction," to *Travels in the Interior*, 22:38; Lloyd, "Translator's Preface," 22:36; Thwaites, "Preface," 22:19.

36. Chardon to P. D. Papin, 28 Nov. 1837, *Papers of the St. Louis Fur Trade*, reel 25, p. 185; Halsey to Pratte Chouteau & Co., 2 Nov. 1837, p. 140; D. D. Mitchell to Papin, 1 Dec. 1837, ibid., pp. 203–204.

37. Larpenteur, *Forty Years a Fur Trader*, 111–112; [Bradley and Culbertson], "Affairs at Fort Benton," 226–227.

38. "New Orleans, *June* 6, 1838," 22:33; Halsey to Pratte Chouteau & Co., 2 Nov. 1837, reel 25, p. 141. Audubon, *Journals*, 2:43.

39. Chardon, *Journal*, 162; Crawford, "Report of the Commissioner of Indian Affairs," 25 Nov. 1838, p. 424; Dollar, "High Plains Smallpox Epidemic," 32; Ray, "Epidemic of 1837–38," 8–13.

40. Lawrence W. White, Robert E. L. Newberne, and Joseph A. Murphy, "Historical Sketch of the United States Indian Medical Service," in George M. Kober, George E. Bushnell, Joseph A. Murphy, Albert B. Tonkin, William H. Baldwin, and Hoyt E. Dearholt, *Tuberculosis among the North American Indians* (Washington: Government Printing Office, 1923), 91–93; U.S. Public Health Service, *Health Services for American Indians* (Washington: Government Printing Office, 1957), 56, 86; Ronald N. Satz, *American Indian Policy in the Jacksonian Era* (Lincoln: University of Nebraska Press, 1975), 151–155; Francis Paul Prucha, *The Great Father: The United States Government and the American Indians* (Lincoln: University of Nebraska Press, 1984); Russell Thornton, "The Demography of the Trail of Tears Period: A New Estimate of Cherokee Population Losses," in *Cherokee Removal: Before and After*, ed. William G. Anderson (Athens: University of Georgia Press, 1991), 75–95; Jeff Henderson, "Native American Health Policy: From US Territorial Expansion to Legal Obligation," *JAMA* 265 (1 May 1991): 2272; Stephen J. Kunitz, "The History and Politics of US Health Care Policy for American Indians and Alaskan Natives," *AJPH* 86 (October 1996): 1464.

41. W. A. Trimble to John C. Calhoun (1818), and J. Morse, "Report to the Secretary of War on Indian Affairs" (1822), both in E. Wagner Stearn and Allen E. Stearn, *The Effect of Smallpox on the Destiny of the Amerindian* (Boston: Bruce Humphries, 1945), 61. Edwin James, *Account of an Expedition from Pittsburg to the Rocky Mountains* (1823), in *Early Western Travels*, 14:37–38, 15:202, 15:208.

42. John J. Heagerty, *Four Centuries of Medical History in Canada* (London: Simpkin, Marshall, Hamilton, Kent, 1928), 1:52. James O. Pattie, *Personal Narrative during an Expedition from St. Louis*, ed. Timothy Flint (1824–1830), in *Early Western Travels*, 18:10–17, 264–285; Sherburne F. Cook, "Smallpox in Spanish and Mexican California, 1770–1845," *Bulletin of the History of Medicine* 7 (February 1939): 177–182.

43. John Dougherty to William Clark, 29 Oct. 1831, in Lewis Cass, "Small Pox Among the Indians: Letter from the Secretary of War, Upon the subject of the Small Pox among the Indian tribes," 30 March 1832, 22d Cong., 1st sess., 220 H. Doc. 190, p. 1; Cass to Andrew Stevenson, 29 March 1832, ibid., p. 1; James Jackson to Cass, 16 March 1832, ibid., p. 2; "An Act to Provide the Means of Extending the Benefits of Vaccination, as a Preventive of the Small-pox, to the Indian Tribes, and thereby, as far as Possible, to Save Them from the Destructive Ravages of that Disease," 5 May 1832, *Statutes at Large*, vol. 4 (1824–1835), 514–515; Cass, "Circular to Indian Agents," 10 May 1832, in Cass, "A report of the Commissioner of Indian Affairs in relation to the execution of the act extending the benefit of Vaccination to the Indian Tribes, &c.," 2 Feb. 1833, 22d Cong., 2d sess., 234

H. Doc. 82, p. 5. See Michael K. Trimble, "The 1832 Inoculation Program on the Missouri River," in *Disease and Demography in the Americas*, ed. Verano and Ubelaker, 257–264.

44. Elbert Herring to Cass, 31 Jan. 1833, in Cass, "A report of the Commissioner," 2 Feb. 1833, pp. 2–4; Herring, "Report from the Office of Indian Affairs," 22 Nov. 1832, 22d Cong., 2d sess., 233 H. Doc. 2, p. 175; Herring, "Report of the Commissioner of Indian Affairs," 29 Nov. 1833, 23d Cong., 1st sess., 254 H. Doc. 1, p. 174; Herring, "Report of the Commissioner of Indian Affairs," 25 Nov. 1834, 23d Cong., 2d sess., 271 H. Doc. 2, p. 258. Stearn and Stearn, *Effect of Smallpox*, 65.

45. Crawford to J. R. Poinsett, 14 Dec. 1838, in Poinsett, "Small-Pox Among the Indians: Letter from the Secretary of War, On the subject of the Small-pox among the Indians," 2 Jan. 1839, 25th Cong., 3d sess., 346 H. Exec. Doc. 51, pp. 1–2; Sylvanus Fansher, "Memorial of Sylvanus Fansher, praying the establishment of a permanent vaccine institution, for the benefit of the army, navy, and Indian department," 18 April 1838, 25th Cong., 2nd sess., 317 S. Doc. 385, pp. 1–9; McCoy, *History of Baptist Indian Missions*, 554.

46. Maximilian, *Travels in the Interior*, 22:286; Catlin, *Manners, Customs, and Condition*, 2:258. Ferch, "Fighting the Smallpox Epidemic of 1837–38," 2; Ferch, "Fighting the Smallpox Epidemic of 1837–38—Conclusion," 8; Trimble, "1832 Inoculation Program," 263; Trimble, "1837–1838 Smallpox Epidemic," 86.

47. Maximilian, *Travels in the Interior*, 22:286; Larpenteur, *Forty Years a Fur Trader*, 109; [Bradley and Culbertson], "Affairs at Fort Benton," 224. Mary C. Gillett, *The Army Medical Department, 1818–1865* (Washington: Government Printing Office, 1987), 134.

48. John H. Eaton (Secretary of War) to John Forsyth (governor of Georgia), 14 Oct. 1829, in Thomas L. McKenney, "Annual Report for 1829 from the Bureau of Indian Affairs," 17 Nov. 1829, 21st Cong., 1st sess., 198 H. Doc. 2, p. 187–188. Sheehan, *Seeds of Extinction*; Michael Paul Rogin, *Fathers and Children: Andrew Jackson and the Subjugation of the American Indian* (1975; New Brunswick: Transaction, 1991); Ronald N. Satz, "Rhetoric versus Reality: The Indian Policy of Andrew Jackson," in *Cherokee Removal: Before and After*, ed. William L. Anderson (Athens: University of Georgia Press, 1991), 31–35.

49. C. A. Harris, "Report from the Commissioner of Indian Affairs," 1 Dec. 1836, 24th Cong., 2d sess., 301 H. Doc. 2, pp. 402, 403. *Damage estimates:* see Ferch, "Fighting the Smallpox Epidemic of 1837–38," 4. President Jefferson and William Todd (who vaccinated Canadian tribes) also had interest in evaluating the vaccine's efficacy: Eldon G. Chuinard, *Only One Man Died: The Medical Aspects of the Lewis and Clark Expedition* (Glendale, Calif.: Arthur H. Clarke, 1979), 102; Ray, "Epidemic of 1837–38," 12–13.

50. Cass to Dougherty, 9 May 1832, quoted in Chardon, *Journal*, 319 n.507.

51. Harris, "Report from the Office of Indian Affairs," 1 Dec. 1837; Chardon, *Journal*, 162; Dollar, "High Plains Smallpox Epidemic," 32.

5. Race to Extinction

1. "The No Ears, Short Man, and Iron Crow Winter Counts," in James R. Walker, *Lakota Society*, ed. Raymond J. DeMallie (Lincoln: University of Nebraska Press, 1982), pp. 127–141; Paul H. Carlson, *The Plains Indians* (College Station: Texas A&M University Press, 1998), 181.

2. "White Priest of Indian Tribes Writes Record of Religious Beliefs," in [unidentified Denver newspaper], 13 Nov. 1918, in *Mythen der Oglala*, ed. Karl A. Nowotny, *Dokumente der Geistesgeschichte* 5 (Vienna: F. Nowotny, 1979), pp. 18–20; Hiram Price, commissioner of Indian affairs, *ARCIA 1883*, xliii; C. P. Luse, Agent, White Earth Agency, *ARCIA 1883*, 96; James R. Walker to W. A. Jones, 27 Nov. 1900, *LRBIA*, 1900–59121; Raymond J. DeMallie and Elaine A. Jahner, "James R. Walker: His Life and Work," in Walker, *Lakota Belief and Ritual*, ed. DeMallie and Jahner (Lincoln: University of Nebraska Press, 1980), 5.

3. *Measles, 1888:* W. W. Anderson, agent, Crow Creek and Lower Brule, *ARCIA 1889*, 137; L. F. Spencer, agent, Rosebud, *ARCIA 1889*, 159; Frederick Treon, "An Epidemic of Malignant Measles among the Sioux Indians," *Cincinnati Lancet-Clinic* 21 (17 Nov. 1888): 581. *Influenza, 1890:* Treon, "Epidemic Influenza among the Sioux Indians," *Cincinnati Lancet-Clinic* 24 (8 Feb. 1890): 161. *Measles, 1893:* Treon, "The Effect of Education on the American Indian," *Medical Record* (New York) 43 (1 April 1893): 390. *Measles, 1896:* L. M. Hardin, physician, Rosebud, *ARCIA 1896*, 299. *Measles, 1899:* John W. Harding, agent, Yankton, *ARCIA 1899*, 380; Hardin, physician, Rosebud, *ARCIA 1900*, 380; Nathan P. Johnson, Agent, Sisseton, *ARCIA 1900*, 387. *Smallpox, 1901:* Ira A. Hatch, agent, Cheyenne River, *ARCIA 1901*, 359; C. L. Woods, physician, Standing Rock, *ARCIA 1901*, 310; Harry D. Chamberlain, agent, Crow Creek, *ARCIA 1901*, 360; Charles E. McChesney, agent, Rosebud, *ARCIA 1901*, 372; Harding, agent, Yankton, *ARCIA 1901*, 377; Hardin, physician, Rosebud, *ARCIA 1902*, 345; Walker, physician, Pine Ridge, *ARCIA 1902*, 339. *Smallpox, 1902:* Z. T. Daniel, physician, Rosebud, *ARCIA 1903*, 315.

4. James H. Stephen, agent, Crow Creek, *ARCIA 1899*, 332; Yankton Agency, *ARCIA 1900*, 387. Russell Thornton, *American Indian Holocaust and Survival: A Population History since 1492* (Norman: University of Oklahoma Press, 1987), 101.

5. Daniel, *ARCIA 1903*, 315. E. Wagner Stearn and Allen E. Stearn, *The Effect of Smallpox on the Destiny of the Amerindian* (Boston: Bruce Humphries, 1945), 59; Joel N. Shurkin, *The Invisible Fire: The Story of Mankind's Victory over the Ancient Scourge of Smallpox* (New York: Putnam, 1979), 203.

6. Daniel, physician, Cheyenne River, *ARCIA 1891*, 392.

7. Royal B. Hassrick, *The Sioux: Life and Customs of a Warrior Society* (Norman: University of Oklahoma Press, 1964); Joseph M. Prince, "Intersection of Economics, History, and Human Biology: Secular Trends in Stature in Nineteenth-Century Sioux Indians," *Human Biology* 67 (June 1995): 389–390; Catherine Price, *The Oglala People, 1841–1879* (Lincoln: University of Nebraska Press, 1996), 21–22; Carlson, *Plains Indians*. For protection from smallpox, see Michael K. Trimble, "The 1837–1838 Smallpox Epidemic on the Upper Missouri," in *Skeletal Biology in the Great Plains: Migration, Warfare, Health, and Subsistence*, ed. Douglas W. Owsley and Richard L. Jantz (Washington: Smithsonian Institution Press, 1994), 87.

8. Francis Paul Prucha, *The Great Father: The United States Government and the American Indians* (Lincoln: University of Nebraska Press, 1984); Reginald Horsman, *Race and Manifest Destiny: The Origins of American Racial Anglo-Saxonism* (Cambridge: Harvard University Press, 1981), 199; Theda Perdue, "The Trail of Tears: Removal of the Southern Indians," in *The American Indian Experience, A Profile: 1524 to the Present*, ed. Philip Weeks (Wheeling, Ill.: Forum Press, 1988),

96–117; Ronald N. Satz, "Rhetoric versus Reality: The Indian Policy of Andrew Jackson," in *Cherokee Removal: Before and After*, ed. William L. Anderson (Athens: University of Georgia Press, 1991), 29–54; Russell Thornton, "The Demography of the Trail of Tears Period: A New Estimate of Cherokee Population Losses," ibid., 75–95; Dee Brown, *Bury My Heart at Wounded Knee: An Indian History of the American West* (New York: Henry Holt, 1970), 5–9.

 9. Gary Clayton Anderson, "Dakota Sioux Uprising, 1862," in *Kinsmen of Another Kind: Dakota-White Relations in the Upper Mississippi Valley, 1650–1862* (Lincoln: University of Nebraska Press, 1984), 261–280; Donald J. Berthrong, "The Bitter Years: Western Indian Reservation Life," in *American Indian Experience*, ed. Weeks, 153–173.

 10. "Report of the Sioux Commission," *ARCIA 1878*, 158; James Irwin, agent at Red Cloud, *ARCIA 1877*, 62; James Cook, agent at Rosebud, *ARCIA 1881*, 50. See also D. C. Poole, *Among the Sioux of Dakota: Eighteen Months Experience as an Indian Agent* (New York: Van Nostrand, 1881), 38; E. M. Marble, acting commissioner of Indian affairs, *ARCIA 1880*, xxviii.

 11. E. A. Hayt, commissioner of Indian affairs, *ARCIA 1879*, iii; J. D. C. Atkins, commissioner of Indian affairs, *ARCIA 1887*, iii; T. J. Morgan, commissioner of Indian affairs, *ARCIA 1890*, v. *Tensions:* V. T. McGillycuddy, agent, Pine Ridge, *ARCIA 1885*, 37. *Wounded Knee:* Morgan, *ARCIA 1891*, 131–141. See also Brown, *Bury My Heart at Wounded Knee*, 431–444; Prucha, *The Great Father*, 2:634–639, 2:726–728; Carlson, *Plains Indians*, 177–180.

 12. Morgan, *ARCIA 1891*, 9. W. A. Jones, commissioner of Indian affairs, *ARCIA 1901*, 6; Jones, *ARCIA 1902*, 2–12. Charles G. Penney, acting agent, Pine Ridge, *ARCIA 1893*, 287. *Droughts:* J. A. Smith, agent, Yankton, *ARCIA 1894*, 303. *Alcohol:* John W. Cramsie, agent, Standing Rock, *ARCIA 1897*, 219. *Land reform:* Ira A. Hatch, agent, Cheyenne River, *ARCIA 1900*, 372.

 13. Virginia Morell, "Mummy Settles TB Antiquity Debate," *Science* 263 (24 March 1994): 1686–1687; Mary Lucas Powell, "Health and Disease in the Late Prehistoric Southeast," in *Disease and Demography in the Americas*, ed. John W. Verano and Douglas H. Ubelaker (Washington: Smithsonian Institution Press, 1992), 41–53; Hans L. Reider, "Tuberculosis among American Indians of the Contiguous United States," *Public Health Reports* 104 (November–December 1989): 654. Paul le Jeune, *Relation of What Occurred in New France in 1633* (1634), *Jesuit Relations*, 5:101; Roger Williams to John Throckmorton, 30 July 1672, in *The Correspondence of Roger Williams*, ed. Glenn W. LaFantasie (Hanover: University Press of New England, 1988), 2:675; Daniel Gookin, *Historical Collections of the Indians in New England* (ca. 1680) (1792; n.p.: Towtaid, 1970), 53. Washington Matthews, "Further Contributions to the Study of Consumption Among the Indians," *Transactions of the American Climatological Association* 5 (1888): 142; Ales Hrdlicka, *Tuberculosis among Certain Indian Tribes of the United States* (Washington: Government Printing Office, 1909), 1.

 14. Thomas S. Williamson, "Diseases of the Dakota Indians" (1873–1874), *Minnesota Medicine* (October 1940): 800; Washington Matthews, "Consumption Among the Indians," *Transactions of the American Climatological Association* 3 (1886): 236; Matthews, "Further Contributions to the Study of Consumption," 143. *Disease lists:* James R. Doolittle, *Conditions of the Indian Tribes* (Washington: Government Printing Office, 1867), 4–5; W. T. Hughes, agent at Standing Rock, *ARCIA 1877*, 74.

15. René Dubos and Jean Dubos, *The White Plague: Tuberculosis, Man, and Society* (1952; New Brunswick: Rutgers University Press, 1987), xxxvii; Paul Farmer, *Infections and Inequalities: The Modern Plagues* (Berkeley: University of California Press, 1999), 5.

16. Prevalence data were compiled from each *Annual Report of the Commissioner of Indian Affairs to the Secretary of the Interior* from 1877 to 1906. For specific descriptions, see Theodore Schwan, acting agent, Cheyenne River, *ARCIA 1878*, 23; E. W. Foster, agent, Yankton, *ARCIA 1890*, 72; Foster, agent, Yankton, *ARCIA 1892*, 476; Frederick Treon, physician, Crow Creek, *ARCIA 1892*, 449; Daniel, physician, Pine Ridge, *ARCIA 1894*, 290; Daniel, *ARCIA 1903*, 316; Walker, physician, Pine Ridge, *ARCIA 1906*, 357.

17. A. Stewart, physician, Devil's Lake, *ARCIA 1891*, 318; T. M. Bridges, physician, Crow Creek, *ARCIA 1893*, 286; Walker, physician, Pine Ridge, *ARCIA 1901*, 367; O. M. Chapman, physician, Yankton, *ARCIA 1906*, 364; Frederick Treon, "Medical Work among the Sioux Indians," *JAMA* 10 (25 February 1888): 224–227; Treon, "Consumption Among the Sioux Indians," *Cincinnati Lancet-Clinic* 23 (10 August 1889): 148–154; Joseph B. Graham, "Scrofula among the Sioux Indians; Its Origin and Nature," *American Practitioner and News* 9 (4 January 1890): 1–5; James R. Walker, "Tuberculosis among the Oglala Sioux Indians," *American Journal of the Medical Sciences* 132 (1906): 600–605.

18. *Report of the Surgeon-General of the Army to the Secretary of War, 1892* (Washington: Government Printing Office, 1892), 48; *Report of the Surgeon-General of the Army to the Secretary of War, 1893* (Washington: Government Printing Office, 1893), 64; George E. Bushnell, *A Study in the Epidemiology of Tuberculosis, with Especial Reference to Tuberculosis of the Tropics and of the Negro Race* (New York: William Wood, 1920), 146; T. M. Bridges, physician, Crow Creek, *ARCIA 1895*, 288; Chapman, physician, Yankton, *ARCIA 1903*, 325; Chapman, physician, Yankton, *ARCIA 1904*, 341; Joseph A. Murphy, "Health Problems of the Indians," *Annals of the American Academy of Political and Social Science* 37 (March 1911): 105.

19. McGillycuddy, agent, Pine Ridge, *ARCIA 1885*, 33; Jason M. Bell, acting agent, Pine Ridge, *ARCIA 1886*, 76; Peter Thompson, "The Fight for Life: New Mexican Indians, Health Care, and the Reservation Period," *New Mexico Historical Review* 69 (April 1994): 153.

20. Records of the Russian Orthodox Church in Alaska show that while Europeans were diagnosed with pneumonia, Alaskan Natives were diagnosed with tuberculosis: J. G. Townsend, Joseph D. Aronson, Robert Saylor, and Irma Parr, "Tuberculosis Control among the North American Indians," *American Review of Tuberculosis* 45 (January 1942): 41; David S. Barnes, "Historical Perspectives on the Etiology of Tuberculosis," *Microbes and Infection* 2 (2000): 431–440. For the old nomenclature, see *ARCIA 1891*, 806–812. For the new nomenclature, see *ARCIA 1892*, 919–925.

21. Treon, "Consumption Among the Sioux," 148. See Georgina D. Feldberg, *Disease and Class: Tuberculosis and the Shaping of Modern North American Society* (New Brunswick: Rutgers University Press, 1995), 11–14, 38, 44–45; Katherine Ott, *Fevered Lives: Tuberculosis in American Cultures since 1870* (Cambridge: Harvard University Press, 1996), 38.

22. A. B. Holder, "Papers on Diseases among Indians," *Medical Record* (New York) 42 (24 September 1892): 358; No-Flesh [Oglala healer], "The Causes of Disease," in James R. Walker, "The Sun Dance and Other Ceremonies of the Oglala

Division of the Teton Dakota," *Anthropological Papers of the American Museum of Natural History* 16 (1917): 161–163, 162; Thomas Tyon, "Gophers are *Wakan (Wahinheya Yuwakanpi),*" in Walker, *Lakota Belief and Ritual,* 169.

23. Bushnell, *Epidemiology of Tuberculosis,* 13–14. On diathesis, see Benjamin Rush, "Thoughts upon the Cause and Cure of Pulmonary Consumption," in *Medical Inquiries and Observations* (1815; New York: Arno, 1972), 2:38; Charles E. Rosenberg, "The Bitter Fruit: Heredity, Disease, and Social Thought in Nineteenth Century America" (1974), in *From Consumption to Tuberculosis: A Documentary History,* ed. Barbara Gutmann Rosenkrantz (New York: Garland, 1994), 154–194; Erwin H. Ackerknecht, "Diathesis: The Word and Concept in Medical History," *Bulletin of the History of Medicine* 56 (Fall 1982): 317–325.

24. Williamson, "Diseases of the Dakota Indians," 800; Holder, "Diseases Among Indians," 180; J. A. Stephan, agent, Standing Rock, *ARCIA 1879,* 48; William W. Anderson, agent, Crow Creek and Lower Brulé, *ARCIA 1887,* 21; James McLaughlin, agent, Standing Rock, *ARCIA 1883,* 51; McLaughlin, *ARCIA 1888,* 63; Penney, *ARCIA 1893,* 289; Charles L. Davis, school superintendent, Devil's Lake, *ARCIA 1904,* 272; Harry D. Chamberlain, agent, Crow Creek, *ARCIA 1905,* 331. See Warwick Anderson, "Excremental Colonialism: Public Health and the Poetics of Pollution," *Critical Inquiry* 21 (Spring 1995): 640–659.

25. Treon, "Consumption Among the Sioux," 148–149; Treon, "Medical Work Among the Sioux," 226; C. H. Kermott, physician, Devil's Lake, *ARCIA 1893,* 232; L. F. Michael, physician, Cheyenne River, *ARCIA 1895,* 284; Graham, "Scrofula among the Sioux," 3; W. H. Harrison, physician, Rosebud, *ARCIA 1904,* 335.

26. Treon, "Consumption Among the Sioux," 152; Daniel, *ARCIA 1903,* 318; Fordyce Grinnell, "The Healing Art, as practiced by the Indians of the Plains," *Cincinnati Lancet and Observer* 17 (March 1874): 146; Holder, "Diseases Among Indians," 179; Hardin, physician, Rosebud, *ARCIA 1900,* 380; Stephan, agent, Standing Rock, *ARCIA 1880,* 58.

27. Hardin, *ARCIA 1900,* 381; Treon, "Medical Work among the Sioux," 225; W. A. Wray, physician, Yankton, *ARCIA 1893,* 313; Treon, "Epidemic Influenza among the Sioux," 160; J. George Wright, agent, Rosebud, *ARCIA 1890,* 57; Stephan, *ARCIA 1879,* 48; Treon, "Consumption Among the Sioux," 149.

28. Richard Irving Dodge, *Our Wild Indians: Thirty-Three Years' Personal Experience among the Red Men of the Great West* (1882) (New York: Archer House, 1959), 314; Matthews, "Further Contributions to the Study of Consumption," 152; Daniel, physician, Pine Ridge, *ARCIA 1894,* 290; J. F. Kinney, agent, Yankton, *ARCIA 1884,* 62; McLaughlin, agent, Standing Rock, *ARCIA 1886,* 91; R. H. Pratt, Carlisle School, *ARCIA 1886,* 22; Ales Hrdlicka, *Physiological and Medical Observations among the Indians of Southwestern United States and Northern Mexico* (Washington: Government Printing Office, 1908), 175; Chapman, *ARCIA 1904,* 342. Paul Farmer has argued that such victim blaming, common in modern discussions of tuberculosis, ignores underlying economic conditions and distracts "attention from the preventable social disorder that exacerbates biological disorders": *Infections and Inequalities,* 4.

29. Ott, *Fevered Lives,* 17–19, 101; Rosenberg, "The Bitter Fruit," 163.

30. Robert Koch, "Ætiology of Tuberculosis," trans. F. Sause (1884), in *From Consumption to Tuberculosis,* ed. Rosenkrantz, 223; Graham, "Scrofula among the Sioux," 4–5. See Marion M. Torcha, "The Tuberculosis Movement and the Race Question, 1890–1950," *Bulletin of the History of Medicine* 49 (Summer 1975): 152–

168; Nancy Krieger, "Shades of Difference: Theoretical Underpinnings of the Medical Controversy on Black/White Differences in the United States, 1830–1870," *International Journal of Health Services* 17 (1987): 259–278.

31. J. F. Kinney, agent, Yankton, *ARCIA 1887*, 64; William McKusick, agent, Sisseton, *ARCIA 1889*, 164; Daniel, *ARCIA 1891*, 393; Walker, physician, Pine Ridge, *ARCIA 1900*, 379; Charles E. Eastman [Ohiyesa], *The Indian To-day: The Past and Future of the First American* (New York: Doubleday, Page, 1915), 139; McChesney, *ARCIA 1901*, 372; Daniel, *ARCIA 1894*, 290.

32. F. O. Getchell, agent, Devil's Lake, *ARCIA 1901*, 298; Walker, "Tuberculosis among the Oglala Sioux," 600; Bushnell, *Epidemiology of Tuberculosis*, 61, 162; Walker, *ARCIA 1903*, 310; W. H. Clapp, acting Agent, Pine Ridge, *ARCIA 1896*, 294.

33. *Hereditary tuberculosis:* J. A. Stephan, agent, Standing Rock, *ARCIA 1881*, 60; Kinney, *ARCIA 1887*, 64; Daniel, physician, Cheyenne River, *ARCIA 1890*, 44–45; Wright, *ARCIA 1890*, 57; Kermott, *ARCIA 1893*, 232; Kermott, physician, Devil's Lake, *ARCIA 1894*, 218; Bridges, *ARCIA 1895*, 288; Daniel, *ARCIA 1903*, 317. *Intermarriage:* McKusick, *ARCIA 1889*, 164; Daniel, *ARCIA 1891*, 393; W. L. Brown, physician, Yankton, *ARCIA 1891*, 433; Daniel, *ARCIA 1894*, 290; Daniel, *ARCIA 1903*, 317. *Fresh Blood:* Daniel, *ARCIA 1894*, 290. *Downplay heredity:* F. O. Getchell, agent, Devils Lake, *ARCIA 1901*, 298. In his 1906 article about Sioux tuberculosis, Walker also downplays the roll of heredity: Walker, "Tuberculosis among the Oglala Sioux," 600. Nonhereditary explanations included: housing behavior, 28 instances; personal habits, 16; climate, 16; food preparation, 16; housing conditions, 13; nursing care, 12; social upheaval, 11; food quality, 9; and poverty, 4.

34. W. J. Stephenson, physician, Winnebago and Omaha agency, *ARCIA 1897*, 179.

35. J. C. Nott and George R. Gliddon, *Types of Mankind* (1854; Miami: Mnemosyne, 1969), 69; Doolittle, *Conditions of the Indian Tribes*, 3; General [James] Carleton, quoted in Doolittle, 4.

36. Henry A. Boller, *Among the Indians: Eight Years in the Far West, 1858–1866*, ed. Milo Milton Quaife (1868; Chicago: Lakeside Press, 1959), 436; McGillycuddy, *ARCIA 1885*, 33; Daniel, *ARCIA 1903*, 317; Treon, quoted in Matthews, "Further Contributions to the Study of Consumption," 143.

37. J. M. Sturtevant and Walter F. Wilcox, both quoted in George M. Fredrickson, *The Black Image in the White Mind: The Debate on Afro-American Character and Destiny, 1817–1914* (Hanover: University Press of New England, for Wesleyan University Press, 1971, 1987), 159, 252, 77, 223, 238–247, 255. On syphilis and African Americans, see Allan M. Brandt, "Racism and Research: The Case of the Tuskegee Syphilis Study," *Hastings Center Report* 8 (1978): 21–23.

38. S. N. Clark, "Memoranda: Importance of the Inquiry," in "Are the Indians Dying Out? Preliminary Observations Relating to Indian Civilization and Education," *ARCIA 1877*, 494.

39. Clark, "Are the Indians Dying Out?" *ARCIA 1877*, 489–493; Clark, "Importance of the Inquiry," 494, 520; J. H. Hammond, superintendent, Dakota superintendency, *ARCIA 1877*, 51; Matthews, "Consumption Among the Indians," 240; Fordyce Grinnell, "Indian Questions from a Medical Standpoint," *Cincinnati Lancet and Observer* 21 (February 1878): 169; W. A. Jones, *ARCIA 1900*, 47–49.

40. Graham, "Scrofula among the Sioux," 5; Dodge, *Our Wild Indians*, 296.

41. Bushnell, *Epidemiology of Tuberculosis*, 159–160; Matthews, "Consumption Among the Indians," 238–240; McLaughlin, agent, Standing Rock, *ARCIA 1887*, 52; Treon, "Consumption among the Sioux," 148; McKusick, *ARCIA 1889*, 164; Getchell, *ARCIA 1901*, 298; Eastman, *Indian To-Day*, 12; Hardin, physician, Rosebud, *ARCIA 1898*, 282.

42. General Sprague, quoted in Doolittle, *Conditions of the Indian Tribes*, 4; Grinnell, "Indian Questions from a Medical Standpoint," 162; Jones, *ARCIA 1904*, 33.

43. Nat McKitterick, quoted in Holder, "Diseases Among Indians," 177; Bushnell, *Epidemiology of Tuberculosis*, 160.

44. Holder, "Diseases among Indians," 177.

45. Treon, "Consumption Among the Sioux," 153; R. H. Pratt, superintendent of the Indian Industrial School at Carlisle Barracks, Pennsylvania, *ARCIA 1885*, 220; Pratt, *ARCIA 1886*, 21–22; Pratt, *ARCIA 1887*, 259; Pratt, *ARCIA 1889*, 365; W. A. Mercer, superintendent of the Carlisle Indian School, *ARCIA 1906*, 338; A. Judson Morris, physician, Rosebud, *ARCIA 1894*, 299; Treon, "Effect of Education on the American Indian," 391; T. M. Bridges, physician, Crow Creek, *ARCIA 1894*, 280; Walker, *ARCIA 1903*, 310; Walker to Paul Kennaday (secretary, tuberculosis committee, Charity Organization Society), 5 Feb. 1906, LRBIA, 1906–13371. For Pratt's uncertainty principle, see *ARCIA 1886*, 22. For background, see David Wallace Adams, "From Bullets to Boarding Schools: The Educational Assault on the American Indian Identity," in *American Indian Experience*, ed. Weeks, 218–239.

46. Graham, "Scrofula among the Sioux," 5; S. R. Riggs to John Eaton, 27 Aug. 1877, in Clark, "Importance of the Inquiry," *ARCIA 1877*, 515; Grinnell, "Indian Questions from a Medical Standpoint," 167; J. M. Woodburn, physician, Rosebud, *ARCIA 1889*, 162; Bridges, Crow Creek, *ARCIA 1893*, 286; James McLaughlin, agent, Standing Rock, *ARCIA 1894*, 228; Charles L. Woods, physician, Standing Rock, *ARCIA 1901*, 310; Eastman, *Indian To-Day*, 136.

47. Riggs to Eaton, *ARCIA 1877*, 515; Getchell, agent, Devil's Lake, *ARCIA 1903*, 230.

6. Impossible Responsibilities

1. Francis Paul Prucha, *The Great Father: The United States Government and the American Indians* (Lincoln: University of Nebraska Press, 1984), 2:610.

2. U.S. Public Health Service, *The Indian Health Program of the U.S. Public Health Service* (Washington: U.S. Department of Health, Education, and Welfare, 1966), 17; "The United States Indian Service: A Sketch of the Development of the Bureau of Indian Affairs and of Indian Policy," *Navajo Yearbook: 1951–1961, A Decade of Progress*, vol. 8 (Window Rock, Ariz.: Navajo Agency, 1961), 578–580. See also Stephen J. Kunitz, "The History and Politics of US Health Care Policy for American Indians and Alaskan Natives," *AJPH* 86 (October 1996): 1464. The terminology for the federal bureaucracies for American Indians has been inconsistent. Established in 1824 as the Bureau of Indian Affairs, it has routinely been called the Indian Office, the Office of Indian Affairs, the Indian Bureau, or the Indian Service. In 1947 the executive branch standardized its nomenclature into a rigid hier-

archy, officially restoring the title of Bureau of Indian Affairs. See Prucha, *The Great Father,* 2:1227–1229.

3. Hiram Price, commissioner of Indian affairs, *ARCIA 1882,* xlviii; T. J. Morgan, commissioner of Indian affairs, *ARCIA 1889,* 12.

4. The official job description can be found on the back of the agency physicians' monthly sanitary report form. See, e.g., Charles A. Eastman, "Monthly Sanitary Report of Sick and Wounded at Pine Ridge Agency, S.D., for November 1892," 23 Dec. 1892, *LRBIA,* 1893–104. A similar list appears in Morgan, *ARCIA 1889,* 13. For vacations, see W. A. Wray, physician, Yankton, *ARCIA 1893,* 313. Prucha, *The Great Father,* 2:646.

5. Morgan, *ARCIA 1890,* xx; Morgan, *ARCIA 1889,* 12. The Sioux reservations provided few opportunities for private practice: Frederick Treon to J. D. C. Atkins, 4 Feb. 1887, *LRBIA,* 1887–4049.

6. W. T. Hughes, agent, Standing Rock, *ARCIA 1878,* 45; John Cook, agent, Rosebud, *ARCIA 1880,* 45; L. F. Spencer, agent, Rosebud, *ARCIA 1887,* 45; Frederick Treon, "Consumption among the Sioux Indians," *Cincinnati Lancet-Clinic* 23 (10 Aug. 1889): 153; A. Judson Morris, physician, Rosebud, *ARCIA 1892,* 300 (he does not describe this treatment); Julius Silberstein, physician, Crow Creek, *ARCIA 1904,* 325. Historian Virginia Allen believed that Indians received better care than most poor, rural whites: "Agency Physicians to the Southern Plains Indians, 1868–1900," *Bulletin of the History of Medicine* 49 (Fall 1975): 330.

7. Hughes, *ARCIA 1878,* 45; V. T. McGillycuddy, agent, Pine Ridge, *ARCIA 1879,* 40; McGillycuddy, *ARCIA 1880,* 42; McGillycuddy, *ARCIA 1881,* 49; J. A. Stephan, agent, Standing Rock, *ARCIA 1880,* 58; Price, commissioner of Indian affairs, *ARCIA 1883,* xliii.

8. L. M. Hardin, physician, Rosebud, *ARCIA 1902,* 345.

9. *Pine Ridge:* "Report of the Sioux Commission," *ARCIA 1878,* 158. *Self-reliance, aided by "Divine Blessing":* John Harries, agent, Lemhi Indian Agency (Idaho), *ARCIA 1882,* 51–52. Reports from Rosebud mentioned a physician in 27 of 30 years; Lower Brulé only mentioned a physician in one of eight years—did a physician not exist the other seven, or was he simply not mentioned? *Agent's complaint:* Jason M. Bell, acting agent, Pine Ridge, *ARCIA 1886,* 76. Morgan, *ARCIA 1890,* v, xx. *Learning curve:* C. A. May, physician, Yankton, *ARCIA 1892,* 479; Price, *ARCIA 1882,* xlviii.

10. Charles E. Eastman [Ohiyesa], *The Indian To-day: The Past and Future of the First American* (New York: Doubleday, Page, 1915), 141; James R. Walker, physician, Pine Ridge, *ARCIA 1898,* 277; Walker to the commissioner of Indian affairs, 15 June 1913, in Central Classified Files, 1907–1939, Bureau of Indian Affairs (CCF-BIA), Pine Ridge, 5685–1936–732 to 88049–1924–734, National Archives and Records Administration, Record Group 75, Records of the Bureau of Indian Affairs, 52038–1913. Required monthly school inspections would have taken Walker eighteen days each month by horseback, or ten by car. J. George Wright, agent, Rosebud, *ARCIA 1890,* 62–63; James Brewster, physician, Standing Rock, *ARCIA 1892,* 367; V. T. McGillycuddy to Hiram Price, 15 March 1883, *LRBIA,* 1883–5649; Z. T. Daniel, physician, Cheyenne River, *ARCIA 1889,* 133; Frederick Treon, "Medical Work Among the Sioux Indians," *Journal of the American Medical Association* 10 (25 February 1888): 227; James G. Reid, agent, Cheyenne River, *ARCIA 1899,* 328.

11. Cicero Newell, agent, Rosebud, *ARCIA 1879*, 42; James McLaughlin, agent, Standing Rock, *ARCIA 1885*, 55; Eastman, *Indian To-Day*, 141; Ralph H. Ross, physician, Standing Rock, 25 Aug. 1898, *ARCIA 1898*, 229; Walker, physician, Pine Ridge, *ARCIA 1904*, 332. Price, *ARCIA 1884*, xxxvi; "Operations against the Sioux Indians," in *Report of the Surgeon-General of the Army, 1891* (Washington: Government Printing Office, 1891), 39; Treon, "Surgery Among the Sioux Indians" (1888), *Journal-Lancet* (Minneapolis) 53 (15 March 1933): 464–465, 474; Treon, "Fibrous Tumor of the Upper Jaw," *Cincinnati Lancet-Clinic* 20 (5 May 1888): 528–529; Daniel, "Amputation of the Leg of a Full-Blooded Sioux Indian," *International Journal of Surgery* 4 (March 1891): 54–55. Daniel, physician, Pine Ridge, *ARCIA 1894*, 290.

12. J. Ashley Thompson, physician, Pine Ridge, *ARCIA 1884*, 211; Treon, "Surgery among the Sioux Indians," 474; Frederick Treon, "An Epidemic of Malignant Measles among the Sioux Indians," *Cincinnati Lancet-Clinic* 21 (17 November 1888): 580; Eastman, *Indian To-day*, 141.

13. W. T. Hughes, agent, Standing Rock, *ARCIA 1877*, 74; James McLaughlin, agent, Standing Rock, *ARCIA 1882*, 46; J. D. C. Atkins, commissioner of Indian affairs, *ARCIA 1887*, li; W. A. Jones, commissioner of Indian affairs, *ARCIA 1904*, 35; Ira A. Hatch, agent, Cheyenne River, *ARCIA 1903*, 299.

14. Treon, "Medical Work Among the Sioux," 227; W. L. Brown, physician, Yankton, *ARCIA 1891*, 434. For a modern critique of behavioral explanations of noncompliance, see Paul Farmer, *Infections and Inequalities: The Modern Plagues* (Berkeley: University of California Press, 1999).

15. McGillycuddy, agent, Pine Ridge, *ARCIA 1884*, 40; Treon, "Medical Work Among the Sioux," 226; Treon, "An Epidemic of Malignant Measles," 580; J. M. Woodburn, physician, Rosebud, *ARCIA 1889*, 162; Eastman, *Indian To-Day*, 142; Walker, "Autobiographical Statement," in Walker, *Lakota Belief and Ritual*, ed. Raymond J. DeMallie and Elaine A. Jahner (Lincoln: University of Nebraska Press, 1980), 46.

16. Fordyce Grinnell to Hiram Price, 28 April 1881, *LRBIA*, 1881–6793; T. J. Saunders to Hiram Price, 13 April 1881, *LRBIA*, 1881–8841; Saunders to Price, 7 May 1881, *LRBIA*, 1881–8841; Memo on Office of Indian Affairs stationery, included with Saunders to Price, 7 May 1881; Grinnell to T. A. Blanel, 8 April 1885, *LRBIA*, 1885–7968; McGillycuddy, agent, Pine Ridge, *ARCIA 1882*, 38; Grinnell to William J. Pollock, 21 Sept. 1882, *LRBIA*, 1882–18772; Grinnell to Pollock, 22 Sept. 1882, *LRBIA*, 1882–18772; Grinnell to Price, 10 May 1883, *LRBIA*, 1883–9101; Pollock, note on back of Grinnell's letter of 22 Sept. 1882; James G. Wright, agent, Rosebud, *ARCIA 1883*, 42; Grinnell to Blanel, 8 April 1885; Wright to J. D. C. Atkins, 31 July 1885, *LRBIA*, 1885–17959; Wright, *ARCIA 1885*, 43.

17. Wright, *ARCIA 1885*, 43; Wright, *ARCIA 1886*, 78; S. S. Bloom to secretary of the interior, 18 June 1886, *LRBIA*, 1886–17343; Bloom to Daniel S. Lamont (secretary to President Cleveland), 26 June 1886, *LRBIA*, 1886–17342; L. F. Spencer to J. D. C. Atkins, 1 Nov. 1886, *LRBIA*, 1886–29816; George Underhill to Atkins, 23 Nov. 1886, *LRBIA*, 1886–32308.

18. William S. Holman (U.S. House of Representatives) to A. B. Lipshaw (deputy commissioner of Indian affairs), ca. Aug. 1886, *LRBIA*, 1886–23646; physicians and citizens of Dearborn County, Ind., to Holman, 18 Aug. 1886, *LRBIA*, 1886–23774; Holman to J. D. C. Atkins, 3 Oct. 1886, *LRBIA*, 1886–26624; see also

J.F.D.C., "Frederick Treon, M.D.," *Journal-Lancet* (Minneapolis) 53 (1 September 1933): 477; James Lamb to "Dr. General," 10 May 1890, *LRBIA*, 1890–14556; Treon, "Consumption Among the Sioux," 153; Treon to T. J. Morgan, 29 Nov. 1890, *LRBIA*, 1890–38475; Treon to Morgan, 29 April 1891, *LRBIA*, 1891–15448; Treon to Morgan, 22 June 1891, *LRBIA*, 1891–23134; Treon to Morgan, 28 July 1891, *LRBIA*, 1891–27424; Treon to Morgan, 22 Oct. 1891, *LRBIA*, 1891–38687; A. P. Dixon to Morgan, 3 Oct. 1891, *LRBIA*, 1891–36306; C. A. May to Morgan, 5 Oct. 1891, *LRBIA*, 1891–36306; William H. DeLacy (acting chief clerk, office of Indian affairs) to Treon, 20 June 1893, *LRBIA*, 1893–22280.

19. "Biographical Note," in Eastman, *Indian To-day*, vi–vii; Raymond Wilson, "Introduction," to Eastman, *From the Deep Woods to Civilization: Chapters in the Autobiography of an Indian* (1916; Lincoln: University of Nebraska Press, 1977), vi–viii; Eastman, "Application for Appointment as Physician," 18 Aug. 1890, *LRBIA*, 1890–25761; Frank Wood to David Dorchester (superintendent of Indian schools), 18 July 1890, *LRBIA*, 1890–24038; "Re. Charles A. Eastman, applicant to Fort Berthold," 18 Aug. 1890, in *LRBIA*, 1890–25605; Eastman to Morgan, 20 Aug. 1890, *LRBIA*, 1890–25761; Eastman to R. V. Bell (acting commissioner of Indian affairs), 9 Oct. 1890, *LRBIA*, 1890–31206. While in Boston, Eastman met Francis Parkman and lectured at Wellesley College about the Pontiac Conspiracy; he does not mention Jeffrey Amherst's smallpox schemes, which Parkman would have known about: Eastman, *Indian To-day*, 20–21; Eastman, *Deep Woods to Civilization*, 72.

20. Eastman, *Deep Woods to Civilization*, vii–ix, 76, 128–135, 131, 134–135, 139, 152, 189; Eastman to Morgan, 27 March 1891, *LRBIA*, 1891–11888; "Indexes of the Letters Received," 1892–22753, 1892–42983; George Le Roy Brown to Morgan, 28 Dec. 1892, *LRBIA*, 1893–102; Brown to Morgan, 3 Jan. [1893], *LRBIA*, 1893–266; Eastman to Morgan, 2 Dec. 1892, *LRBIA*, 1893–1069; H. L. Dawes (U.S. Senate) to Frank Wood, 31 Dec. 1892, *LRBIA*, 1893–3339; secretary of the interior to the commissioner of Indian affairs, 5 Jan. 1893, *LRBIA*, 1893–486; Eastman to Morgan, 1 Jan. 1893, *LRBIA*, 1893–794; Brown to Morgan, 23 Jan. 1893, *LRBIA*, 1893–2949.

21. Raymond J. DeMallie and Elaine A. Jahner, "James R. Walker: His Life and Work," in Walker, *Lakota Belief and Ritual*, 5–6; James R. Walker, "Tuberculosis among the Oglala Sioux Indians," *American Journal of the Medical Sciences* 132 (1906): 600–605.

22. Walker to Paul Kennaday (secretary, tuberculosis committee, Charity Organization Society), 5 Feb. 1906, LRBIA, 1906–13371, pp. 3–5; Walker, physician, Pine Ridge, *ARCIA 1905*, 339; Walker, physician, Pine Ridge, *ARCIA 1906*, 356; Walker, "Tuberculosis among the Oglala Sioux," 604–605.

23. Walker to Francis E. Leupp, 14 Feb. 1906, *LRBIA*, 1906–16389, pp. 2–3; John R. Brennan, agent, Pine Ridge, *LRBIA*, 1906–16389, p. 6 verso; Walker, "Tuberculosis among the Oglala Sioux," 605; DeMallie and Jahner, "Walker: His Life and Work," 12–13; Don Southerton, "Dr. James R. Walker and His Campaign against Tuberculosis at the Pine Ridge Indian Reservation, 1896–1908," *South Dakota History*, forthcoming. On Walker's anthropological interests, see Walker, *ARCIA 1902*, 339; James R. Walker, "The Sun Dance and Other Ceremonies of the Oglala Division of the Teton Dakota," *Anthropological Papers of the American Museum of Natural History* 16 (1917): 53–221; Walker to Clark Wissler, 25 Feb. 1916, in DeMallie and Jahner, "Walker: His Life and Work," 38; ibid., 9–44.

24. Ibid., 6; Mary-Ellen Kelm, *Colonizing Bodies: Aboriginal Health and Healing in British Columbia, 1900–50* (Vancouver: University of British Columbia Press, 1998), 132. For reform efforts, see Hiram Price, 6 Jan. 1882, in Chester A. Arthur, "Message from the President of the United States, transmitting a letter from the Secretary of the Interior with draft of a bill to create the office of Medical Inspector for the United States Indian service," 18 Jan. 1882, 47th Cong., 1st sess., 1987. S. Doc. 59, p. 2; Eastman, *Deep Woods to Civilization*, 78–79; Eastman, *Indian To-Day*, 140.

25. McGillycuddy, *ARCIA 1882*, 38; McGillycuddy, *ARCIA 1884*, 40; McGillycuddy, *ARCIA 1885*, 36; Charles E. McChesney, agent, Cheyenne River, *ARCIA 1889*, 133; Morgan, *ARCIA 1890*, xx; Walker, *ARCIA 1898*, 277; Hardin, physician, Rosebud, in *ARCIA 1900*, 381; Walker, *ARCIA 1905*, 339; Morgan, *ARCIA 1892*, 100–102; Treon, agent, Crow Creek, *ARCIA 1897*, 266.

26. Hughes, *ARCIA 1877*, 74; Newell, *ARCIA 1879*, 42; McLaughlin, *ARCIA 1882*, 46; Price, *ARCIA 1883*, xliii–xliv; Atkins, *ARCIA 1886*, xli; John H. Oberly, commissioner of Indian affairs, *ARCIA 1888*, lxxiii; Morgan, *ARCIA 1890*, cxli; P. C. Barbour, physician, Cheyenne River, *ARCIA 1887*, 19; Woodburn, *ARCIA 1889*, 162. See also Paul Starr, *The Social Transformation of American Medicine* (New York: Basic Books, 1982), 145–179; Charles E. Rosenberg, *The Care of Strangers: The Rise of America's Hospital System* (Baltimore: Johns Hopkins University Press, 1987), 5, 97–121.

27. Morgan, *ARCIA 1892*, 63; McChesney, agent, Rosebud, *ARCIA 1901*, 372; McLaughlin, agent, Standing Rock, *ARCIA 1890*, 39; George H. Bingenheimer, agent, Standing Rock, *ARCIA 1901*, 310; Bingenheimer, *ARCIA 1902*, 271; "Report of the Superintendent of the Indian Insane Asylum," in Chapman, *ARCIA 1903*, 325; John F. Turner, asylum physician, in "Report of the Superintendent of the Indian Insane Asylum," *ARCIA 1903*, 326. For histories of this asylum, see Frank N. Willis, Larry M. Dean, and Larry Larsen, "The First Mental Hospital for American Indians, 1900–1934," *Bulletin of the Menninger Clinic* 45 (1981): 149–154; John M. Spaulding, "The Canton Asylum for Insane Indians: An Example of Institutional Neglect," *Hospital and Community Psychiatry* 37 (October 1986): 1007–1011.

28. Brown, *ARCIA 1891*, 434; Frederick Treon, Agent, Crow Creek and Lower Brulé, 15 Aug. 1895, *ARCIA 1895*, 285–287; Ales Hrdlicka, *Tuberculosis among Certain Indian Tribes of the United States* (Washington: Government Printing Office, 1909), 33–35; Henry R. Wheeler, "Tuberculosis," *ARCIA 1900*, 460; J. G. Bulloch, physician, the Cherokee school, North Carolina, "What Steps Should be Taken to Bring Tuberculosis Under Control," July 1902, in *ARCIA 1902*, 423. See Diane Therese Putney, "Fighting the Scourge: American Indian Morbidity and Federal Policy, 1897–1928" (Ph.D. diss., Marquette University, 1980), 83–85.

29. Treon to Morgan, 7 Aug. 1890, *LRBIA*, 1890–24620; Treon, "An Epidemic of Malignant Measles," 149–150; A. P. Dixon, agent, Crow Creek and Lower Brulé, *ARCIA 1892*, 437; Treon, physician, Crow Creek, *ARCIA 1892*, 448; I. N. Hughey, physician, Lower Brulé, *ARCIA 1892*, 460; Brown, agent, Pine Ridge, *ARCIA 1892*, 454; Charles G. Penney, acting agent, Pine Ridge, 9 Oct. 1893, *ARCIA 1893*, 287; Treon, agent, Crow Creek and Lower Brulé, *ARCIA 1894*, 275; Treon, *ARCIA 1895*, 287; "The No Ears, Short Man, and Iron Crow Winter Counts," in Walker, *Lakota Society*, ed. Raymond J. DeMallie (Lincoln: University of Nebraska Press, 1982), p. 153. See also Prucha, *The Great Father*,

2:648–669; Barbara Gutmann Rosenkrantz, "The Trouble with Bovine Tuberculosis," *Bulletin of the History of Medicine* 59 (1985): 155–175.

30. Treon, quoted in Frank H. Creamer, "Tuberculosis among the American Indians," *Journal-Lancet* 32 (1912): 438; Eastman, *Indian To-day*, 135.

31. Prevalence reached 187/1,000 at Standing Rock in 1880 and 214/1,000 at Sisseton in 1885. Representative mortality: 68 percent of 84 deaths at Yankton in 1880; 80 percent of 111 deaths at Standing Rock in 1881; 61 percent of 54 at Yankton, and 15 percent of 191 at Standing Rock in 1891; 50 percent of adult deaths at Pine Ridge in 1901; 64 percent of all deaths at Standing Rock and 50 percent of 39 at Yankton in 1902; 75 percent of 184 at Pine Ridge and 40 percent of 68 at Yankton in 1903. See Thomas McKeown, *The Role of Medicine: Dream, Mirage, or Nemesis?* (Princeton: Princeton University Press, 1979); Amy L. Fairchild and Gerald M. Oppenheimer, "Public Health Nihilism vs. Pragmatism: History, Politics, and the Control of Tuberculosis," *AJPH* 88 (1998): 1105–1117.

32. Price, *ARCIA 1884*, xviii; Prucha, *The Great Father*, 2:717–718. Woodburn, *ARCIA 1889*, 162; Treon to Morgan, 10 Dec. 1891, *LRBIA*, 1891–44875; A. P. Dixon to Laura E. Tileston, 11 Dec. 1891, *LRBIA*, 1891–44875.

33. Ralph Hall, agent, Devil's Lake, 1 Sept. 1894, *ARCIA 1894*, 217; Hardin, *ARCIA 1902*, 345; Daniel, *ARCIA 1903*, 315; McChesney, *ARCIA 1889*, 133; Woodburn, *ARCIA 1889*, 162; F. O. Getchell, agent, Devil's Lake, *ARCIA 1903*, 230.

34. Grinnell, in Wright, *ARCIA 1884*, 47; "Operations against the Sioux Indians," in *Report of the Surgeon-General 1891*, 37–38; Morgan, *ARCIA 1890*, xxi; Robert Valentine, commissioner of Indian affairs, *ARCIA 1912*, 20–21.

35. Richard Irving Dodge, *Our Wild Indians: Thirty-Three Years' Personal Experience among the Red Men of the Great West* (1882; New York: Archer House, 1959), 640; Chapman, physician, Yankton, *ARCIA 1905*, 350; John N. Alley, "The Responsibility of the Profession in the Campaign against Tuberculosis among the American Indians," *Northwest Medicine* 4 (October 1912): 305–306; Margaret W. Koenig, *Tuberculosis among the Nebraska Winnebago: A Social Study on an Indian Reservation* (Lincoln: Nebraska State Historical Society, 1921), 44–45.

36. Creamer, "Tuberculosis among the American Indians,"436.

37. J. F. Kinney, agent, Yankton, 23 Aug. 1886, *ARCIA 1886*, 102; Ralph Hall, agent, Devil's Lake, 26 Aug. 1895, *ARCIA 1895*, 229; Chapman, *ARCIA 1902*, 350; Hrdlicka, *Tuberculosis among Certain Indian Tribes*, 13.

38. Charles L. Davis, superintendent, Devil's Lake, *ARCIA 1905*, 294; Chapman, *ARCIA 1905*, 350; Joseph A. Murphy, "Health Problems of the Indians," *Annals of the American Academy of Political and Social Science* 37 (March 1911): 108.

39. "Tuberculosis and the Indians," unidentified newspaper, excerpted in [Walker], *Mythen der Oglala*, ed. Karl A. Nowotny, Dokumente der Geistesgeschichte 5 (Vienna: F. Nowotny, 1979), 22; Murphy, "Health Problems of the Indians," 103.

40. Jones, *ARCIA 1904*, 34–38; Hrdlicka, *Tuberculosis among Certain Indian Tribes*, 3–5, 12–36. See Putney, "Fighting the Scourge," 41–44, 83–85; Prucha, *The Great Father*, 2:846.

41. Leupp, quoted in Prucha, *The Great Father*, 2:848; Leupp, commissioner of Indian affairs, *ARCIA 1908*, 26; Murphy, "The Prevention of Tuberculosis in the Indian Schools," *Addresses and Proceedings, National Education Association of the United States* (1909): 919–923; Creamer, "Tuberculosis among the American Indi-

ans," 439. See Putney, "Fighting the Scourge," 90; Prucha, *The Great Father,* 2:848; Robert A. Trennert, *White Man's Medicine: Government Doctors and the Navajo, 1863–1955* (Albuquerque: University of New Mexico Press, 1998), 99–100.

42. William H. Taft, "Special Message to Congress," 12 Sept. 1912, in Valentine, *ARCIA 1912,* 17–19.

43. Murphy, "Health Problems of the Indians," 103; Taft, "Special Message to Congress," 18; George M. Kober, George E. Bushnell, Joseph A. Murphy, Albert B. Tonkin, William H. Baldwin, and Hoyt E. Dearholt, *Tuberculosis among the North American Indians* (Washington: Government Printing Office, 1923), 43; Valentine, *ARCIA 1912,* 17; Eastman, *Indian To-day,* 136; Prucha, *The Great Father,* 2:842–843. Prucha traced the growing interest to the efforts of Indian inspector William J. McConnell, Trennert traced it to the placement of the tribes under federal protection on reservations, while Stephen J. Kunitz and Jerrold E. Levy stressed the importance of the new appreciation for Indian population decline: Trennert, *White Man's Medicine,* 63; Kunitz and Levy, "Dances with Doctors: Navajo Encounters with the Indian Health Service," in *Western Medicine as Contested Knowledge,* ed. Andrew Cunningham and Bridie Andrews (New York: Manchester University Press, 1997), 95–104.

44. Robert H. Wiebe, *The Search for Order, 1877–1920* (New York: Hill and Wang, 1967), xiv, 114–116; Trennert, *White Man's Medicine,* 63.

7. Pursuit of Efficacy

1. Walsh McDermott, in "Minutes of the Navajo Tribal Council," 2 June 1959, *WMP*/11/7, p. 2.

2. James R. Walker, "Tuberculosis among the Oglala Sioux Indians," *American Journal of the Medical Sciences* 132 (1906): 600–605; Joseph A. Murphy, "The Prevention of Tuberculosis in the Indian Schools," *Addresses and Proceedings, National Education Association of the United States* (1909): 919. See Diane Therese Putney, "Fighting the Scourge: American Indian Morbidity and Federal Policy, 1897–1928" (Ph.D. diss., Marquette University, 1980), 104, 108–109, 170–185, 198, 309; Francis Paul Prucha, *The Great Father: The United States Government and the American Indians* (Lincoln: University of Nebraska Press, 1984), 2:850–855; Robert A. Trennert, *White Man's Medicine: Government Doctors and the Navajo, 1863–1955* (Albuquerque: University of New Mexico Press, 1998), 74–75, 136–138.

3. George E. Bushnell, *A Study in the Epidemiology of Tuberculosis* (New York: William Wood, 1920), 163; George M. Kober, George E. Bushnell, Joseph A. Murphy, Albert B. Tonkin, William H. Baldwin, and Hoyt E. Dearholt, *Tuberculosis among the North American Indians* (Washington: Government Printing Office, 1923), 42.

4. Kober et al., *Tuberculosis,* 1; Lewis Meriam, Ray A. Brown, Henry Roe Cloud, Edward Everett Dale, Emma Duke, Herbert R. Edwards, Fayette Avery McKenzie, Mary Louise Mark, W. Carson Ryan, Jr., and William J. Spillman, *The Problem of Indian Administration* (Baltimore: Johns Hopkins University Press, 1928), 3, 204; H. J. Warner, "The Incidence of Tuberculous Infection among School-Children on Five Montana Indian Reservations," *American Review of Tuberculosis* 26 (July–December 1932): 507–515; Horace DeLien and Arthur W. Dahlstrom, "Tuberculosis Control among American Indians," *Journal-Lancet* 70 (April 1950): 131.

5. *Health surveys:* Ales Hrdlicka, *Physiological and Medical Observations among the Indians of Southwestern United States and Northern Mexico* (Washington: Government Printing Office, 1908); Joseph W. Mountin and J. S. Townsend, *Observations on Indian Health Problems and Facilities* (Washington: Government Printing Office, 1936); Herbert Hoover, *The Hoover Commission Report on Organization of the Executive Branch of Government* (New York: McGraw-Hill, Inc., 1949), 461–471. *Physicians' publications:* Isaac W. Brewer, "Tuberculosis among the Indians of Arizona and New Mexico," *New York Medical Journal* 84 (1906): 981–983; Ralph M. Alley, "Tuberculosis among Indians," *Diseases of the Chest* 6 (February 1940): 44–46; Albert Reifel, "Tuberculosis among Indians of the United States," *Diseases of the Chest* 16 (August 1949): 234–247; Fred T. Foard, "Health Services for the North American Indians," *Medical Woman's Journal* 57 (November 1950): 10–12. *Flawed data:* Stephen J. Kunitz, *Disease Change and the Role of Medicine: The Navajo Experience* (Berkeley: University of California Press, 1983), 70; J. Nixon Hadley, "Health Conditions among Navajo Indians," *Public Health Reports* 70 (September 1955): 832–833.

6. Robert Valentine, commissioner of Indian affairs, *ARCIA 1912*, 17; DeLien and Dahlstrom, "Tuberculosis Control," 131; U.S. Public Health Service, *Health Services for American Indians* (Washington, D.C.: Government Printing Office, 1957), 40, 44, 57.

7. Walsh McDermott, "Demography, Culture, and Economics and the Evolutionary Stages of Medicine," in *Human Ecology and Public Health*, ed. Edwin D. Kilbourne and Wilson G. Smilie, 4th ed. (London: Macmillan, 1969), 9.

8. Hrdlicka, *Physiological and Medical Observations*, 210–211; Herbert A. Burns, "Tuberculosis in the Indian," *American Review of Tuberculosis* 26 (July–December 1932): 498–499; Foard, "Health Services for the North American Indians," 12; Hadley, "Health Conditions among Navajo Indians," 835.

9. Clyde Kluckhohn and Dorothea Leighton, *The Navajo* (1946), rev. ed. (Cambridge: Harvard University Press, 1974), 23; Frank S. French, James R. Shaw, and Joseph O. Dean, "The Navajo Health Problem, Its Genesis, Proportions and a Plan for Its Solution," *Military Medicine* 116 (June 1955): 451–454; René Dubos, *Mirage of Health: Utopias, Progress, and Biological Change* (New York: Harper, 1959), 3; Stephen J. Kunitz and Jerrold E. Levy, "Dances with Doctors: Navajo Encounters with the Indian Health Service," in *Western Medicine as Contested Knowledge*, ed. Andrew Cunningham and Bridie Andrews (New York: Manchester University Press, 1997), 95–105; Trennert, *White Man's Medicine*.

10. Sydney J. Tillim, "Medical Annals of Arizona: Health Among the Navajos," *Southwestern Medicine* 20 (July–November 1936): 273; Stephen Kunitz, "Underdevelopment, Demographic Change, and Health Care on the Navajo Indian Reservation," *Social Science and Medicine* 15A (1981): 177; Kunitz, "The Social Philosophy of John Collier," *Ethnohistory* 18 (Summer 1971): 213–229.

11. J. A. Krug, *The Navajo: A Long Range Program for Navajo Rehabilitation* (Washington: U.S. Government Printing Office, 1948), vii, 1–9; Ruth M. Underhill, *The Navajos* (Norman: University of Oklahoma Press, 1956), 252–259.

12. Mountin and Townsend, *Observations on Indian Health*, 10; Robert W. Young, *The Navajo Yearbook: 1951–1961, A Decade of Progress*, vol. 8 (Window Rock, Ariz.: Navajo Agency, 1961), 67; Abraham B. Bergman, David C. Grossman, Angela M. Erdich, John G. Todd, and Ralph Forquera, "A Political History of the Indian Health Service," *Milbank Quarterly* 77 (1999): 578.

13. Hrdlicka, *Physiological and Medical Observations*, 131, 141, 155; Hrdlicka, "Disease, Medicine and Sorcery Among the American Aborgines," *JAMA* 99 (12 Nov. 1932): 1661; J. A. Carroll, quoted in Brewer, "Tuberculosis Among the Indians of Arizona and New Mexico," 982; New Mexico State Department of Health, quoted in Kober et al., *Tuberculosis*, 31; Tillim, "Health among the Navajos," 311; Aidan Cockburn, *Infectious Diseases: Their Evolution and Eradication* (Springfield, Ill.: Charles C. Thomas, 1967), 105. For an example of other genetic explanations, see Irvine H. Page, Lena A. Lewis, and Harvey Gilbert, "Plasma Lipids and Proteins and their Relationship to Coronary Disease among Navajo Indians," *Circulation* 13 (May 1956): 678.

14. Kober et al., *Tuberculosis*, 4; Burns, "Tuberculosis in the Indian," 501; J. G. Townsend, Joseph D. Aronson, Robert Saylor, and Irma Parr, "Tuberculosis Control among the North American Indians," *American Review of Tuberculosis* 45 (January 1942): 46; Alley, "Tuberculosis Among Indians," 45; Warner, "Incidence of Tuberculous Infection," 511–512; J. Arthur Myers and Virginia L. Dustin, "Albert Reifel and Tuberculosis among the American Indians," *Hygeia* 25 (April 1947): 319; J. A. Myers, "Editorial: Tuberculosis among American Indians," *Diseases of the Chest* 16 (August 1949): 248.

15. René Dubos and Jean Dubos, *The White Plague: Tuberculosis, Man, and Society* (1952; New Brunswick: Rutgers University Press, 1987), 191; Tillim, "Health Among the Navajos," 277; Myers and Dustin, "Albert Reifel and Tuberculosis," 322; Burns, "Tuberculosis in the Indian," 499.

16. Lewis J. Moorman, "Tuberculosis on the Navaho Reservation," *American Review of Tuberculosis* 61 (April 1950): 588; Mountin and Townsend, *Observations on Indian Health*, 13; Foard, "Health Services for the North American Indians," 13; Reifel, "Tuberculosis among Indians," 239. See also Joseph Murphy, "Health Problems of the Indians," *Annals of the American Academy of Political and Social Science* 37 (March 1911): 106–107; Kober et al., *Tuberculosis*, 2, 29–37; Myers and Dustin, "Albert Reifel and Tuberculosis," 272–273; Krug, *Long Range Program*, 35.

17. W. A. Jones, commissioner of Indian affairs, *ARCIA 1904*, 33–38; Brewer, "Tuberculosis among the Indians of Arizona and New Mexico," 981–982; Kober et al., *Tuberculosis*, 29–37; Tillim, "Health Among the Navajos," 391; Alley, "Tuberculosis among Indians," 45; Dubos and Dubos, *White Plague*, xxxviii.

18. *Navajo theories:* Alexander H. Leighton and Dorothea C. Leighton, *The Navaho Door: An Introduction to Navajo Life* (Cambridge: Harvard University Press, 1945), 24–37; *The People's Health*, 4–13; Kunitz and Jerrold E. Levy, "Traditional Navajo Health Beliefs and Practices," in Kunitz, *Disease Change*, 118–127. *Specific explanations:* Hrdlicka, *Physiological and Medical Observations*, 23; Cara Richards Dobyns, "Report on Research of the Resident Anthropologist, Navajo-Cornell Field Health Research Project, 1958–1958," 19 Dec. 1959, *NCFHPP/*1, pp. 89–91; Hoskie Cronemeyer, quoted in "Minutes of the Navajo Tribal Council," 5 Jan. 1953, *WMP/*11/7, p. 12; Wauneka, quoted in Kurt Deuschle, "Tuberculosis among the Navajo: Research in Cross-Cultural Technologic Development in Health," *American Review of Respiratory Diseases* 80 (August 1959): 201.

19. Deuschle, "Tuberculosis among the Navajo," 201; "Minutes of the Navajo Tribal Council," 12 Feb. 1954, *WMP/*11/7, pp. 10, 18; Manuelito Begay, quoted in Deuschle, "Tuberculosis among the Navajo," 200; *The People's Health*, 34–35, 47;

Begay, quoted in "Minutes of the Navajo Tribal Council" (1954), 10; Begay, quoted in *The People's Health*, 42; Deuschle, "Tuberculosis among the Navajo," 201.

20. John Adair, "Physicians, Medicine Men and Their Navaho Patients," in *Man's Image in Medicine and Anthropology*, ed. Iago Galdston (New York: International Universities Press, 1961), 243; Kluckhohn and Leighton, *The Navajo*, 220; *The People's Health*, 5–6, 13.

21. Kober et al., *Tuberculosis*, 4.

22. USPHS, *Health Services for American Indians*, 90–92; U.S. Public Health Service, *The Indian Health Program of the U.S. Public Health Service* (Washington: U.S. Department of Health, Education, and Welfare, 1966), 18–19; Jeff Henderson, "Native American Health Policy: From U.S. Territorial Expansion to Legal Obligation," *JAMA* 265 (1 May 1991): 2272; Trennert, *White Man's Medicine*, 117–121; Bergman et al., "Political History of the IHS," 591 (Snyder Act). Hospital construction on the reservations lagged behind construction among the general population: Paul Starr, *The Social Transformation of American Medicine* (New York: Basic Books, 1982), 145–179; Charles E. Rosenberg, *The Care of Strangers: The Rise of America's Hospital System* (Baltimore: Johns Hopkins University Press, 1987), 5, 97–121.

23. Burns, "Tuberculosis in the Indian," 506; Reifel, "Tuberculosis among Indians," 234; Moorman, "Tuberculosis on the Navaho Reservation," 589; Moorman, quoted in "Hearings on H.R. 303: An Act to Transfer the Maintenance and Operation of Hospital and Health Facilities for Indians to the Public Health Service," 28–29 May 1954, in Congressional Hearings, Senate, Interior and Insular Affairs, 83rd Cong., 2d sess., 1953–1954, vol. 14, 83 S. 1085-10, p. 101; James E. Perkins, quoted ibid., 51; Lewis Orme, assistant secretary of the interior for Indian affairs, ibid., 2.

24. Burns, "Tuberculosis in the Indian," 498; Townsend et al., "Tuberculosis Control," 41–52; Joseph D. Aronson, Charlotte F. Aronson, and Helen C. Taylor, "A Twenty-Year Appraisal of BCG Vaccination in the Control of Tuberculosis," *Archives of Internal Medicine* 101 (1958): 881–893.

25. "Report of the Commissioner of Indian Affairs," 1920, quoted in Kober et al., *Tuberculosis*, 88; Alley, "Tuberculosis among Indians," 45; Leighton and Leighton, *Navaho Door*, 48; USPHS, *Health Services for American Indians*, 88.

26. Elinor D. Gregg, *The Indians and the Nurse* (Norman: University of Oklahoma Press, 1965), 24; Putney, "Fighting the Scourge," 255–285; Meriam et al., *Problem of Indian Administration*, 287–298, 303; USPHS, *Health Services for American Indians*, 91 (reluctance).

27. Foard, "Health Services for the North American Indians," 12; French et al., "Navajo Health Problem," 453; Moorman, "Tuberculosis on the Navaho Reservation," 588; Foard, "Health Services for the North American Indians," 13; DeLien and Dahlstrom, "Tuberculosis Control," 132.

28. Dorothea Leighton and Clyde Kluckhohn, *Children of the People: The Navajo Individual and his Development* (Cambridge: Harvard University Press, 1947), 232; Mountin and Townsend, *Observations on Indian Health*, 13; USPHS, *Health Services for American Indians*, vii.

29. "Report to Accompany H.R. 4627: Authorizing an Appropriation for the Immediate Relief of the Navajo and Hopi Indians," 5 Dec. 1947, 80th Cong., 1st sess., 11123 H. Rep. 1156, p. 1; William E. Warne, quoted in "Report to accom-

pany S. 1407: Rehabilitation of the Navajo and Hopi Tribes," 2 June 1949, 81st Cong., 1st sess., 11293 S. Rep. 550, p. 5. On postwar enthusiasm, see James T. Patterson, *Grand Expectations: The United States, 1945–1970* (New York: Oxford University Press, 1996).

30. Krug, *Long Range Program*, v–x; BIA, "Summary of Navajo Development," 8 April 1949, in "Report to accompany S. 1407," p. 9; French et al., "Navajo Health Problem," 453; "An Act to Promote the Rehabilitation of the Navajo and Hopi Tribes of Indians and a Better Utilization of the Resources of the Navajo and Hopi Indian Reservations, and for Other Purposes," Public Law 474, *United States Code*, 81st Cong., 2nd sess., 1950, pp. 44–45. See also Kunitz, *Disease Change*, 26–43.

31. Robert W. Young, *The Navajo Yearbook of Planning in Action*, vol. 4, 1954 (Window Rock: Navajo Agency, 1955), 17; ibid., vol. 5, 1955 (Window Rock: Navajo Agency, 1955), 22; Krug, *Long Range Program*, 38.

32. Kober et al., *Tuberculosis*, 44; USPHS, *Health Services for American Indians*, 93–94. Orme Lewis, Written Statement, 5 May 1953, in "Report to Accompany H.R. 303: Transferring the Maintenance and Operation of Hospital and Health Facilities for Indians to the Public Health Service," 17 July 1953, 83rd Cong., 1st sess., 11667 H. Rep. 870, p. 10; Senate, "Hearings on H.R. 303," 15; Stephen J. Kunitz, "The History and Politics of US Health Care Policy for American Indians and Alaskan Natives," *AJPH* 86 (October 1996): 1465.

33. Hoover, *Organization of the Executive Branch*, 471; "Report to Accompany H.R. 303," 8; Senate, "Hearings on H.R. 303," 98–107, 103; Wauneka, Written Statement, 2 Nov. 1953, read in the Senate, "Hearings on H.R. 303," 43.

34. Orme, in "Hearings on H.R. 303," 2; Fred Foard, ibid., 17–18; House, "Report to Accompany H.R. 303," 6–7; USPHS, *Health Services for American Indians*, 95–96. Hoover, *Organization of the Executive Branch*, 471; "Report to Accompany H.R. 303," 2; "Report to Accompany H.R. 303: Transferring the Maintenance and Operation of Hospital and Health Facilities for Indians to the Public Health Service," 13 May 1954, 83rd Cong., 2nd sess., 11729 S. Rep. 1530, p. 2; "An Act to Transfer the Maintenance and Operation of Hospital and Health Facilities for Indians to the Public Health Service, and for Other Purposes," Public Law 568, *United States Code*, 83rd Cong., 2nd sess., 1954.

35. USPHS, *Health Services for American Indians*, 39–57, 230–232.

36. Meriam et al., *Problem of Indian Administration*, viii.

37. Dubos and Dubos, *White Plague*, xxxviii; *The People's Health*, 50.

38. Harry F. Dowling, *Fighting Infection: Conquests of the Twentieth Century* (Cambridge: Harvard University Press, 1977); Allan M. Brandt, *No Magic Bullet: A Social History of Venereal Disease in the United States since 1880* (New York: Oxford University Press, 1987); R. Y. Keers, *Pulmonary Tuberculosis: A Journey down the Centuries* (London: Baillière Tindall, 1978); Frank Ryan, *The Forgotten Plague: How the Battle against Tuberculosis Was Won—and Lost* (Boston: Little, Brown, 1992); Allan M. Brandt and Martha Gardner, "The Golden Age of Medicine?" in *Medicine in the Twentieth Century*, ed. Roger Cooter and John Pickstone (Amsterdam: Harwood Academic, 2000), 24; Scott Podolsky, *Serotherapy, Pneumonia, and the Rise of Scientific Medicine, 1890–1940*, unpublished manuscript.

39. Paul B. Beeson, "Walsh McDermott, October 24, 1909–October 17, 1981," *Biographical Memoirs, National Academy of Sciences*, vol. 59 (Washington:

National Academy Press, 1990), 284–286; Walsh McDermott, "Oral History Transcript" (ca. 1977), *OHT*, pp. 1–15; McDermott, "Early Days of Antimicrobial Therapy," *Antimicrobial Agents and Chemotherapy* 8 (1968): 5–6; McDermott, "The Story of INH," *Journal of Infectious Diseases* 119 (June 1969): 678–683.

40. McDermott, "Oral History Transcript," 9. There is a gap in the transcript; "war" makes most sense.

41. *NIH Factbook*, 1st ed. (Chicago: Marquis Academic Media, 1976); Starr, *Social Transformation*, 347; Walsh McDermott, "Antimicrobial Therapy," *Proceedings of the Institute of Medicine of Chicago* 18 (15 Jan. 1950): 2–12.

42. H. Corwin Hinshaw, "Antibacterial Drug Therapy in TB," *Bulletin of the National Tuberculosis Association* 35 (1948): 119–120, 132; Carl Muschenheim, Walsh McDermott, and Richard B. Maxwell, "The Therapy of Miliary and Meningeal Tuberculosis: Review of a Five Year Experience," *Transactions of the American Clinical and Climatological Association* 63 (1951): 257–265; Lawrence B. Hobson and McDermott, "Criteria for the Clinical Evaluation of Antituberculous Agents," *Annals of the New York Academy of Sciences* 52 (1949): 784–786; "Practitioners' Conference: Principles of Treatment of Pulmonary Tuberculosis," *New York Medicine* 8 (1952): 16, 49; Ralph Tompsett, McDermott, and John G. Kidd, "Tuberculostatic Activity of Blood and Urine from Animals Given Gliotoxin," *Journal of Immunology* 65 (1950): 59–63; Charles A. Werner, Tompsett, Muschenheim, and McDermott, "The Toxicity of Viomycin in Humans," *American Review of Tuberculosis* 63 (January 1951): 49–61; Charles A. LeMaistre, Thompsett, Muschenheim, James A. Moore, and McDermott, "Effects of Adrenocorticotropic Hormone and Cortisone in Patients with Tuberculosis," *Journal of Clinical Investigation* 30 (1951): 445–456.

43. "Medicine: War Booty," *Time Magazine*, 21 Nov. 1949, pp. 98–99; Corwin Hinshaw and McDermott, "Thiosemicarbazone Therapy of Tuberculosis in Humans," *American Review of Tuberculosis* 61 (January 1950): 145–157; Carl Muschenheim, DuMont F. Elmendorf, William D. Cawthon, and McDermott, "Failure of Para-Isobutoxybenzaldehyde Thiosemicarbazone as an Antituberculous Drug in Man," *American Review of Tuberculosis* 68 (November 1953): 791–793.

44. National Tuberculosis Association, "Press Conference," 21 Feb. 1952, *CMP/2/6*; [McDermott], "Annual Report of the Division [of Infectious Disease, NYH], 1952," *WMP/11/5*; Dowling, *Fighting Infection*, 167–171. Although isoniazid had been synthesized in 1912, its antituberculous properties went unrecognized until 1951.

45. Hobson and McDermott, "Criteria for Clinical Evaluation," 782–783; J. Yerushalmy, L. H. Garland, J. T. Harkness, H. C. Hinshaw, E. R. Miller, S. J. Shipman, and H. B. Zwerling, "An Evaluation of the Role of Serial Chest Roentgenograms in Estimating the Progress of Disease in Patients with Pulmonary Tuberculosis," *Chest* 64 (September 1951): 225–248; Charles M. Clark, Dumont Elmendorf, William Cawthon, Carl Muschenheim, and McDermott, "Isoniazid (Isonicotinic Acid Hydrazide) in the Treatment of Miliary and Meningeal Tuberculosis," *American Review of Tuberculosis* 66 (October 1952): 406, 407; Werner et al., "Toxicity of Viomycin," 55.

46. [McDermott], "Annual Report of the Division, 1952"; Dumont Elmendorf, William Cawthon, Carl Muschenheim, and Walsh McDermott, "The Absorption, Distribution, Excretion and Short-term Toxicity of Isonicotinic Acid

Hydrazide (Nydrazid) in Man," *American Review of Tuberculosis* 65 (April 1952): 441.

47. [McDermott], "Annual Report of the Division, 1952"; McDermott, "Conversation with Jane K. Zaidi (CUMC Archivist)," 7 Feb. 1972, *WMP*/11/5, p. 1 ("ethnic"); McDermott, "Early Days of Antimicrobial Therapy," 2 ("ethical"). It is unclear whether "ethnic" in the oral history reflects McDermott's intent or a transcription error.

48. Moorman, "Tuberculosis on the Navaho Reservation," 590; [McDermott], "Annual Report of the Division, 1952"; Frederick Woltman, "The Medicine Men Accept Our Healing," *World-Telegram and Sun Saturday Magazine*, 22 Jan. 1955, p. 4.

49. McDermott, "Early Days of Antimicrobial Therapy," 2; *The People's Health*, 95.

8. Experiments at Many Farms

1. *The People's Health*, 50, 95; Walsh McDermott, Kurt Deuschle, John Adair, Hugh Fulmer, and Bernice Loughlin, "Introducing Modern Medicine in a Navajo Community: Physicians and Anthropologists Are Cooperating in This Study of Changing Patterns of Culture and Disease," *Science* 131 (22 January 1960): 197–205, 280–287; McDermott, Deuschle, and Clifford R. Barnett, "Health Care Experiment at Many Farms," *Science* 175 (7 January 1972): 23–31.

2. Frederick Woltman, "The Medicine Men Accept Our Healing," *World-Telegram and Sun Saturday Magazine*, 22 Jan. 1955, p. 4; Steven M. Spencer, "They're Saving Lives in Navajo-Land," *Saturday Evening Post*, 23 April 1955, p. 92; [McDermott], "Annual Report of the Division [of Infectious Disease, NYH], 1952," *WMP*/11/5; Mickey [Charles LeMaistre] to McDermott, 31 Dec. 1951, *WMP*/11/5.

3. Spencer, "Saving Lives in Navajo-Land," 92; Walsh McDermott, Kurt Deuschle, Edwin Kilbourne, and David Rogers, "Interim Report on Indian Health, Committee on American Indians," 30 June 1959, *WMP*/10/2, p. 68; McDermott, "Conversation with Jane K. Zaidi (CUMC Archivist)," 7 Feb. 1972, *WMP*/11/5, p. 1; McDermott, "Early Days of Antimicrobial Therapy," *Antimicrobial Agents and Chemotherapy* 8 (1968): 2; "Medicine: Good News from the West," *Time Magazine*, 21 July 1952, p. 55.

4. Spencer, "Saving Lives in Navajo-Land," 92–94; "Medicine: Good News from the West," 55; DuMont F. Elmendorf, William U. Cawthon, Carl Muschenheim, and Walsh McDermott, "The Absorption, Distribution, Excretion and Short-term Toxicity of Isonicotinic Acid Hydrazide (Nydrazid) in Man," *American Review of Tuberculosis* 65 (April 1952): 441 n.7.

5. National Tuberculosis Association, "Press Conference," 21 Feb. 1952, *CMP*/2/6; "Medicine: TB—and Hope," *Time Magazine*, 3 March 1952, p. 42. McDermott, "Oral History Transcript," ca. 1977, *OHT*, p. 17; McDermott, "Conversation with Zaidi (Archivist)," 2; "Minutes of the Navajo Tribal Council," 25 April 1952, *WMP*/11/7. Charles M. Clark, Dumont Elmendorf, William Cawthon, Carl Muschenheim, and McDermott, "Isoniazid (Isonicotinic Acid Hydrazide) in the Treatment of Miliary and Meningeal Tuberculosis," *American Review of Tuberculosis* 66 (October 1952): 406; "Minutes of the Navajo Tribal Coun-

cil," 5 Jan. 1953, WMP/11/7, pp. 1, 5; "Minutes of the Navajo Tribal Council," 12 Feb. 1954, WMP/11/7, pp. 12–14, 19; *The People's Health*, 36–40.

6. Annie D. Wauneka, "Helping a People to Understand: A Navajo Leader Taught Herself and Then Others How to Fight Tuberculosis," *American Journal of Nursing* 62 (July 1962): 88; Kurt Deuschle, "Tuberculosis among the Navajo: Research in Cross-Cultural Technologic Development in Health," *American Review of Respiratory Diseases* 80 (August 1959): 201; [McDermott], "Annual Report of the Division, 1952"; *The People's Health*, xiv.

7. *Data:* John Adair, Kurt Deuschle, and Walsh McDermott, "Patterns of Health and Disease among the Navahos," *Annals of the American Academy of Political and Social Science* 311 (May 1957): 85, 88–90; McDermott et al., "Introducing Modern Medicine," 203; *The People's Health*, 15, 43. *Explanations:* McDermott, "Conversation with Zaidi," 3, 5; Adair et al., "Patterns of Health and Disease," 84–85; *The People's Health*, 15, 21; Spencer, "Saving Lives in Navajo-Land," 92; McDermott et al., "Interim Report on Indian Health," 83.

8. John Etling, *The Germ of Laziness: Rockefeller Philanthropy and the Public Health in the New South* (Cambridge: Harvard University Press, 1981); C. C. Ch'en, "The Rural Public Health Experiment in Ting Hsien, China," *Milbank Memorial Fund Quarterly Bulletin* 14 (January 1936): 66–80; Shula Marks, "South Africa's Early Experiment in Social Medicine: Its Pioneers and Politics," *AJPH* 87 (March 1997): 452–459; Sidney L. Kark, Emily Kark, and J. H. Abramson, "Commentary: In Search of Innovative Approaches to International Health," *AJPH* 83 (November 1993): 1533–1536. *The People's Health*, vii, 49.

9. "Minutes of the Navajo Tribal Council" (1954), 13, 23; Sam Akeah, in "Minutes of the Navajo Tribal Council," 13 Jan. 1955, *WMP/11/7*, p. 7; Robert W. Young, *The Navajo Yearbook of Planning in Action*, vol. 5, 1955 (Window Rock, Ariz.: Navajo Agency, 1955), 25; McDermott, "Conversation with Zaidi," 2, 7; *The People's Health*, 47, 50–52.

10. "Navajo-Cornell Field Health Research Grant Report," 1 March 1959, *WMP/10/9*, pp. 4–8; McDermott et al., "Introducing Modern Medicine," 199.

11. *The People's Health*, 50–56, 60; McDermott, "Conversation with Zaidi," 7.

12. Walsh McDermott, Kurt Deuschle, Hugh Fulmer, and John Adair, "The Navajo-Cornell Field Health Research Project at Many Farms," 30 Jun. 1958, *NCFHPP/1*, pp. 2–3; Deuschle, Adair, and Fulmer, "The Navajo-Cornell Field Health Research Project at Many Farms," *Navajo Yearbook* 7 (1958): 44–45; Bernice W. Loughlin and Ellen Mansell, "Training Health Workers on the Navajo Indian Reservation," *Nursing Times* (30 January 1959); McDermott et al., "Health Care Experiment," 24; Edward Taylor, "Transcript of Interview with Jane K. Zaidi (CUMC Archivist)," 16 March 1972, *OHT*, pp. 1–4.

13. McDermott, "Conversation with Zaidi," 4, 8; Kurt Deuschle and John Adair, "An Interdisciplinary Approach to Public Health on the Navajo Indian Reservation: Medical and Anthropological Aspects," *Annals of the New York Academy of Sciences* 84 (8 December 1960): 889; "Minutes of the Navajo Tribal Council" (1954), 10, 18; *The People's Health*, 34–35, 47, 64–65.

14. McDermott, "Conversation with Zaidi," 4; John Adair, "Physicians, Medicine Men and Their Navaho Patients," in *Man's Image in Medicine and Anthropology*, ed. Iago Galdston (New York: International Universities Press, 1961), 247–250; *The People's Health*, 12; *The People's Health (1988)*, 161–177.

15. Ellen Mansell and Bernice W. Loughlin, "The Navajo Health Visitor," *Practical Nursing* 8 (April 1958): 13–15; Loughlin, Kenneth Dennison, Mansell, Hugh Fulmer, and Health Committee for the Navajo Tribal Council, "Syllabus for Teachers in Navajo Health," 1960, *WMP*/10/10; Adair, "The Indian Health Worker in the Cornell-Navaho Project," *Human Organization* 19 (Summer 1960): 59–63; Deuschle and Adair, "Interdisciplinary Approach," 899; Deuschle, "Training and Use of Medical Auxiliaries in a Navajo Community," *Public Health Reports* 78 (June 1963): 461–469; *The People's Health*, 67–92.

16. Adair and Deuschle, "Some Problems of the Physicians on the Navajo Reservation," *Human Organization* 16 (Winter 1958): 20; Herbert Landar, "The Language of Pain in Navaho Culture," in *Studies in Southwestern Ethnolinguistics: Meaning and History in the Languages of the American Southwest*, ed. Dell H. Hymes and William E. Bittle (Paris: Mouton, 1967), 119–144; *The People's Health*, 108–127.

17. Adair et al., "Patterns of Health and Disease," 89; "Navajo-Cornell Field Health Research Grant Report," 14, 22; Deuschle and Adair, "Interdisciplinary Approach," 895; *The People's Health*, 16, 106; Deuschle, "Tuberculosis among the Navajo," 203; McDermott et al., "Health Care Experiment," 27.

18. Deuschle and Adair, "Interdisciplinary Approach," 903; John Hayslett, James McCarroll, Eileen Brady, Kurt Deuschle, Walsh McDermott, and Edwin D. Kilbourne, "Endemic Influenza: I. Serologic Evidence of Continuing and Subclinical Infection in Disparate Populations in the Post-Pandemic Period," *American Review of Respiratory Diseases* 85 (January 1962): 1–8; Deuschle and Adair, "Interdisciplinary Approach," 902; McDermott et al., "Introducing Modern Medicine," 280; David Rabin, Clifford Barnett, William D. Arnold, Robert H. Freiberger, and Gyla Brooks, "Untreated Congenital Hip Disease: A Study of the Epidemiology, Natural History, and Social Aspects of the Disease in a Navajo Population," *AJPH* 55 (1965): 1–44; *The People's Health*, 133–135. For a partial bibliography, see *The People's Health (1988)*, 263–266; for a more extensive list, see David S. Jones, "Rationalizing Epidemics: Historical Accounts of American Indian Health Disparities" (Ph.D. diss., Harvard University, 2001), 637–656.

19. McDermott, "Conversation with Zaidi," 7, 8, 12; McDermott et al., "Health Care Experiment," 24; Young, "Foreword," in *The People's Health (1988)*, xiv; *The People's Health*, 55, 61. On recent controversies about treatment and research, see Marcia Angell, "The Ethics of Clinical Research in the Third World," *New England Journal of Medicine* 337 (1997): 847–849; David J. Rothman, "The Shame of Medical Research," *New York Review of Books* (30 November 2000): 60–64.

20. *Reports:* Clark et al., "Isoniazid in the Treatment of Miliary and Meningeal Tuberculosis," 391–415; Kurt Deuschle, Louise Ormond, DuMont Elmendorf, Carl Muschenheim, and Walsh McDermott, "The Course of Pulmonary Tuberculosis during Long-term Single-drug (Isoniazid) Therapy," *American Review of Tuberculosis* 70 (August 1954): 228–265, 240; McDermott, Ormond, Muschenheim, Deuschle, McCune, and Tompsett, "Pyrazinamide-Isoniazid in Tuberculosis," *American Review of Tuberculosis* 69 (March 1954): 319–333; Roger Des Prez, Clarence Jordahl, Deuschle, Muschenheim, and McDermott, "Streptovaricin and Isoniazid in the Treatment of Pulmonary Tuberculosis," *American Review of Respiratory Diseases* 80 (September 1959): 431–433; Jordahl, Des Prez, Deuschle, Muschenheim, and McDermott, "Ineffectiveness of Nicotinamide and Isoniazid in

the Treatment of Pulmonary Tuberculosis," *American Review of Respiratory Diseases* 83 (June 1961): 899–900. *Concerns:* McDermott, "Antimicrobial Therapy of Pulmonary Tuberculosis," *Bulletin of the World Health Organization* 23 (1960): 427–461; McDermott, "The Chemotherapy of Tuberculosis," *American Review of Respiratory Diseases* 86 (September 1962): 335.

21. Loughlin et al., "Syllabus for Teachers in Navajo Health," 102b; Kurt Deuschle, Clarence Jordahl, and Gladys L. Hobby, "Clinical Usefulness of Riboflavin-Tagged Isoniazid for Self-Medication in Tuberculous Patients," *American Review of Respiratory Diseases* 82 (July 1960): 9; McDermott et al., "Introducing Modern Medicine," 283. For a more extensive discussion, see David S. Jones, "Technologies of Compliance: Attempts to Improve Self-Administration of Tuberculosis Treatment, 1956–1966," *History and Technology* 17 (Winter 2001): 279–318.

22. Daniel N. Mohler, David G. Wallin, and Edward G. Dreyfus, "Studies in the Home Treatment of Streptococcal Disease: I. Failure of Patients to Take Penicillin by Mouth as Prescribed," *New England Journal of Medicine* 252 (30 June 1955): 1116–1118; Peter Stradling and Graham Poole, "Self-medication in Tuberculosis," *Lancet* ii (15 November 1958): 1066; Wallace Fox, "The Problem of Self-administration of Drugs; with Particular Reference to Pulmonary Tuberculosis," *Tubercle* 39 (1958): 269.

23. McDermott et al., "Introducing Modern Medicine," 282; Cedric Northrop, John H. Fountain, and Daniel W. Zahn, "The Practical Management of the Recalcitrant Tuberculous Patient," *Public Health Reports* 67 (September 1952): 894–898; Barron H. Lerner, "New York City's Tuberculosis Control Efforts: The Historical Limitations of the 'War on Consumption,'" *AJPH* 83 (May 1993): 758–766; Lerner, *Contagion and Confinement: Controlling Tuberculosis along the Skid Road* (Baltimore: Johns Hopkins University Press, 1998); Stradling and Poole, "Self-medication," 1066; Ronald Bayer and David Wilkinson, "Directly Observed Therapy for Tuberculosis: History of an Idea," *Lancet* 345 (17 June 1995): 1545–1548.

24. Deuschle et al., "Clinical Usefulness of Riboflavin-Tagged Isoniazid," 1; Gladys Hobby and Deuschle, "The Use of Riboflavin as an Indicator of Isoniazid Ingestion in Self-Medicated Patients," *American Review of Respiratory Diseases* 80 (September 1959): 415; Richard W. Roberts and Deuschle, "Comparative Study of Urine Tests for the Detection of Isoniazid," *American Review of Respiratory Diseases* 80 (December 1959): 904; "Navajo-Cornell Field Health Research Grant Report," 36.

25. Thomas Moulding, "Preliminary Study of the Pill Calendar as a Method of Improving the Self-Administration of Drugs," *American Review of Respiratory Diseases* 84 (August 1961): 284; Moulding, "Proposal for a Time-Recording Pill Dispenser as a Method for Studying and Supervising the Self-Administration of Drugs," ibid. 85 (May 1962): 754–756.

26. McDermott et al., "Introducing Modern Medicine," 283; Moulding, "Proposal for a Time-Recording Pill Dispenser," 756. This regime of distrust and surveillance emerged during the height of the Cold War. The initial blush of postwar victory (antibiotics over infectious disease) had given way to the recognition that the battle would continue against an indolent enemy (tuberculosis). Mutual distrust (between patients and doctors) required constant surveillance (pill calendars, urine testing). Some hoped that radiation (Moulding's dispenser) would save the day.

27. See Michel Foucault, *Discipline and Punish: The Birth of the Prison* (1975), trans. Alan Sheridan (New York: Vintage, 1995).

28. Paul B. Beeson, "Walsh McDermott, October 24, 1909–October 17, 1981," *Biographical Memoirs, National Academy of Sciences*, vol. 59 (Washington: National Academy Press, 1990), 297; Carl Muschenheim, "Albert Lasker Award, Draft of Acceptance Speech," 1955, *CMP/2/13*.

29. Adair and Deuschle, "Problems of the Physicians on the Navajo Reservation," 19; IHS nurses, in Doris Schwartz, "Notes on Three Weeks at the Cornell-Navajo Field Health Project: Manyfarms, Arizona," 1956, *DSP/1/3*, pp. 3–4; IHS nurse, in *The People's Health*, 147. For the limited impact, see Stephen J. Kunitz, "Underdevelopment, Demographic Change, and Health Care on the Navajo Indian Reservation," *Social Science and Medicine* 15A (1981): 186; Kunitz, *Disease Change and the Role of Medicine: The Navajo Experience* (Berkeley: University of California Press, 1983), 201 n.1; *The People's Health (1988)*, 246 n.2.

30. Alexander H. Leighton, *Human Relations in a Changing World: Observations on the Use of the Social Sciences* (New York: Dutton, 1949), 11, 13, 327; Clyde Kluckhohn and Dorothea Leighton, *The Navajo* (1946), rev. ed. (Cambridge: Harvard University Press, 1974), 25.

31. *The People's Health*, vii, xiv–xv; McDermott et al., "Introducing Modern Medicine," 287; Cara E. Richards, "Cooperation between Anthropologists and Medical Personnel," *Human Organization* 19 (Summer 1960): 64–67.

32. For claims of success, see *The People's Health*, 144; Bernice Loughlin and Kenneth Dennison, "A Report on the Demographic Studies During the Past Five Years," *Navajo Yearbook* 8 (1961): 115; "Navajo-Cornell Field Health Pilot Project (CH 00007), 1957–1952, Final Report," ca. 1962, *WMP/11/10*, p. 3; McDermott, "Conversation with Zaidi," 13. For the project as a model, Deuschle, "Cross-Cultural Medicine," 182; Alan L. Silver and David N. Rose, "Kurt W. Deuschle and Community Medicine: Clinical Care, Statistical Compassion, Community Empowerment," *Mount Sinai Journal of Medicine* 59 (November 1992): 440. For tensions, see *The People's Health*, 152–158, 163, 168.

33. George Rosen, *A History of Public Health* (1958), expanded ed. (Baltimore: Johns Hopkins University Press, 1993), 460–461; World Health Organization, *The First Ten Years of the World Health Organization* (Geneva: World Health Organization, 1958), 192–194; Elizabeth W. Etheridge, *Sentinel for Health: A History of the Centers for Disease Control* (Berkeley: University of California Press, 1992); Javed Siddiqi, *World Health and World Politics: The World Health Organization and the UN System* (London: Hurst, 1995), 56–57, 123–133, 142.

34. McDermott et al., "Introducing Modern Medicine," 197; *The People's Health*, xiii, xv; McDermott et al., "Interim Report on Indian Health," 64; Deuschle, "Cross-Cultural Medicine," 176; Young, "Foreword," in *The People's Health (1988)*, xii; McDermott, in Bert Jerger, "Medicine Men to the Navajo: Inside an Indian Reservation with Modern Medics," *Think* 25 (January 1959): 15.

35. Taylor, "Interview with Zaidi," 2; Deuschle, "Cross-Cultural Medicine," 177; Kenneth G. Johnson, "Reaching Out to the Community: Responses by Medicine," *Daedalus* 115 (Spring 1986): 161; McDermott, "The Role of Biomedical Research in International Development," *Journal of Medical Education* 39 (July 1964): 667; Arthur J. Rubel and Linda C. Garro, "Social and Cultural Factors in the Suc-

cessful Control of Tuberculosis," *Public Health Reports* 107 (November–December 1992): 632; Silver and Rose, "Kurt W. Deuschle," 440.

36. *The People's Health*, 142; Young, "Foreword," in *The People's Health (1988)*, xiv; *The People's Health (1988)*, 145–147, 153–155; Deuschle, "Tuberculosis among the Navajo," 202–205; McDermott et al., "Introducing Modern Medicine," 203; Loughlin et al., "Syllabus for Teachers in Navajo Health," 102a; Kunitz, *Disease Change*, 76. Tuberculosis mortality among the Navajo peaked at 300/100,000 in 1939. It declined to 150/100,000 by 1952. During the Many Farms project it fell to 40/100,000, moving from the leading cause of death to the sixth cause of death. It is not clear which, if any, of the project's interventions (isoniazid, off-reservation sanatoria, education) contributed to the continuing decline.

37. McDermott et al., "Health Care Experiment," 25–27; *The People's Health (1988)*, 157–159; McDermott, "Draft of Chapter II," undated, *WMP/11/6*, p. 12.

38. Walsh McDermott, "Environmental Factors Bearing on Medical Education in the Developing Countries: A. Modern Medicine and the Demographic-Disease Pattern of Overly Traditional Societies: A Technologic Misfit," *Journal of Medical Education* 41 supp. (1966): 155; McDermott, "Conversation with Zaidi," 11, 13; McDermott et al., "Health Care Experiment," 27–28; McDermott et al., "Interim Report on Indian Health," 175.

39. McDermott et al., "Health Care Experiment," 23, 30; McDermott, "Medicine: The Public Good and One's Own," *Perspectives in Biology and Medicine* 21 (Winter 1978): 169; McDermott, "Absence of Indicators on the Influence of Its Physicians on a Society's Health: Impact of Physician Care on Society," *American Journal of Medicine* 70 (1981): 839–841.

40. David Rogers, "The Early Years: The Medical World in Which Walsh McDermott Trained," *Daedalus* 115 (Spring 1986): 2; McDermott with Rogers, "Social Ramifications of Control of Microbial Disease," *Johns Hopkins Medical Journal* 151 (1982): 302–312; McDermott, "Medical Institutions and Modification of Disease Patterns," *American Journal of Psychiatry* 122 (June 1966): 1403–1405; McDermott et al., "Health Care Experiment," 30. The ideas that sophisticated healthcare is a luxury and that developing countries should limit themselves to "appropriate technologies" have been challenged by the work of Paul Farmer. For a discussion, see Tracy Kidder, *Mountains beyond Mountains* (New York: Random House, 2003).

41. Walsh McDermott, "Evaluating the Physician and His Technology," *Daedalus* (Winter 1977): 135–157; Thomas McKeown, *The Role of Medicine: Dream, Mirage, or Nemesis?* (Princeton: Princeton University Press, 1979); Robert G. Evans, Morris L. Barer, and Theodore R. Marmor, eds., *Why Are Some People Healthy and Others Not? The Determinants of Health of Populations* (New York: Aldine de Gruyter, 1994); Richard Wilkinson, *Unhealthy Societies: The Afflictions of Inequality* (London: Routledge, 1996).

42. McDermott, "Conversation with Zaidi," 16; *The People's Health (1988)*, 145.

43. McDermott to Anna Wauneka, 16 Nov. 1977, *WMP/11/3*; McDermott, "Oral History Transcript," 20; Alfred E. Clark, "Walsh McDermott, Medical Researcher, Dies," *New York Times*, 19 Oct. 1981, p. D15; Beeson, "Walsh

McDermott," 283–307; McDermott, chairman, "A Free Choice Program for American Indians: Report of the President's Task Force on American Indians," Dec. 1966, *WMP*/11/9.

44. Kurt Deuschle, Hugh Fulmer, M. J. McNamara, and Jesse W. Tapp Jr., "The Kentucky Experiment in Community Medicine," *Milbank Memorial Fund Quarterly* 44 (January 1966): 9–22; Alan L. Silver and David N. Rose, eds., "Urban Community Medicine: The Mount Sinai Experience Honoring the Work of Kurt W. Deuschle," *Mount Sinai Journal of Medicine* 59 (November 1992): 439–468. Thomas Moulding, G. David Onstad, and John A. Sbarbaro, "Supervision of Outpatient Drug Therapy with the Medical Monitor," *Annals of Internal Medicine* 73 (October 1970): 559–564; Moulding, "The Medication Monitor for Studying the Self-administration of Oral Contraceptives," *American Journal of Obstetrics and Gynecology* 110 (15 August 1971): 1143–1144; Moulding, "The Medication Monitor for Treating Tuberculosis in Developing Countries," *Tropical Doctor* 9 (July 1979): 106–109. McDermott, "Memorial [to Carl Muschenheim]," 8 Feb. 1979, *WMP*/ 39/7, p. 4. Dubos, *Mirage of Health: Utopias, Progress, and Biological Change* (New York: Harper, 1959), 3–4. Abdel Omran and Bernice Loughlin, "An Epidemiologic Study of Accidents among the Navajo Indians," *Journal of the Egyptian Medical Association* 55 (1972): 1–22; Omran, "The Epidemiologic Transition: A Theory of the Epidemiology of Population Change," *Milbank Memorial Fund Quarterly* 49 (October 1971): 509–538. Eric Pace, "John Adair, 84, Anthropologist Who Studied Navajo Culture," *New York Times*, 29 Dec. 1997, p. B8.

45. Fred L. Soper, "Problems to Be Solved if the Eradication of Tuberculosis Is to Be Realized," *AJPH* 52 (May 1962): 734–745. U.S. Public Health Service, *The Indian Health Program of the U.S. Public Health Service* (Washington: U.S. Department of Health, Education, and Welfare, 1966), 5–7; Stephen Kunitz, "The History and Politics of US Health Care Policy for American Indians and Alaskan Natives," *AJPH* 86 (October 1996): 1466. McDermott to Peter McDonald, chairman of Navajo Tribal Council, 10 Oct. 1977, *WMP*/11/3; McDermott to Forrest Gerard, Commissioner of Indian Affairs, 10 Oct. 1977, *WMP*/11/3; MacDonald to McDermott, ca. 1 Nov. 1977, *WMP*/11/3; McDermott, "Oral History Transcript," 20–21. Had he returned in 2000, McDermott might have been less impressed: 50 percent of the population in some areas remained without running water (personal observations, Indian Health Service, Navajo Area, Crownpoint Service Unit, New Mexico, May 2000).

46. Everett R. Rhoades, "The Major Respiratory Diseases of American Indians," *American Review of Respiratory Diseases* 141 (March 1990): 596.

47. Navajo Health Authority, "Position Paper and Statement of the Navajo Health Authority," c. 1974, *WMP*/11/1, pp. 1–4; Navajo Health Authority, "Summary of Program Components," ca. 1974, *WMP*/11/1, p. 4; Navajo Health Authority, "Capsules of Navajo Health History," in "Summary of Program Components," p. 19; Richard Nixon, "Message to Congress," 8 July 1970, ibid., p. 19; Wauneka to Elliot Richardson, 1 July 1971, ibid., p. 19. For the political background, see Abraham B. Bergman, David C. Grossman, Angela M. Erdich, John G. Todd, and Ralph Forquera, "A Political History of the Indian Health Service," *Milbank Quarterly* 77 (1999): 575, 588.

48. Navajo Health Authority, "Position Paper," cover sheet, 1–2.

49. Navajo Health Authority, "Position Paper," 2–5; Navajo Health Authority,

"Press Release: American Indians Announce First Medical School: *Pan-Indian University Planned in Navajo Nation,*" 3 June 1974, *WMP*/11/1, pp. 1–2.

    50. Navajo Health Authority, "Position Paper," 5–6.

Epilogue and Conclusions

    1. Navajo Health Authority, "Press Release: American Indians Announce First Medical School: *Pan-Indian University Planned in Navajo Nation,*" 3 June 1974, *WMP*/11/1, p. 2.

    2. Ibid., 2; Navajo Health Authority, "Position Paper and Statement of the Navajo Health Authority," ca. 1974, *WMP*/11/1, pp. 3–5; Navajo Health Authority, "Summary of Program Components," ca. 1974, *WMP*/11/1, pp. 4, 12.

    3. Navajo Health Authority, "Press Release," 1–2; Walsh McDermott to David Rogers, Margaret Mahoney, and Mrs. Shuster, 14 June 1974, *WMP*/11/1. Rogers agreed to consider funding improvements to existing institutions: Calvin Bland to Robert Kalinowski, 5 Dec. 1975, *WMP*/11/1. Training programs were established with the University of New Mexico, Navajo Community College, Northern Arizona University, Fort Lewis College, the College of Ganado, and the Health Professionals Schools in Arizona, Colorado, New Mexico, and Utah: Navajo Health Authority, "Position Paper," 4–5; "Summary of Program Components," 4.

    4. Paul le Jeune, *Relation of What Occurred in New France in 1633* (1634), in *Jesuit Relations,* 5:237.

    5. Navajo Health Authority, "Press Release," 1; "Position Paper," 4. The Native Healing Sciences Program hoped to "Develop and promote the full utilization, preservation, education, and practice of the Navajo healing sciences appropriate to the future health education needs of the people . . . and to incorporate such arts into the health care education and delivery systems." See Navajo Health Authority, "Summary of Program Components," 9.

    6. Many archeologists estimate a precontact North American population of 1.8 million: Douglas H. Ubelaker, "North American Indian Population Size: Changing Perspectives," in *Disease and Demography in the Americas,* ed. John W. Verano and Ubelaker (Washington: Smithsonian Institution Press, 1992), 169–176. The 2000 census for the United States reported nearly 2.5 million American Indians (self-identified race as American Indian or Alaskan Native alone), and over 4 million who claimed Indian ancestry (American Indian or Alaskan Native, alone or in combination with other races): U.S. Census Bureau, *Census 2000,* www.census.gov.

    7. Richard S. Steckel and Jerome C. Rose, *The Backbone of History: Health and Nutrition in the Western Hemisphere* (Cambridge: Cambridge University Press, 2002); David S. Jones, "Virgin Soils Revisited," *William and Mary Quarterly* 60 (October 2003): 703–742.

    8. Allan M. Brandt, "Racism and Research: The Case of the Tuskegee Syphilis Study," *Hastings Center Report* 8 (1978): 21–29; Susan E. Lederer, *Subjected to Science: Human Experimentation in America before the Second World War* (Baltimore: Johns Hopkins University Press, 1995); David J. Rothman, "The Shame of Medical Research," *New York Review of Books* (30 Nov. 2000): 60–64.

    9. Walsh McDermott, "Environmental Factors Bearing on Medical Educa-

tion in the Developing Countries: A. Modern Medicine and the Demographic-Disease Pattern of Overly Traditional Societies: A Technologic Misfit," *Journal of Medical Education* 41 supp. (1966): 155; U.S. Public Health Service, *Indian Health Service: A Comprehensive Health Care Program for American Indians and Alaska Natives* (Washington: U.S. Department of Health and Human Services, 1989); Abraham B. Bergman, David C. Grossman, Angela M. Erdich, John G. Todd, and Ralph Forquera, "A Political History of the Indian Health Service," *Milbank Quarterly* 77 (1999): 574.

10. Stephen J. Kunitz, "The History and Politics of US Health Care Policy for American Indians and Alaskan Natives," *AJPH* 86 (October 1996): 1464–1473; Kevin Gover, "Ceremony Acknowledging the 175th Anniversary of the Bureau of Indian Affairs," 8 Sept. 2000, *www.doi.gov/bia/as-ia/175gover.htm*.

11. Roy M. Nakamura, Richard King, Ernest H. Kimball, Robert K. Oye, and Steven D. Helgerson, "Excess Infant Mortality in an American Indian Population, 1940–1990," *JAMA* 266 (23/30 October 1991): 2244–2248; David C. Grossman, James W. Krieger, Jonathan R. Sugarman, and Ralph A. Forquera, "Health Status of Urban American Indians and Alaska Natives: A Population-Based Study," *JAMA* 271 (16 March 1994): 845–850; U.S. Department of Health and Human Services, *Healthy People 2010: Understanding and Improving Health*, 2nd ed. (Washington: Government Printing Office, 2000), 12; Marsha F. Goldsmith, "American Indian Medicine Aims to Add Physicians, Improve Health," *JAMA* 254 (11 October 1985): 1871–1876.

12. Jeff Henderson, "Native American Health Policy: From US Territorial Expansion to Legal Obligation," *JAMA* 265 (1 May 1991): 2272–2273; Kunitz, "US Health Care Policy for American Indians," 1464–1473; Joseph G. Jorgensen, "Comment: Recent Twists and Turns in American Indian Health Care," *AJPH* 86 (October 1996): 1362–1364; Indian Health Service, "Year 2001 Profile," at www.ihs.gov/PublicInfo/PublicAffairs/PressReleases/Press_Release_2001/fy%202001%20ihs%20profile.pdf.

13. Jeff Benedict, *Without Reservation: The Making of America's Most Powerful Indian Tribe and Foxwoods, the World's Largest Casino* (New York: HarperCollins, 2000); W. Dale Mason, *Indian Gaming: Tribal Sovereignty and American Politics* (Norman: University of Oklahoma Press, 2000); Joan Stephenson, "For Some American Indians, Casino Profits Are a Good Bet for Improving Health Care," *JAMA* 275 (19 June 1996): 1783–1785; "Indians Losing in Gambling Business," *Seattle Post-Intelligencer*, 4 Sept. 2000, web ed.; "Special Report: Indian Casinos," *Time Magazine* 160 (8 December 2002): 44–58.

14. Marsha F. Goldsmith, "First Americans Face Their Latest Challenge: Indian Health Care Meets State Medicaid Reform," *JAMA* 275 (19 June 1996): 1786–1788.

15. Stephen Kunitz, "Globalization, States, and the Health of Indigenous Peoples," *AJPH* 90 (2000): 1531. Life expectancy for indigenous populations compared to the general public is 71.1 versus 75.5 in the United States, and 60.4 versus 77.7 in Australia (p. 1532). Kunitz and Maggie Brady, "Health Care Policy for Aboriginal Australians: The Relevance of the American Indian Experience," *Australian Journal of Public Health* 19 (1995): 549–558; Randall M. Packard, *White Plague, Black Labor: Tuberculosis and the Political Economy of Health and Disease in South Africa* (Berkeley: University of California Press, 1989), 299–301; Solomon

Benatar, "Health Care Reform in the New South Africa," *New England Journal of Medicine* 336 (20 March 1997): 891–895.

16. World Health Organization, International Conference on Primary Health Care, Alma-Ata, USSR, "Declaration of Alma-Ata," 12 Sept. 1978; Oscar Gish, "The Political Economy of Primary Care and 'Health by the People': An Historical Exploration," *Social Science and Medicine* 13C (1979): 203–211.

17. G. Parayil, "The 'Kerala Model' of Development: Development and Sustainability in the Third World," *Third World Quarterly* 17 (December 1996): 941–957; K. R. Thankappan and M. S. Valiathan, "Country Profile: India: Health at Low Cost: The Kerala Model," *Lancet* 351 (25 April 1998): 1274–1275; N. R. Menon, "The Health Status of Kerala," *Health for the Millions* 26 (March–April 2000): 11–13; Per Ashorn, Teija Kulmala, and Merimaaria Vaahtera, "Health For All in the 21st Century?" *Annals of Medicine* 32 (2000): 87–89; Lynn Morgan, *Community Participation in Health: The Politics of Primary Care in Costa Rica* (Cambridge: Cambridge University Press, 1993).

18. Gregory Pappas, Susan Queen, Wilbur Hadden, and Gail Fisher, "The Increasing Disparity in Mortality between Socioeconomic Groups in the United States, 1960 and 1986," *New England Journal of Medicine* 329 (8 July 1993): 103–109; Amartya Sen, *Development as Freedom* (New York: Anchor, 1999), 21, 97–98, 104; Richard Wilkinson, *Unhealthy Societies: The Afflictions of Inequality* (London: Routledge, 1996); John W. Lynch, George A. Kaplan, Elsie R. Pamuk, Richard D. Cohen, Katherine E. Heck, Jennifer L. Balfour, and Irene H. Yen, "Income Inequality and Mortality in Metropolitan Areas of the United States," *AJPH* 88 (July 1998): 1074–1080; Norman Daniels, Bruce Kennedy, and Ichiro Kawachi, eds., *Is Inequality Bad for Our Health?* (Boston: Beacon Press, 2000); Health and Human Services, *Healthy People 2010*, 2, 11.

19. This has been well demonstrated by the work of Partners in Health in Haiti and Peru. See Tracy Kidder, *Mountains beyond Mountains* (New York: Random House, 2003).

Index